Anthropology of Infectious Disease

Honoring his landmark contributions to the anthropological study of infectious disease and to the biocultural synthesis that has guided such work, this book is dedicated to the memory and inspiration of George J. Armelagos, 1936–2014.

MERRILL SINGER

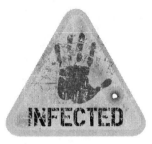

The
ANTHROPOLOGY
of
INFECTIOUS
DISEASE

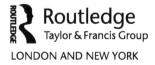

Routledge
Taylor & Francis Group

LONDON AND NEW YORK

First published 2015 by Left Coast Press, Inc.

Published 2016 by Routledge
2 Park Square, Milton Park, Abingdon, Oxon OX14 4RN
711 Third Avenue, New York, NY 10017, USA

Routledge is an imprint of the Taylor & Francis Group, an informa business

Library of Congress Cataloging-in-Publication Data

Singer, Merrill.
    Anthropology of infectious disease / Merrill Singer.
        pages cm
    Includes bibliographical references and index.
    ISBN 978-1-62958-043-2 (hardback)—
    ISBN 978-1-62958-044-9 (paperback)—
    ISBN 978-1-62958-045-6 (institutional ebook)—
    ISBN 978-1-62958-046-3 (consumer ebook)
    1. Communicable diseases.   2. Medical anthropology.   I. Title.
    RA643.S56 2015
    616.9—dc23
                                                                        2014030349

ISBN-13: 978-1-62958-043-2 (hbk)
ISBN-13: 978-1-62958-044-9 (pbk)

Cover design by Piper Wallis
Cover photo by Laura R. Wagner

CONTENTS

ILLUSTRATIONS

FIGURES

TABLES

ACKNOWLEDGEMENT

Deep appreciation is extended to Jennifer Collier Jennings, my editor at Left Coast Press. I would be a very rich man if I had a dollar for all of the suggested changes she provided for this book.

INTRODUCTION

Anthropology and the Large
Impact of Small Worlds

> Breathe in. Feel the air pass through your nostrils and move into your nose. Your diaphragm contracts, pulling the air deep into your chest. Oxygen floods into tiny cavities in your lungs and travels into your capillaries, ready to fuel every cell in your body. You're alive. So is that breath you just took. When we inhale, our nostrils capture millions of invisible particles: dust, pollen, sea spray, volcanic ash, plant spores. These specks in turn host a teeming community of bacteria and viruses.
>
> *Nathan Wolfe, microbiologist (2013)*

With these words, Stanford microbiologist Nathan Wolfe, founder of Global Viral and author of *The Viral Storm*, draws attention to the intimate relationship between our species and a host of tiny organisms, most too small to see with our own eyes, a relationship "we still understand precious little about" (Wolfe 2012). Humans have been keenly aware of the existence of microorganisms since the invention of the microscope about 350 years ago; long before that some people suspected their existence. But we discovered some forms of microbes, such as *viruses*, little more than a century ago, and only much more recently are we beginning to appreciate fully their abundance and complex variety, the diverse niches they occupy in almost all environments, their natural ecology, and the full role they play in human health. In fact, we now believe that all life forms on Earth, including humans, are descendants of microbes called Archaea, or "ancient ones." Archaea are still around in some unexpected locations—volcanic vents on the ocean floor, for example.

Just how important are microbes? Microbes are responsible for producing about half of the oxygen we need to survive (plants account for much of the rest of it). Within the human body they are more numerous than human cells. Each of us is more than a distinct individual—we are composed of an internal community of organisms that function together in various forms of mutual dependency. Although most of the microbes inside of us have little or no impact on us (that we have yet discovered), some, as we will see in Chapter 2, help us digest food, absorb nutrients, produce needed vitamins, yield vital anti-inflammatory

Anthropology of Infectious Disease, by Merrill Singer, 11–19. © 2015 Left Coast Press, Inc. All rights reserved.

proteins, protect our skin, and serve other body functions that contribute to human well-being. In return, we have a lot to offer microbes:

> A human host is a nutrient-rich, warm, and moist environment, which remains at a uniform temperature and constantly renews itself. It is not surprising that many microorganisms have evolved the ability to survive and reproduce in this desirable niche (Albers et al. 2004:1486).

Of course, our commune with microbes is not all mutual affection. In the pages of *National Geographic,* a magazine that brims with pride over the triumph of the human species over every corner of the planet and even into outer space, Nathan Wolfe offers this more ominous assessment: "behind our world is a shadow world of microbes—and they are often calling the shots" (2012). Some microbes—a fairly small percentage, actually—are pathogenic: they cause human diseases or diseases of other species that may evolve to affect humans. Infectious pathogens, or disease-causing organisms, include some types of viruses, *bacteria, fungi,* and *protozoa* as well as multicellular parasites and an aberrant set of proteins known as *prions.* Despite their miniscule size and relatively small number of varieties, the toll they take on human life and well-being is staggering (see Figure I.1).

Worldwide, *infectious diseases* are the leading cause of death of both children and adolescents and one of the leading causes of death in adults. They have claimed hundreds of millions of human lives throughout history and remain primary sources of morbidity and mortality globally, especially in developing countries but also in highly developed industrial countries. Of the top ten

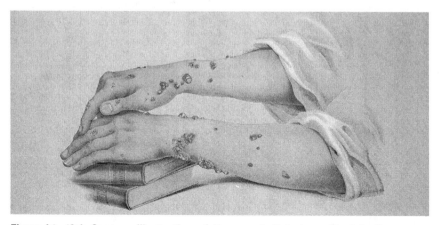

Figure I.1 19th Century illustration of Herpes gladiatorium skin infection. (Image from the History of Medicine)

causes of death in the world, three are infectious diseases; these account for about 16 percent of all deaths each year (Center for Strategic and International Studies 2012). Consider just one of the infectious diseases discussed in this book: *tuberculosis*. The World Health Organization (2011) estimates that the microorganism that causes tuberculosis infects one person in the world every second and that every twenty seconds one person dies as a result. This microbe travels by air; other pathogenic microbes have evolved an array of strategies for transmission. For example, rabies, which humans have contended with for millennia, is spread through the bites and scratches of infected animals. Our understanding of microbes may be recent, but we have long understood this route of disease transmission: written descriptions of how to control the spread of this disease date to more than three thousand years ago (Albers et al. 2004).

Unfortunately we are discovering new infectious diseases every year. Among the most important new diseases of the twentieth century, of course, is *HIV disease*. So far I have distinguished the microbe that causes a disease from the disease itself, but in reality the dividing line between the *infection* by a pathogen and the *disease* that develops is arbitrary. I use the term "HIV disease" to avoid imposing an artificial line between infection with the HIV virus and the development of a disease called AIDS. A growing list of other emergent and reemergent infectious diseases includes the well-publicized *severe acute respiratory syndrome (SARS), swine flu,* and *avian flu*. A few new infectious diseases, notes anthropologist George Armelagos, are "so bloodcurdling and bizarre that descriptions of them bring to mind tacky horror movies. Ebola virus, for instance, can in just a few days reduce a healthy person to a bag of teeming flesh spilling blood and organ parts from every orifice." After decades of believing that we would triumph over infectious disease, treatment-resistant infections, covered in Chapter 5, have significantly heightened public concern about infectious diseases in the contemporary world. In the United States infectious diseases killed 58 percent more people in 1992 than in 1980 (Armelagos 1997:24). The impact of infectious diseases in the United States has continued to grow since then. As stressed by the Institute of Medicine (Smolinski, Hamburg, and Lederberg 2003:21),

> Infectious diseases unknown in this country just a decade ago, such as West Nile encephalitis and hantavirus pulmonary syndrome, have emerged to kill hundreds of Americans—and the long-term consequences for survivors of the initial illnesses are as yet unknown. Other known diseases, including measles, multi-drug-resistant tuberculosis, and even malaria, have been imported and transmitted within the United States in the last 10 years.

New research on the relationship between the environment and health is enhancing our understanding of infectious disease. *Global warming,* for example, contributes to the spread of water-borne and vector-borne *infectious agents* (see Chapter 4). Researchers are also taking a more multidimensional approach focused on *syndemics,* which entails examining pathogenic microbes not only in isolation but also in their complex relationship to other, noninfectious diseases and sociocultural and economic conditions, such as poverty. The conceptualization of syndemics, examined in Chapter 6, was a major contribution of *medical anthropology* that has diffused to other health-related disciplines in recent years.

Of particularly keen interest to anthropology is the way in which diverse human behaviors contribute directly and indirectly to the threat pathogens pose—we are overdosing on antibiotics, changing the planet's climate, occupying new terrains, developing new residence patterns, and adopting new food production and handling strategies. Consequently, as Wolfe (2012) stresses,

> As we learn more about the relationships between ourselves and our microbes—and their own complex relationships with one another—scientists are coming to see the microbiome the way ecologists have long viewed an ecosystem: not as a collection of species but as a dynamic environment, defined by the multitude of interactions among its constituents.

In other words, infectious diseases are *never only biological in their nature, course, or impact.* What they are and what they do are deeply entwined with human sociocultural systems, including the ways humans understand, organize, and treat each other (see, in particular, Chapter 7). Infectious diseases are at once biological realities and social constructions that reflect both biological and social relationships and interactions. Ultimately, in spite of our ingrained habit of treating them as distinct and even opposing forces, biology and culture are inseparable. This fact makes anthropology particularly well suited to understand and generate key insights about infectious disease.

Consider again HIV disease. As we all know, biomedical treatments for this condition have improved enormously over the last thirty years, contributing to astonishing advances in the health of people living with the disease. Yet three stubborn challenges endure:

- People are often diagnosed late and, as a result, cannot receive the optimal benefits from existing antiretrovial therapies.
- For various reasons, some people drop out of treatment.
- Some people are uneven in their adherence to day-to-day treatment requirements.

Why? Leading HIV researchers explain: "Although an emphasis on testing and treatment sounds primarily biomedical, the three challenges depend on behavioral, social system and [social] structural factors" (Morin et al. 2011:175). Nevertheless, the vast majority of researchers and research dollars are still focused on the biological aspects of infectious diseases rather than the ways their emergence and spread reflect human activities, modes of production and residence, beliefs and attitudes, governance and structures of social relation, and environmental transformations.

Given their significant and enduring role in human life and death—and hence their influence on human societies both subtle and monumental—infectious diseases have become an important concern within anthropology, particularly in the subfield known as medical anthropology. This book explores the nature of infectious diseases and how our coexistence with them shapes the human condition, contributing in ways small and large to making us who we are biologically, culturally, and socially as well as influencing our individual life experiences. As increasing numbers of medical anthropologists study biocultural and biosocial processes in *health, illness,* and treatment, including environmentally mediated factors in human health and well-being, they are generating important new concepts and research questions. This book explores these intriguing questions on the frontier of infectious disease research:

- How does the human world look different if we move beyond thinking of human communities as collections of interacting people and instead recognize that we live in multispecies communities that include disease vectors and zoonotic pathogens that regularly "jump" from animal hosts to humans?
- How does our understanding of ourselves change if we recognize that every person is, in fact, a community of interacting species?
- How does our conception of health change if we think of health not as an individual state but instead as a reflection of human social relationships mediated by the environment?
- Why, in an era of miraculous improvements in health interventions, do infectious diseases remain the leading cause of death in developing nations?
- Why, even in highly developed and comparatively wealthy nations with advanced and costly medical systems, such as the United States, are infections the third leading cause of human mortality?
- How do human activities and understandings (e.g., cultural conceptions of "plague" and stigmatization) contribute to the spread of infectious

diseases, the emergence of new infectious diseases, the course of infectious disease epidemics, and the magnitude of human suffering?

- How are broader forces of globalization likely to affect the spread of infectious diseases and their overall health consequences?
- How are our cultural understandings of disease changing through time, and how will these changes affect social responses to infectious disease?
- How does anthropology contribute to the understanding of the role of infectious diseases in human communities?

This book advances an anthropologically framed approach to disease and contagion transnationally by integrating the natural history of infection with human social behavior and structures of social relation. It is informed by *ecosocial theory*, a term coined by epidemiologist Nancy Krieger (2007) to describe a multilevel framework that integrates social and biologic reasoning along with a dynamic, historical, and ecological perspective to understand population distributions of disease and social inequalities in health. To this framework, anthropology brings evolutionary depth, investigating humans as a species that has evolved in constant interaction with other species; an ethnographically informed focus on the processes and pathways of biocultural and biosocial interaction; and a growing focus on the interface of local sociocultural and environmental settings with wider fields of social force and exchange in a globalizing world.

In recent years the anthropological approach has demonstrated its value to understanding and responding to HIV, ebola, SARS, tuberculosis, malaria, influenza, kuru, and numerous other infectious diseases by analyzing their role in the creation of lived experiences and as reflections in physical bodies of conflicts and points of tension in social bodies as well as by identifying and assessing human behaviors linked to prevention and treatment. Anthropology can nest everyday, on-the-ground activity within the encompassing frame of social groups and communities and, beyond this, within the big picture of global processes and international social relationships. Its scope broadens even further to explore the linkages—not readily apparent yet critically important—between microscopic entities and the political and economic structures of human societies by identifying the pathways that connect human bodies, cultural and social systems, and health.

The anthropological approach to HIV disease demonstrates its particular contribution to the larger multidisciplinary study of infectious diseases. International health programs invest considerable effort into two areas. First, they examine risk behaviors, focusing on individuals as rational decision makers and interpreting behavior as a direct outcome of an individual's characteristics or capacities. For example, whether someone is likely to engage in sexual behaviors considered more risky for contracting HIV is analyzed in terms of an individual's characteristics, like sexual orientation, knowledge, attitudes, and perceived ability to prevent infection. Second, they look at the structural vulnerabilities of entire populations, such as the role of poverty in risk behavior. By contrast, one important focus of anthropology has been the relationship between individual agency and structural factors in health. This is the level that encompasses social groups, interpersonal networks, and communities. Moreover, anthropologists move beyond the simplistic understanding of individuals as rational decision-making agents, recognizing instead that people's behaviors are not the direct product of their individual characteristics, decisions, or capacities; behavior, including action that puts people at risk of infection, "is always itself social, imbued with meaning, rich in significance, and the outcome of a variety of forces" (Kippax et al. 2013:1368). One of those forces is people's involvement in social groups, which are critical influences on their identities, values, knowledge, health status, and activities. For example, groups that view the primary role of sex as procreation do not receive favorably public health messages promoting the use of condoms to prevent HIV infection. Group membership also mediates awareness of and attitudes toward particular infectious diseases as well as appropriate behaviors to avoid or treat them, however they are understood, which may have nothing to do with notions of microbial infection. Group membership also influences the emergence of social responses to infectious diseases, such as the kind of community organizing that has emerged worldwide around HIV disease.

USING THEORY

This discussion underlines the importance of theory in the anthropology of infectious disease. Medical anthropologists concerned with health issues have utilized and combined various theoretical perspectives in their work. *Medical ecological theory* stresses the ways societies respond to the challenges and opportunities presented by the physical environments and climatic conditions they face, including the local presence of particular infectious agents. Within this theoretical framework the health of a population is seen as a complex reflection of the group's degree of success in meeting these challenges, including those generated in the social environment.

Exemplary is anthropologist Edward Green's (1999) argument that indigenous beliefs about disease contagion around the world are not necessarily the result of the influence of biomedicine but often are rooted in far older cultural ideas about body pollution. Such beliefs, he suggests, are adaptive in that they lead to behaviors that reduce the spread of infectious diseases. If a man, for example, avoids having sexual intercourse with many partners or with commercial sex workers to protect himself from uncleanliness and mystical pollution, he reduces his exposure to pathogenically transmitted diseases associated with sexual intercourse even if he is unaware of bacteria or viruses. In other words, in the course of human history beliefs about pollution-based contagion developed, and these had adaptive value in lowering rates of infection and were retained in various cultural systems up to the present. Moreover, indigenous ethnomedical systems are not, as some might see them, "superstition, meaningless pseudo-psychological mumbo-jumbo, which is positively harmful" to health (Nthato Motlana quoted in Freeman and Motsei 1992:186); rather, although containing some practices that may be harmful, on the whole they are historic adaptive systems that have contributed to human survival in varied environments.

Phenomenological and related meaning-centered approaches draw attention to the subjectivities of illness and the ways it is experienced, interpreted, and made meaningful in human societies. For example, in her research in Indonesia, anthropologist Karen Kroeger (2008:343) found AIDS rumors shared among people "are a kind of 'somatization' of pathology in the Indonesian body politic, a metaphorical expression of concerns that Indonesians have about the break-down of the social order and the power of the Indonesian state." Participation in spreading AIDS rumors—such as tales of unknown assailants sticking people with infected syringes—involves drawing on existing cultural symbolism in Indonesia in the midst of an epidemic to express growing social (dis)ease and a sense of vulnerability in a tense and conflicted society.

A final theoretical perspective, discussed more fully in Chapter 7, is known as *critical medical anthropology.* This framework, which is conceptually linked to ecosocial theory in epidemiology, views health as an expression of social relations within society, especially the ways that social inequality structures health disparities and vulnerability, patterns morbidity and mortality, and contributes to the social distribution of disease-related social suffering but also to health-related resilience, agency, and social action. Commonly social relations in society are mediated by environmental conditions, including anthropogenic impacts on the environment, such as the contributions of greenhouse gas emissions to global warming and, consequently, to warming-related dissemination of infectious diseases. Critical medical anthropology seeks to focus attention on the complex of interactions between the local and the global, the sociocultural and the biological, the human and nonhuman environments, and the rich and poor in infectious diseases. From the perspective of critical medical anthropology, we cannot understand the global pandemic of HIV disease independent of the international, national, regional, and local structures of unequal social relationships, and processes of social challenge and conflict have helped to determine who gets infected, under what conditions as well as what is their access to treatment and the consequences of infection.

The first chapter of this book lays a foundation for the anthropology of infectious diseases, presenting some key lessons of biocultural and biosocial understanding as well as core concepts and special attributes anthropology brings to comprehending disease in human societies. Chapter 2 focuses on microbes as entities in the world. The chapter emphasizes the unexpected complexity of these organisms; their origins, variety, considerable impact on the world around them, their social interactions with each other; and both beneficial and malevolent interactions with humans. Chapter 3 delves more deeply into the implications of the fact that our species does not live separately from other species and their infectious diseases. It reports current knowledge on the development of both HIV and Lyme disease as examples of the biosocial nature of infectious diseases.

The role of the environment and dramatic human impacts on the environment in the nature and spread of infectious disease is addressed in Chapter 4. This discussion extends a central theme of the book: the complexities of our entwinement with the world around us and the ways our actions rebound on our health. Chapter 5 highlights critical changes in today's world of infectious agents and disease, including the emergence, reemergence, and drug resistance of pathogens as well as health implications for humans. The following chapter concentrates on infectious disease syndemics and the social conditions that foster pathogen concentration and adverse interaction. The last chapter explores the multiple ways imbalances of power produce savage inequalities in the distribution and health consequence of infectious diseases. A primary message of the chapter is that you cannot understand infectious disease in the world independent of the way social structures produce significant disparities in living conditions and other aspects of daily existence. Together the chapters in this book show the benefits of turning the anthropological lens on infectious diseases, revealing clearly the biosocial and biocultural nature of these conditions that significantly impact all life on Earth.

CHAPTER ONE

Defining the Anthropology of Infectious Disease
Toward a Biocultural/Biosocial Understanding

> I believe that there is no dichotomy between the natural world and the human environment
>
> *Juliet Clutton-Brock (1994:23)*

HUMANS AND PATHOGENS

The human species evolved in a world already populated by *pathogens*. Surviving bone material of our distant hominid ancestors dating to over a million years ago shows evidence of infectious diseases. Our attempts to understand infection and the human relationship with infectious disease systematically is far younger. Younger still is anthropological work on the topic, which dates only to the mid-twentieth century. In this short time, however, we have learned some key lessons about the biocultural and biosocial nature of infectious disease. This chapter explores these lessons as well as core concepts in the anthropology of infection, the special contributions of anthropology to our understanding of infectious diseases, and the biosocial/biocultural and political ecological vision the discipline brings to this domain of research and practice. It underlines the importance of understanding infectious disease as a multistranded intersection of biology—both our own and that of pathogens—and human social and cultural systems in a globalizing and environmentally disrupted world. The chapter then identifies some of the research methods anthropology brings to the study of infectious diseases and concludes with several questions for further discussion.

DEVELOPING AN ANTHROPOLOGY OF INFECTIOUS DISEASE

Most anthropological research on infectious disease occurs within the subfield of medical anthropology, a domain concerned with health in social and cultural context. Marcia Inhorn and Peter Brown, whose volume *The Anthropology of Infectious Disease* was a benchmark for the new field, define it as "the broad area which emphasizes the interaction between sociocultural, biological, and ecological variables relating to the etiology and prevalence of infectious disease" (1990:91). This definition can usefully be broadened to read: *the anthropology of infectious disease is the arena of applied and basic anthropological research that focuses on the interaction among sociocultural, biological, political, economic, and ecological variables involved in the etiology, prevalence, experience, impact, cultural understanding, prevention, and treatment of infectious diseases.*

The first focused anthropological work on infectious disease began in the post–World War II period of the 1950s, in a new era characterized by international development aimed to assist less developed countries achieve Western/Japanese levels of technological and civic development. Although Western countries framed these initiatives in humanitarian terms, they had other motives as well. As a result of the war and the national liberation movements that arose after movement in succeeding decades, many former colonies, for example in Africa and Southeast Asia, gained independence. The coalition between the United States, Europe, and the Soviet Union, tenuously held together in opposition to Germany and the Axis powers during World War II, quickly dissolved into Cold War rivalries. The postwar passion for international development was strongly driven by worry in the West that underdeveloped nations would turn to communism rather than capitalism. Although then billed as a humanitarian effort the huge mobilization for development had a definite political subtext.

What is commonly referred to as the Western model has guided development initiatives of the United States and Europe. This model was a "top-down" approach to development that reflected the goals and values of the industrialized nations. One of its tenets was the "conviction that enhanced economic growth automatically brings with it increased prosperity and a better way of life for all—not only the already affluent but, in the long run, the disadvantaged members of society as well" (Millen, Irwin, and Kim 2000:6). This belief, which reflects Western cultural ideals, was hardly questioned at the time; indeed, the array of cultural patterns in countries targeted for development was seen as an obstacle to acceptance of the Western model. In this context, the idea emerged among international development professionals that anthropological research on cultural patterns and on planned cultural change could be useful in implementing development programs.

Practitioners of development working within the Western model sought to eliminate all barriers to economic expansion, and disease and unsanitary conditions were quickly identified as significant obstacles. Thus, part and parcel of the Western model was the idea that biomedicine, the Western approach to addressing health issues, was a critical component of the normal development process. Biomedicine, now a globally dominant medical system, is based on natural-science principles. Its particular understandings of human anatomy and the causes and clinical treatment of diseases are institutionalized around hospital-based or -linked treatment, a hierarchy of specialized clinical practitioners, and, with reference to infectious diseases, a supportive set of ideas and actions regarding identification of pathogens, hygiene, sanitation, and pharmaceutical intervention. It is widely held that biomedicine is universal and acultural, in contrast to *ethnomedicine,* for example, which implies that a medical system is embedded within a specific cultural tradition.

In recent decades anthropologists have been critical of the distinction, highlighting the sociocultural nature of biomedicine and viewing it as a Western ethnomedical tradition that gained worldwide distribution through its historic connections to colonialism and corporate globalization. But in the post–World War II period anthropologists were invited to engage in new development-driven health promotion programs that implemented centralized biomedical treatment in urban areas. In short, anthropologists' first involvement with infectious disease work supported Western-oriented development in roles that the discipline itself later criticized as being subordinated handmaidens of biomedicine (Browner 1999).

Anthropologists in the postwar period found, in fact, that attempts to export biomedical ideas often did not work as planned. One example is the experience of Edward Wellin, who was sent to southern Peru in the early 1950s as a graduate student through a Rockefeller Foundation program on health promotion. He observed an effort designed to get people to boil drinking water to avoid infection. Wellin wrote about two of the Peruvians he worked with in the town of Los Molinos:

> Although Mrs. F and her daughter have attended several . . . [hygiene promotion] talks, they remain unreceptive to the notion of bacteriological contamination and unconvinced of the need to boil their drinking water. . . . How, she argues, can microbes fall into water? Are they fish? If they are so small that they cannot be seen or felt, how can such delicate things survive in water? Even in the clean water they would have no chance, let alone in dirty water. . . . There are enough real threats in the world to worry about—"cold" [as in hot/cold imbalance], [bad] "airs", poverty and hunger—without bothering oneself about animals one cannot see hear, touch or smell. (1955:92)

After two years of water-boiling promotion efforts to reduce water-borne infections, only eleven housewives were convinced to boil water. Benjamin Paul effectively articulated anthropology's key insight into this kind of biocultural encounter with infectious disease:

If you wish to help a community improve its health, you must learn to think like the people of that community. Before asking a group of people to assume new health habits, it is wise to ascertain the existing habits, how these habits are linked to one another, what functions they perform [for society], and what they mean to those who practice them. (1955:1)

Although anthropologists today might wince at the phrase "learn to think like the people," Paul's emphasis on seeking to understand the emic—or insider's—perspective remains a core lesson. But the question of exactly what role anthropologists should play in health development remains controversial.

The World Health Organization (WHO) arose as a leading player in health development during a period (1950s–1980s) now known as the Era of International Health. During these decades campaigns to improve world health were largely dominated by biomedicine and, except for water and sanitation projects, focused on narrowly defined programs and individual patients rather than on broader social and economic issues in underdeveloped nations, including issues of poverty; unequal access to basic resources; discrimination based on class, ethnicity and gender; and, ultimately, the structure of unequal relations between wealthy and poor nations.

During the 1970s, the World Health Organization created the Tropical Disease Research program (TDR), which further opened the door for a number of anthropologists to become involved in infectious disease research. It was during this period that infectious disease research finally "won its spurs" as a legitimate topic for anthropology. In subsequent years the TDR adopted an aggressive emphasis on addressing the infectious diseases of the poor and disadvantaged, harmonizing with anthropology's biocultural view of health and the inseparability of disease and society.

For a brief period following the signing of the 1978 Alma Ata Declaration by WHO member nations, international health advocates rallied around the recognition that health should be addressed as a fundamental human right. They paid particular attention to the social origins of disease and the implementation of horizontal (participatory) rather than vertical (top-down) programming. These ideas, embraced by many medical anthropologists, were a direct challenge to the status quo and biomedical reductionism. Unfortunately the "health-for-all initiative," as it came to be known, was undermined at every turn, and by the 1980s the World Health Organization had returned to its former strategy of focusing on primary health care with narrowly targeted interventions.

In the midst of these struggles, anthropologists strengthened their own biocultural approaches and professional networks. In 1980, just before the dawn of the HIV disease era, a group of anthropologists working on infectious disease formed the Working Group on Anthropology and Infectious Disease; subsequently the International Health and Infectious Disease Study Group and the AIDS and Anthropology Research Group were created. Although only the latter group survives within the Society for Medical Anthropology, anthropological involvement in infectious disease research and the application of research to health improvement continues to grow unabated. Today there are anthropologists working on infectious disease issues all around the world.

The post–World War II rise of international development was an endeavor so massive that it is frequently referred to as the "development-industrial complex" and has had a major role in shaping the twentieth-century world order. Beyond its involvement in international development issues, the anthropology of infectious disease has been influenced by a number of other factors, academic, socioeconomic, and political in nature. A review of six of these additional influencing factors that have played a role in the emergence of the anthropology of infectious diseases follows below. This mosaic of influences laid the foundation for a major subfield of research and application that lies on the cusp between biological and cultural anthropology.

PALEOPATHOLOGY

Paleopathlogy is the study of the diseases suffered by people who lived in the past as revealed through archeological excavation. The term unites "paleo," meaning ancient, with pathology, which is the study of disease processes. Marc Armand Ruffer, who named the field, often is credited with being the first paleopathologist based on his discovery and description of the parasitic disease urinary schistosomiasis among Egyptian mummies, which he published early in the twentieth century. After the Second World War concern about the role of disease in shaping ancient societies grew significantly within archaeology, the branch of anthropology that deals with understanding past societies and their change over time and across geographical contexts. Human remains, primarily skeletal materials, record the impact of various diseases and provide clues to the health challenges of prehistory. In addition, ancient DNA of infectious agents can be recovered from human remains that are hundreds of years old.

By examining the skeletal remains of populations that lived in different environments, paleopathology researchers have been able to gain new insights concerning the long-term interrelationships among human biology, cultural practices, and infectious diseases. For example, paleopathology has helped to reveal changes in patterns of infectious diseases in human populations that accompanied the transition from hunting and gathering to agriculture. In this transition people became more sedentary, increasing the likelihood of infectious disease exposure, and they began to spend more time around domesticated animals, creating opportunities for pathogens to move from animals to people. Signs of infection in human remains increased as settlements grew in size and became more permanent.

Mycobacterial diseases that have been a factor in human history for millennia have particular interest for paleopathologists "because they afford opportunity to examine the interactions between an infectious agent and human migration and settlement patterns" as well as between diet and infectious disease (Wilbur et al. 2008:963). For example, paleopathologists have contributed important research to our biocultural understanding of tuberculosis and leprosy. In the case of tuberculosis, bone and joint changes can occur, usually in adulthood, three to five years after infection. In excavated skeletons tuberculosis commonly is identified by the presence of lesions, often in the vertebrae of the spine, although other skeletal indications, like pitting and new bone formation on rib surfaces, have also been linked to tuberculosis. Additionally, ancient DNA of the bacterial agent that is the immediate cause of tuberculosis has been recovered in archeological finds (Murphy et al. 2009). Although there was a long dispute about whether tuberculosis was only introduced to the New World with the arrival of Europeans, recent research has documented tuberculosis in skeletons from Point Hope in Alaska that date as far back as over two thousand years ago (Dabbs 2009).

Paleopathology investigation of the skeletons excavated at Naestved, the site of a medieval leprosy hospital in Denmark (Møller-Christensen 1978), found that most of the individuals exhibited cribra orbitalia—small holes in the bone ridges under the eyebrows caused by the body's effort to produce more red blood cells in bone marrow nourished by an iron-deficient diet. This finding is interpreted as evidence that people who were most susceptible to leprosy were the poor. As Manchester observes, "The possibility of chronic intestinal parasitic infestation in infancy contributing to this anemia may also suggest a poor general health status and level of poverty" (1991:28). This research supports recognition that leprosy is most commonly a disease of poverty, associated with overcrowding—as the pathogen is transmitted through breathing in the exhalation of an infected individual—and socially compromised *immune systems*. This kind of work on the diseases of ancient societies adds historical depth to the anthropological understanding of the intersection of infections and human societies through time and place.

CHILDREN'S SURVIVAL INITIATIVE

In the 1980s, in the wake of the International Year of the Child, UNICEF launched the Child Survival Initiative. Initially its efforts focused on oral rehydration for diarrhea disease, which usually has an infectious proximal origin, and on immunization against common infectious agents. Numerous anthropologists worked on these programs and became knowledgeable about infectious diseases. An early document that came out of this initiative emphasized the fact that "more than 40,000 young children have died from malnutrition and infection. And for everyone who has died, six now live on in . . . hunger and ill-health which will be forever etched upon their lives" (Grant 1982:4). It proceeded to make the case for a global push for socially appropriate programs to promote child survival. Recognition of the importance of malnutrition in the spread of infection, which draws attention to issues of poverty, access to food, and the causes of food insecurity, further affirmed a biosocial perspective in addressing infectious diseases.

Malaria has long been a major cause of child death in affected areas. In response, through the Children's Survival Initiative, anthropological consultation was solicited to ensure that prevention efforts would be effective in light of local cultural beliefs and behaviors. In Gambia, for example, where insecticide-treated bed nets were being distributed, anthropologists provided program managers with ethnographic information on family sleeping patterns, attitudes, and preferences regarding net use, strategies for protecting children in the poorest households, and ways to train local health educators. Anthropologists provided additional input on the design of health education approaches that build on indigenous conceptions and how to most effectively distribute preventive chloroquine tablets through existing village organizational structures, including how to best involve people from the most socially marginal households. During this process an anthropologist first systematically documented perceived side-effects of taking chloroquine reported by community members (MacCormack 1985).

HIV DISEASE

When the HIV disease pandemic emerged, the disease was expressed differently across countries and groups, and "risk behaviors" were poorly understood. This created a demand for anthropological research domestically and internationally, drawing hundreds of anthropologists over the years into the study of infectious disease. Individuals whose first involvement in infectious disease research was work on HIV disease went on to investigate a range of other infectious diseases, a domain further broadened by the students of these researchers. To the study of HIV disease, anthropologists, as indicated in numerous studies discussed in this book, brought a focus on comprehending both local and wider social and cultural contexts that facilitate disease transmission, an emphasis on accessing community knowledge about and emotional responses to the *epidemic,* and a recognition that structures of inequality in society tend to be replicated through identifiable pathways in patterns of disease transmission and course.

Exemplifying the kinds of work anthropologists have done on HIV disease, in 2003 anthropologists affiliated with the Hispanic Health Council, a community-based service and research institute in Hartford, Connecticut, were funded by the federal Office of AIDS Policy to implement a *rapid ethnographic assessment* of factors contributing to the epidemic that existing prevention programs were not addressing (Singer and Eiserman 2007). Discussions with community representatives and members of the research team led to a decision to examine late-night risk in the city, as there were no prevention efforts going on after city health offices and community organizations closed for the evening. As part of the project team's data-collection strategy, interviewers were sent to sites around the city where high-risk behaviors (e.g., drug use, commercial sex transactions) had been observed in prior research. Team members approached people on the street and asked them whether they would be willing to participate in a brief interview that addressed (1) a participant's major sociodemographic characteristics (e.g., age, gender, employment status), (2) knowledge about places around town where high-risk behaviors occur, (3) knowledge about groups of people who could be found on the street during late-night hours, (4) types of late-night risk behaviors that occurred locally, (5) the participant's degree of exposure to HIV prevention materials, and (6) perception of HIV-related needs in Hartford. In total sixty-seven short walk-up interviews were completed. These were followed by in-depth interviews with individuals who fell into one of four groups engaged in risk behaviors: drug users, drug sellers, commercial sex workers, and men who have unprotected sex with other men. The field team conducted thirty-one in-depth interviews. Based on the data collected from these approaches, the project concluded that people who are active on the street during late-night hours tend to engage in more risk behavior (e.g., sex without a condom, injection drug use, commercial sex) than people who can be contacted on the street during the day. The study also found that people who sleep during the day but are active on the street at night have less contact with HIV prevention services than their counterparts who are active during the day. Consequently the researchers urged the city of Hartford to support late-night prevention efforts (e.g., education and condom distribution) targeted at specific "hot spots" around the city where there was a concentration of after-hours risk behavior. The city responded favorably to this recommendation, and funds were directed toward the implementation of late-night street efforts intended to stem the spread of HIV disease.

NEW AND REEMERGING DISEASES

Today previously controlled diseases are reemerging, in part because of HIV-involved syndemics, and there is growing awareness of new, emergent infectious diseases such avian flu, swine flu, and SARS. In 1989 a conference on viruses, sponsored by Rockefeller University, the National Institute of Allergy and Infectious Diseases, and the Fogarty International Center, sparked interest in the emergence and resurgence of all classes of pathogens. It brought together researchers who shared a growing concern regarding a perceived "complacency in the scientific and medical communities, the public, and the political leadership of the United States toward the danger of emerging infectious diseases and the potential for devastating epidemics" (Lederberg, Shope, and Oaks 1992:vi). New attention focused on the concept of "emerging infectious diseases," a term that developed within biomedicine and diffused from medical circles into general scientific discourse and from there to the lexicon of the mass media during the 1990s (Washer 2010). This created the conceptual space for a multidisciplinary array of approaches to infectious disease, including those formulated within anthropology. This opening was facilitated by recognition that biology alone could not account for the changing world of infectious diseases and human behaviors, such as the cutting down of forests, the overuse of antibiotics, and the human-generated changes in climate, all of which were playing fundamental roles in new and renewed infectious disease epidemics.

GLOBAL WARMING

Anthropological attention to human engagement with the environment has a deep history within the discipline. During the 1950s, with the insightful contributions of Julian Steward (1955), a new ecologically informed perspective began to emerge in anthropology. In this new approach to the human relationship to the rest of nature, a heightened awareness of the widespread impact of human activities on the world replaced an older environmental determinism perspective. More recently, in what has come to be called environmental anthropology, an applied "study of the human-environmental relationship [has been] driven largely by environmental concern" about climate change, natural disasters, loss of biological diversity, the spread of infectious diseases, and related issues of sustainability (Shoreman-Ouimet and Kopnina 2011:1). It is becoming clear that climate change is having serious political-economic, sociocultural, and health impacts on societies that have never before in human history faced an environmental threat on this scale and complexity in such a compressed time frame. Belatedly, researchers have awakened to the role of global warming in the spread of infectious diseases through the movement of *water-borne, vector-borne,* and wind-blown *pathogens.* Singer (2013b), for example, examines various physical interactions between global warming and air pollution in the exacerbation and increasing frequency of global respiratory diseases such as asthma. Similarly Armelagos and Harper (2010:303) observe that various infectious vector-borne diseases, such as dengue and chikungunya, are on the rise in part due to global warming. Anthropology thus far has contributed only a limited amount of work on this topic, but given the grave risk involved and the discipline's strength in developing biocultural understandings of ecology, culture, and health, global warming is another impetus for anthropological work on infectious disease (Baer and Singer 2009, 2014).

GLOBAL HEALTH

During the 1990s the leading paradigm in health development shifted from "international health" to "global health." The rise of the concept of global health paralleled the rise of the new economic term "global economy," which recognized the advancing and systemic economic globalization of human communities on our planet. The global health concept also reflected a shift in perspective from a focus on health issues within nations and regions to the understanding that factors that affect health transcend national borders and are deeply entwined with issues of socioeconomic class, ethnicity, gender, and culture. To put this another way, the shift involved recognition of the fundamental importance to health of flows of capital, people, infectious agents and diseases, medicines, commodities, ideas, and practices that move relatively readily across our culturally constructed political boundaries and that differentially affect the health of everyone. This notion coincides with anthropological attention to global flows in other subfields of the discipline (Appadurai 1990).

As a result of the various influences discussed above, in increasing numbers medical anthropologists are working on infectious disease issues in various roles within the World Health Organization, the Centers for Disease Control, other government bodies, domestic and international *nongovernment organizations (NGOs),* and in other scholarly and applied venues. In addition, an impressive body of literature in the field has developed (e.g., Hesser 1982; Inhorn and Buss 2010; Larsen and Milner 1994; Manderson 2012; Mascie-Taylor 1993). In some ways, however, the anthropology of infectious disease remains an emergent arena of research and applied work because it has yet to consolidate into a subfield with established concepts, theoretical frameworks, conferences, journals, and a distinct identity among participants or to have acquired other common markers of disciplinary institutionalization. The field is somewhat scattered and lacks an organizational core, although the contributions of the anthropological approach are known to varying degrees in other health-related disciplines. Still, as Barry and Bonnie Hewlett (2008) observe with reference to their work on ebola, initially it never occurred to anyone combating the disease at the World Health Organization to involve anthropologists; it was only through their own initiative that anthropologists gained a useful role in research and prevention efforts with this deadly infectious disease. This is because, despite important conceptual developments discussed in this section, biomedicine remains the dominant tendency in global health work on infectious disease, with only secondary consideration given to the fact that these diseases are shaped by and, in turn, shape the societies and cultural systems in which they are found.

Challenges to the traditional approach have grown in recent years as recognition that infectious disease is not simply a consequence of the presence of pathogens or even the interaction of pathogens and the human immune system. Microbes in the environment become the immediate source of human infectious diseases and have shifting distributions and changing levels of virulence because of human activities, social structures, and cultural configurations. So too the way communities respond to the presence of infection, including behaviors that promote and limit the spread of disease, the manner in which others treat infected individuals, and campaigns to control or eliminate infectious agents are all social and not narrowly biological in nature. These factors open doorways for the further development and expanded contributions of the anthropology of infectious diseases.

This book invites you to explore questions that remain somewhat open: What is the anthropology of infectious disease, and what does this field offer to the broader human engagement with communicable disease?

KEY CONCEPTS IN THE ANTHROPOLOGY OF INFECTIOUS DISEASE

Within anthropology in recent years there has been a fundamental shift in perspective that has been labeled the biocultural synthesis. A paper authored by George Armelagos and colleagues (1992) signaled the need for this development. The paper was written in response to recognition that the field of medical anthropology at the time was bifurcated into cultural and biological wings, with limited communication across these dominant orientations. Those who came to the study of health with a cultural focus tended to emphasize ethnomedical research that examined cultural patterns of defining disease and described local social responses to it. Those with a biological orientation paid closest attention to the interactions of a population, identifiable disruptions of bodily organs and process, and the environment factors at the core of the disease process. The lack of a biocultural integration, these authors lamented, was hindering the systematic analysis of health and disease across societies. Building on an idea originally proposed by the biological anthropologist Paul Baker, they urged adoption of an ecological model informed by an integrated biocultural understanding of the disease process to addresses this problem. This approach led to the publication of the paradigm-framing volume *Building A New Biocultural Synthesis* (Good and Leatherman 1998), which brought together the work of biological, cultural, and archeological anthropologists. It also contributed to the development of a number of university medical anthropology training programs that emphasize a biocultural approach to health issues, such as Emory University, the University of Alabama, University of Washington, the University of Connecticut, and the University of Massachusetts, Amherst.

Within this context, central to the emergent field of the anthropology of infectious disease is a *biocultural* or *biosocial* conceptualization. This is the understanding that both cultural and social factors in environmental context significantly mediate the impact of infectious agents on humans. Although the dominant approach to health in society is biomedical—and involves a conceptualization that attempts to isolate and identify biological causation—the anthropological biocultural or biosocial approach is instead integrative, insisting that biological life simply does not exist in isolation from social and cultural life.

The starting point for a biocultural/biosocial conceptualization of infectious disease is recognition that infection is *always more than just biology* in that it is a product of interaction on various levels. One of these levels, assuredly, is biological. Infectious agents, be they viruses, bacteria, protozoa, helminths, fungus, or other pathogens, are necessary for infectious disease to occur. So too are the bodies of the *hosts* they infect, including their immune systems, which have evolved over millions of years as biomechanisms for limiting the harm done by pathogens. Although pathogens are necessary for infection, their presence is not sufficient to explain how and why infection occurs at particular times and places and with particular outcomes. To address these issues we must consider cultural and social factors, often as mediated by environmental conditions. As Niewöhner (2011:289–290) writes, the human body is "heavily impregnated by its own past and by the social and material environment within which it dwells. It is a body that is imprinted by evolutionary and transgenerational time, by 'early-life,' and a body that is highly susceptible to changes in its social and material environment."

Although many anthropologists blend the cultural and social aspects of human life, using terms like "sociocultural processes," there is heuristic value in maintaining conceptual differentiation. The term cultural factors, as used in this book, refers to the beliefs, meanings, norms, values, and stylistics of local behavior that give a distinctive pattern to the various human lifeways. Interpretations of HIV disease as evidence of witchcraft or punishment from God, which are specific local understandings of the nature and causes of this infectious disease, are examples of cultural conceptualizations. So too is the traditional folk belief in Sweden that cholera was spread by an agent of the king to limit the populations of the poor or the Haitian belief during the contemporary cholera epidemic that the disease was introduced by nongovernment organizations as a way to raise money. Many cultural beliefs—such as what is edible or desirable to eat, what a dwelling structure should look like and be made of, whose responsibility it is to acquire water—can shape exposure to agents of infectious disease.

It is also analytically valuable to distinguish the social origins and outcomes of infectious disease. In this case we are concerned with questions such as: Why do infectious diseases tend to cluster among the poor? How do social structures, like the global operations of transnational corporations, promote the spread of diseases? How does war spread infectious disease? These are questions about the biosocial nature of infectious diseases. Social systems can incorporate peoples with diverse cultures. In the contemporary world, the Ju/'hosani—indigenous people of southern Africa who have a tradition of living by hunting and gathering—sheep herders on the grasslands of the Tibetan Plateau, mine workers in Bolivia, and the readers of this book may have quite different cultures, but all are significantly affected by their incorporation within the global capitalist economy, which is a social structure. This book is concerned with both biocultural and biosocial interactions; it recognizes that cultural and social processes and structures are entwined in the real world but that it is useful to separate them for heuristic purposes.

What do biocultural and biosocial understandings of an infectious disease actually look like? Tuberculosis provides an example. It is known to be linked to the bacteria *Mycobacterium tuberculosis*. Yet the presence of these bacteria alone does not explain why only 25 to 50 percent of people exposed to it become infected or why only 10 percent of those who are infected develop full-blown tuberculosis, with adverse consequences if untreated (Dutt and Stead 1999). Based on a review of the literature, Ming-Jung Ho (2004), a cultural anthropologist, has identified key cultural and social factors that help explain these patterns as well as the fact that tuberculosis is disproportionately common among disadvantaged populations and has had a resurgence in developed countries since the late 1970s. For example, communal water-pipe smoking, a custom practiced in a number of African and Asian countries that also has defused to the West, is now recognized as a cultural practice that promotes the spread of tuberculosis (Knishkowy 2005). According to Rania Siam, professor of microbiology at the American University in Cairo,

"Shisha" [smoking] is Egyptian culture, where people smoke tobacco and inhale directly from this device. If I smoke "shisha", some bacteria may reside in it. When you go to a fancy bar, they do change the mouthpiece, but what about the tube of the pipe? And the water? You still have water in the container where the bacteria resides. (quoted in Fuchs 2008)

Communal water-pipe use could potentially transmit numerous other pathogens, including hepatitis C, *herpes simplex*, Epstein-Barr virus, and various respiratory viruses (Knishkowy 2005). Another cultural factor identified in Pakistan, the folk belief that tuberculosis medicines are ineffective during pregnancy (Nichter 2008), could contribute to treatment cessation and disease progression among pregnant women.

In an important set of studies William Dressler and coworkers (e.g., Dressler and Bindon 2000, Bindon 2007) have developed the concept of cultural consonance as a tool for assessing the degree to which individuals in their daily lives are able to conform to locally defined cultural models for a "successful lifestyle" and the health consequences (e.g., experience of stress and elevated blood pressure) of lack of consonance. Building on this idea, McDade (2002) developed a biocultural analysis of societal change, stress, and infectious disease among adolescents in Samoa. Traditionally Samoa youth were taught to be highly respectful of elders and strongly family oriented; they recognized that one's personal status was closely linked to one's position in their extended family and the position of their family in the community. Customary status determinants, however, have been rocked by the introduction of Western lifestyles, ideas, commodities, education, wage labor, universal suffrage, migration off-island for jobs and the sending of monetary remittance to one's family, and other dramatic changes. One consequence is what McDade calls *status incongruity*, a tension between the social status an individual holds using the traditional cultural model versus the social status they acquire as a result of their involvement in introduced Western cultural patterns. He found that youth in Samoa often feel caught between conflicting social pressures to adhere to both traditional and emergent cultural systems, and he linked this incongruity to both rising adolescent suicide rates and the uncertainty and confusion adolescent participants often express in social science research. McDade used a combination of semi-structured interviews, psychosocial information, and blood samples to assess immune function. He tested for the presence of antibodies against Epstein-Barr virus (EBV); immunological response to this herpes virus has been shown to be a consistent immunological marker of chronic stress. In other words, individuals infected with EBV harbor the virus for the rest of their lives, but it is typically kept in a latent state by cell-mediated immune function. Stress, however, can compromise this immune function and allow EBV to switch to an active state, in which it releases viral antigens that can trigger a humoral antibody response. Consequently EBV antibody level is defined as a biomarker of psychosocial stress (a higher level of antibodies indicates lower immunity). McDade found a significant association between elevated antibody levels and status incongruity in adolescents, suggesting reduced cell-mediated immune function and a higher burden of psychosocial stress. Thus, this study revealed how social and cultural changes that produce stressful life experiences are linked to the transition from latent to active infections, further revealing a fundamental aspect of biocultural/biosocial interaction in the making of infectious disease.

Some cultural patterns, by contrast, may inhibit disease transmission. In his research, Norbert Vecchiato (1997) found that the Sidama of Ethiopia believed that overwork, excessive exposure to the sun, or carrying heavy loads could cause tuberculosis (locally known as *balamo*). They also believed that "avoiding contact with a patient" was the best prophylactic measure against contracting this disease. It also has been found that certain cultural practices may affect wealthy and poor sectors of a hierarchical society differently. Brown (1998), for example, describes how the traditional social organization of the grape harvest in Bosa, Sardinia, an autonomous region of the Italian Republic, provided protection to the social elites from malaria. During the malaria season the land-owning families of Bosa moved to summer homes on high ground so they could supervise the harvest. The working class, however, remained living in lower areas where infected mosquitoes were most numerous.

Social factors, including issues of social hierarchy and inequality, the exercise of power, and diverse forms of abuse are absolutely critical to the spread and impact of infectious diseases. Chagas disease is a vector-borne infection transmitted by *triatomins* (kissing bugs) that can produce initial symptoms like fever, fatigue, body aches, rash, and nausea and may lead to more severe outcomes, including congestive heart failure and cardiac arrest. It is most rampant among the poor and happens to be one of the most neglected diseases internationally: "its unequal distribution illustrates the complex interaction of sociocultural, biological and environmental factors" (Ventura-Garcia et al. 2013). For example, during the 1980s in the Amazon region, governments supported economic policies that enhanced industrial production, international trade, and globalization; promoted road building, land expropriations, and deforestation (to support pasturing and beef exploration); forced migration of families to cities; and expanded poorly remunerated wage labor. These changes "altered the traditional conditions that had controlled transmission of the infection to humans" (Briceño-León 2007:36). Triatomins, previously located in more wooded areas, began occupying domestic spaces, and household infestation increased, an incursion facilitated by crowded and impoverished living conditions and shoddy housing construction characterized by cracks and crevices in walls and roofs where tiatomines could find shelter (Coimbra 1988). In short, social factors significantly changed the domain of Chagas disease, resulting in spiraling rates of infection.

But cultural and social factors do not just influence what pathogens can *do*; biocultural/biosocial approaches show us that cultural and social processes affect what pathogens actually *are*. Pathogens constantly evolve in response to changes in the conditions of hosts, such as the development and use of antibiotics, shifting dietary practices, alterations in lifestyle, and so on. The reverse is also true: the presence of infectious diseases shape cultural and social systems. For example, in *Armies of Pestilence: The Impact of Disease on History,* R. S. Bray (2004) reviews the multiple ways diseases such as plague, cholera, smallpox, typhus, yellow fever, influenza, and AIDS have affected the course of history, the configuration of human beliefs and behaviors, and the organization of social systems.

One of the primary ways medical anthropologists think about the actions and effects of infectious diseases is in terms of the environment. This line of thinking, more broadly known as the *EcoHealth perspective,* is concerned with how changes in human ecology, including both naturally occurring and human-promoted changes in Earth's ecosystems, affect human health. For example, emissions from factories, vehicles, and other technologies that burn fossil fuels wind up as large quantities of carbon dioxide in the oceans. Heavy dosing of agricultural areas with fertilizers has led to the run-off of potent chemicals, including nitrates and phosphates, into the oceans. Atmospheric CO_2, also from emissions, in turn, is contributing to heating up the oceans. One result of all of these changes in the composition and temperature of ocean waters is the presence along US coasts of harmful *red tides* comprised of algae and infectious bacteria. *Karenia brevis,* a microscopic marine algae found in red tide, can trigger eye and respiratory irritation that, in people with severe respiratory conditions, may provoke strong adverse reactions. Although they were once unusual, today red tides have become common and annually contribute to illness and death among those who consume contaminated fish and shellfish. As this example suggests, humans are having an ever more dramatic adverse impact on the environment, including behaviors that boost the spread and human exposure to infectious diseases.

Pulling the various threads of this discussion together, the biocultural/ biosocial conceptualization of infectious disease recognizes that in all cases a complex interplay of biological, social, cultural, and environmental factors underlies the appearance, natural history, virulence, and outcomes of agent-related disease. There is a real sense in which there is an inseparability of environmental, social, cultural, and biological factors. All of these participate in an ongoing co-evolutionary transformation.

As a result, it is not really quite accurate to assert, despite its frequent appearance in various health texts, that "tuberculosis is an infectious disease caused by a bacterium called *Mycobacterium tuberculosis*" or "AIDS is a disease caused by a virus called HIV (human immunodeficiency virus)." As we have seen, neither of these diseases spread randomly in populations; patterns of infection change over time and place, and even the virulence or actual disease expressions of infectious agents varies in terms of both location and era of occurrence. Over time infectious agents, cultural systems, and social structures continually undergo reactive changes in response to each other and to changes in the environment, which are often caused by sociocultural changes.

Despite recognition that biology is only one aspect of infection, a necessary but insufficient explanation of its cause—it is important for anthropologists working in this area to have a solid grounding in relevant biological factors, including an understanding of the behavioral ecology of pathogens and vectors; how these are influenced by the physical environment, including anthropogenically impacted environments; other species in the environment; *pathogen-host* and *pathogen-pathogen interactions*; and the functioning of the multilayered human immune system. These are issues of primary concern to other health disciplines like epidemiology. Consequently anthropologists working on infectious disease issues often have broad, multidisciplinary training. Medical anthropologists frequently work in collaboration with epidemiologists, other kinds of social and behavioral scientists, nurses, physicians, and people trained in allied health fields. For example, in studies of HIV risk and strategies for hepatitis B (HBV) vaccination among street injection drug users, the author of this book worked with broad multidisciplinary teams of epidemiological and other researchers (e.g., Grau et al. 2009; Singer et al. 2011).

In sum, as displayed in Table 1.1, from the anthropological perspective, an infectious event is composed of a suite of interlocked components and cannot be reduced to any one of them. Critical to the assessment of such an event is the development of an understanding of the interaction among these components, how they affect each other, not simply their nature as isolated features. As Lock (2001:484) observes, "knowledge about biology is informed by the social and the social is in turn informed by the reality of the material."

Another way to describe the anthropological approach to infectious disease is in terms of an infectious disease formula that identifies key heuristic components in an interactive and interdependent process:

Table 1.1 Components of the Anthropology of Infectious Disease

Biological Factors
Pathogens
Human Immune System
Overall health (nutrition, stress, chronic health problems, other infections)
Pathogen/host interaction

Environmental Factors
Food and water availability
Weather/Climate

Sociocultural Factors
Sociocultural systems seen as local or broader organized sets of knowledge, experience, attitudes, norms and behaviors that generate understanding of and respond to disease
Sociocultural systems seen as forces and energy systems that impact environments
Sociocultural systems as historically rooted forces that structure social relationship, exposure to disease, and access to resources
Patterns of globalization and the flow of commodities, people and disease

As this formula and the arrows within it suggest, infectious disease health status is a reflection of dynamic interrelations among biological, environmental, and social and cultural factors.

Infectious agents ◀▶ Environmental factors ◀▶ Transmission Factors (types of diffusion mechanisms) ◀▶ Immune Factors ◀▶ Social and Cultural Factors = Infectious Disease Health Status.

Infection, of course, is one type of a broader category of conditions that we label *disease.* The term refers to conditions that impair normal tissue function. Medical anthropology commonly differentiates *disease,* as a clinically identified biological condition, from *illness,* which refers to the culturally shaped experience and meaning of being sick. Another way of phrasing this differentiation is that sufferers and their social networks construct illnesses based on immediate sensations and lived experiences and in terms of their cultural understandings. Clinicians, by contrast, construct diseases based on patient reports of symptoms as well as signs of biological disruptions provided by laboratory tests or direct observations and in terms of their medical knowledge.

From an anthropological perspective it is possible to have a disease and not experience illness. An example of this is found with sexually transmitted infections like chlamydia. *Chlamydia trachotais* is a bacteria that enters the body through sexual contact and in many cases spreads without producing experienced symptoms. This stealth factor is the source of the bacteria's name, which is derived from the Greek word for "cloak." It is estimated that three-quarters of all infected females and half of infected males are unaware they have been infected, although, if left untreated, chlamydia can cause pelvic inflammatory disease, ectopic pregnancy, and infertility (Watson et al. 2002). Conversely, it is possible to be ill but undiseased. A classic example is described by Baars (1997:104), who notes that "medical students who study frightening diseases for the first time routinely develop vivid delusions of having the 'disease of the week'—whatever they are currently studying." Upon first learning of the localized symptoms of pneumonia, students may report feeling discomfort in possible sites of pneumonia infection and become convinced, at least temporarily, that they have pneumonia.

It is also important to clarify the difference between infection and infectious disease. The human body can be infected with the strains of *mycobacteria* that have the capacity to cause tuberculosis but then not develop the disease because a healthy immune system prevents the development of active tuberculosis disease. An individual with latent tuberculosis cannot transmit the bacteria to others. If the individual's immune system subsequently is compromised by other diseases, chemotherapy, malnutrition, aging, or other factors, latent tuberculosis can become active and damaging to the sufferer's health and be transmitted to others. In other words, one can be infected with the pathogen that causes tuberculosis and not suffer the disease. The term infection also is often used to refer to very local manifestations of pathogen activity, such as occurs around a small paper cut on a finger, that does not reach the adequate scale of spread and damage to the body to be considered a disease. On a biological level the basic processes are the same, but there is a cultural differentiation made on the basis of perceived threat.

The labeling of one pathogen-related condition as an infection and another as a disease also reflects other sociocultural factors. Historically, for example, infections transmitted through intimate contact were labeled sexually transmitted diseases (STDs). Given the cultural meanings and emotions evoked by the word disease, including social stigmas that may lead sufferers to avoid treatment, there has been a strong push in biomedicine and public health to replace the use of STD with sexually transmitted infection (STI).

One challenge posed by the anthropological definition and, indeed, all definitions of disease is that it is impossible to establish fully what normal tissue function is. Complex conditions influence body tissue, including diet, genetics, stress, toxic exposure, pathogens, environmental conditions, and social factors. In defining health, many people follow the World Health Organization's (1946) statement that health is a state of complete physical, mental, and social well-being and not merely the absence of disease or infirmity. Although it is useful to have this kind of starting point, it too leaves open what a complete state of well-being would be and whether it is in fact achievable. At a minimum it is possible to recognize states of greater and lesser health and of the role that infectious disease plays in our level of health at various scales (individual through global) at any point in time.

Within biomedicine and beyond there has reigned a culturally rooted imagery and lexicon of war in our understanding of infectious disease. As anthropologist Emily Martin (1990:421) observes, "As immunology describes it, bodies are imperiled nations continuously at war to quell alien invaders. These nations have sharply defined borders in space, which are constantly besieged and threatened." Bruce Albers and colleagues (2002:1487), for example, state, "The development of the exquisitely precise adaptive immune system in vertebrates . . . was an important escalation in the arms race that has always existed between pathogens and their hosts." There is nothing "natural," however, about viewing our relationship with pathogens as a kind of military struggle to defend the homeland. Martin notes that one component of our immune system, the *macrophage* white blood cell, consumes microbes. She argues, "If the view that microorganisms serve as food for macrophages were given prominence, we could see this process as a food chain, linked by mutual dependencies" in a world in which all organisms are dependent on others for food. In this world we consume other organisms, and they consume us at various scales. These are natural processes that connect all life forms in complex ecological relationships.

Another way of thinking about infectious diseases is to view them in terms of more immediate and more distal causes. As states of disrupted health, infectious diseases involve impaired tissue function that is immediately or directly caused by biological agents. In order to cause disease, pathogens must be able to enter a person's body, adhere to specific cells therein, colonize body tissues, avoid or subvert the host's immune system, and inflict damage on these tissues as part of normal and natural processes of pathogen consumption and reproduction. Although the growth of pathogen densities may be enough to cause tissue damage in some cases, the production of toxins or destructive enzymes by the pathogen or by the immune response the body mounts often causes the damage. For example, when the pathogen *Mycobacterium tuberculosis* enters a person's body, usually by inhaling the exhale of an already infected individual, as noted above, macrophages detect and consume the bacterium. But rather than being destroyed in this process, the microbe releases a substance known as cyclic AMP, which allows it to avoid destruction and assume a protected dormant state only to become active if the host's immune system subsequently is weakened. Yet this is only a proximate understanding of the situation. Nelson Mandela, who spent twenty-seven years in prison for his efforts to overthrow the racist apartheid government of South Africa, contracted tuberculosis while in prison, where it is a common threat to health. Notably, Mandela announced his condition during the 15th International AIDS Conference because tuberculosis, which kills almost 2 million people each year, is a leading cause of death for people with HIV infection because it weakens the immune system. In his remarks Mandela (quoted in Nakashima 2004) noted, "My friends objected to me sharing my personal affairs," referencing the stigma attached to tuberculosis in many countries, where it is seen as a disease of the poor. As this example suggests, ultimate causes, like the use of imprisonment to control oppressed populations and cultural factors like stigmatization of disease, are not only of keen interest to anthropologists but also critical components of tuberculosis infection as well as other infection diseases. They are, as Geoffrey Rose (1992) expressed it, "the causes of the causes"—the distal factors that enable the proximal causes. More distal and proximate causes of infectious disease comprise an *ecological web of causation* that includes social, cultural, environmental, and biological components (Mayer 2000).

Paul Brown and colleagues (2012) maintain that human social and cultural systems have three fundamental roles in determining the patterns of disease and death in a population: (1) they shape behaviors, such as diet, sexual practice, and land use, that expose people to infections or shield them from them; (2) they reshape the physical environment in ways that affect human susceptibility to infections; and (3) they influence human responses to infectious disease and both facilitate health improvements and exacerbate disease burdens. To this list, two additional items can be added: (4) they have evolutionary impacts on our bodies that influence our interaction with infectious diseases, as discussed below with regard to the role of culture in reductions in our hairiness and exposure to ectoparasites, and (5) they play a role in changing pathogens, and these changes, in turn, rebound on us in our continued interaction with them.

WHAT COUNTS IN INFECTIOUS DISEASE?

How important are infectious diseases in human health? The ways we understand this question and respond to it also reflect sociocultural practices. Looking a two profoundly important current infectious diseases, according to the World Health Organization (2013a), almost 70 million people worldwide have been infected with the HIV virus, and about 35 million of them have died of HIV disease. At the end of 2011 it was estimated that there were 34.0 million people in the world living with HIV infection, or 0.8 percent of adults aged fifteen to forty-nine years, with considerable variance between countries and regions. The World Health Organization (2012a) also reports that the global tuberculosis rates have been falling for several years and decreased by a rate of 2.2 percent between 2010 and 2011. At the country level the World Health Organization points to Cambodia as an example of what can be achieved in a low-income and high-burden country, as Cambodia reports a 45 percent decrease in tuberculosis prevalence since 2002.

We are very familiar with health statistics like those reported above. They regularly show up in mass media accounts of epidemics and other health issues. They are used in this public venue to affirm how significant a health problem has become or that substantial health improvements have been achieved. The epidemiological and public health reporting of infectious disease outbreaks and prevalences, in terms of precise numbers of cases and related quantitative information about the characteristics of sufferers or regional distributions, reflects a social reliance on seemingly objective figures and processes of enumeration. Although tallies like those for HIV and tuberculosis reported above are used in decision making about where to direct limited resources in public health programming and what issues to focus on in public health education, from an anthropological perspective, based on on-the-ground experience in the study of infectious outbreaks and epidemics, questions are raised about the production of official statistics: Where do the numbers come from? How are they compiled, by whom, under what conditions, with what uniformity, and using what criteria? And, in light of these other questions, what do the numbers actually mean?

Here is an example of the importance of being cautious about official statistics. Mary Dixon-Woods and colleagues (2012) conducted an ethnographic study in England on central-line infections, a hospital-acquired bacterial infection most commonly seen in intensive care patients with catheters inserted close to their hearts. They found notable variation in social practices of data collection and reporting across hospitals, which, simply put, "were not counting the same things in the same way" (Dixon-Woods et al. 2012:580). These variations reflected a number of factors, such as whether hospital staff, who bore burdensome workloads and needed to prioritize their efforts, viewed detailed record keeping as a legitimate use of their limited available time. Long-established and entrenched work patterns as well as clinician preferences also contributed to considerable variability in case reporting.

In another take on the reliability of quantitative infectious disease data, Kathleen Gallagher and colleagues (2003) compared information on over two hundred HIV infection cases reported to the Massachusetts Department of Public Health to the original medical records for these cases at the site of patient diagnosis. They found that although routine AIDS surveillance data were reliable for demographic variables (e.g., patient age, gender), they were less reliable for information about clinical events, laboratory findings, or, especially, treatments patients had received. In infectious disease epidemics numbers often are based on what is known as "passive reporting," which is based on cases seen in health facilities. But passive reporting is burdened with multiple shortcomings. As the World Health Organization (2013b) recognizes with reference to epidemic-prone infectious diseases, in various places in the world there is inadequate access to health care facilities. Many people become sick and die without ever visiting a health care facility, so their cases are never reported. Additionally, many diseases are underrecognized. This is especially the case with diseases with nonspecific symptoms or those that are new to a region. These problems are magnified by the fact that in lesser-developed countries the level of laboratory support needed for diagnosis is poor, clinical and laboratory staff may be underpaid and overworked, and training is limited. As a result, considerable variation can be found in the quality of reporting systems from country to country and between urban and more rural areas, reflecting the significant effects on official statistics of economic, social, cultural, and epidemiological factors.

This discussion reveals that health statistics are more than what they seem because they always are socially produced and, hence, are influenced by a wide array of human, cultural, institutional, structural, and situational factors. As anthropologist Didier Fassin (2004:169) emphasizes, health problems "are not only biological realities that specialists elucidate, they are also epidemiological facts that they construct." In assessing statistics on infectious disease it is not possible to parse biology from cultural conditions and social influences. In HIV disease, for example, the way health professionals had defined "AIDS" early in the epidemic precluded the counting of many cases among women, who suffered from *opportunistic infections* that were not recognized as "AIDS related." Consequently, from an anthropological perspective it is always necessary to not take the numbers or even the categories used in epidemiological reporting on infectious diseases at face value as neutral statements about objective realities. Subjecting the numbers as well as what is being counted (and not counted) to scrutiny in light of the influence of social and cultural factors is routine anthropological practice.

THE WIDER CONTEXTS OF INFECTIOUS DISEASE OUTBREAKS

There is an identifiable relationship between infectious diseases—including who gets which disease, how sick they get, and the outcomes of their sickness—and the hierarchy of social relationships structured by inequalities in wealth and power within and across societies (Baer, Singer, and Susser 2013; Farmer 1999). HIV disease, for instance, has tended to spread "along the fault lines of . . . society" (Bateson and Goldsby 1988:2). Although first identified among gay men in the United States, HIV disease soon became disproportionately frequent in low-income and socially subordinated communities of color. This pattern of disease spread was not random, nor was it the consequence of biology; rather, it reflects the fact that infectious disease spread is socially determined. HIV infection interacts with human societies and the social relationships that constitute them to create the global "HIV disease pandemic," which is the worldwide pattern of distribution of the disease and the social responses that have developed around it in particular groups and populations. Glaring social disparities between dominant versus subordinate groups and wealthy versus impoverished populations in the distribution of HIV disease as well as in access to available treatment have typified the pandemic. The relationship between poor health and poverty is a consequence of multiple biocultural/biosocial factors, including "weakened immunity and neurophysiological development because of malnutrition, ease of spread of pathogens because of insalubrious living conditions, and the precariousness of social support networks" (Nguyen and Peschard 2003:449) (see Figure 1.1).

Beyond poverty, other forms of social discrimination, marginalization, structural violence, and assaults on human dignity also are essential factors in the development and spread of infectious diseases, as discussed in greater detail in Chapter 7. Further, as Shirley Lindenbaum (2001:380) comments, the study of infectious disease epidemics "provides a unique point of entry for examining

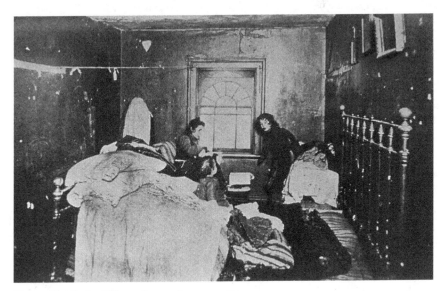

Figure 1.1 Early 20ᵗʰ century urban poverty.

the relationships among cultural assumptions, particular institutional forms, and states of mind," an issue addressed below.

CULTURAL WINDOWS ON INFECTION

People everywhere suffer from infectious disease, and because humans characteristically respond to and understand life experience using socially acquired cultural frameworks, all societies have developed local knowledge about infection and healing practices, including culturally constructed understandings that may differ from biomedical models of infection. Even in the West, the broad adoption of the biomedical germ theory model of infection took time and, in some ways, remains less than fully complete, a fact revealed in times of infectious disease panics.

For example, during a global *pandemic* of *influenza* in the early twentieth century that killed as many as 50 to 100 million people worldwide, countless local health strategies were used to try to protect or cure people. In Utah, which had the third highest rate of death of US states, archival records show that people made use of a mixture of home and doctor remedies. Alcohol, normally banned in the largely Mormon state, was sold to doctors to treat patients. Some parents hung bags of herbs around children's necks to prevent influenza (Department of Health and Human Services n.d.). Many people understood from health authorities that "germs" caused the disease but were not completely sure what germs were or how they were transmitted from one person to another. To feel safe, families locked themselves in their homes and sealed their keyholes and the cracks around their doors with cotton. Utah public health officials enacted laws requiring citizens to wear gauze masks. Some towns required anyone entering their municipalities to possess a certificate signed by a doctor affirming that they were symptom-free. Railroads were warned not to accept passengers without such a certificate, and all passengers wore masks; streetcar conductors were told to limit their passengers; and stores were banned from holding sales. Following a ban on public assemblies, police began making arrests of people for gathering together in small groups (e.g., to play a game of cards). In the town of Cedar City a parade celebrating the end World War I featured a statue of Lady Liberty wearing a mask to publicize this strategy for controlling the spread of disease. Although we know that such masks do not prevent infection, even today graphic news coverage of disease outbreaks around the world reveals the widespread belief that they are protective.

Anthropologists are demonstrating the great diversity of beliefs about disease as well as the many kinds of treatments people use outside of clinical settings. In a study of Hispanic HIV infection patients receiving care at a biomedical clinic in New Jersey, for example, Mariana Suarez and coworkers (1996) found that three quarters of the seventy-six participants in their study believed in good and evil spirits. Among those who did, almost half reported that the spirits had a causal role in their infection, either alone or in conjunction with the human immunodeficiency virus. Most participants engaged in folk healing practices developed within the religious traditions of spiritualism and santeria. People do not just stand by idly when infectious disease strikes but instead take actions that are attuned with their culturally acquired beliefs about the world in both its physical and supernatural aspects, about disease as they understand it, and in light of their traditional healing practices. Such practices are not irrational, regardless of whether they are effective, but rather reflect meaningful cultural constructions of the world.

SOCIAL WINDOWS ON INFECTION

Anthropologist Ronald Frankenberg (1980) advocated examining the "making social of disease." This work entails revealing both the structures of social relationships that shape the making of disease as well as the social roles, behaviors, locations, and messages involved in turning individual experience of symptoms into socially accepted disease events. In part, understanding the making social of disease involves an analysis of "the social construction of medicine as practice, as institution, and as ideology, including the social functions of medicine in society" (Singer 2004:16–17). It also involves investigating the negotiation of disease among health professionals and patients, as Erin Koch did in her analysis of tuberculosis in the post-Soviet country of Georgia (Koch 2013a, Koch 2013b). In 1993 the World Health Organization declared tuberculosis a global health emergency and began promoting a program, known as DOTS (directly-observed treatment, short-course), that involved the direct viewing of patients taking a prescribed short course of tuberculosis medication. DOTS soon became the global standard of tuberculosis control, and Georgia, a "hot spot" in the global resurgence of tuberculosis, with crumbling medical infrastructure, became a center of global assessment of DOTS implementation. At stake was far more than the effective treatment of tuberculosis; external funders and international NGOs implementing DOTS wanted to transition the Georgian health care system away from a Soviet to a market-based model. Included in this transition was an emphasis on shifting to a narrow focus on the clinical aspects of tuberculosis while diminishing attention to the biosocial perspective of the disease embraced by local doctors, nurses, laboratory technicians, and health administrators who were trained under the Soviet model. The market-based medical model ushered in along with DOTS included a biomedical focus on clinical issues isolated from their social contexts.

As a consequence of its crumbling health care system, by the mid-2000s Georgia began to see a growing rate of tuberculosis patients defaulting from fixed treatment regimes. In response, the DOTS program emphasized the creation of "DOTS Spots," which were locations in general polyclinics where nurses could distribute antibiotics to patients and observe that medications were ingested, in accordance with World Health Organization protocols. In studying this approach, which significantly decreased the loss of patients to treatment, Koch found that what often was critical was the social interaction among nurses and patients and the support patients felt they received from treatment providers (Koch 2013b). Despite a programmatic emphasis on clinical procedures and antibiotic distribution, social factors appeared to be crucial to the success of DOTS. This example teaches a broad lesson about the importance of social factors in infectious diseases.

PARASITE-STRESS THEORY OF SOCIALITY

Corey Fincher, Randy Thornhill, and colleagues have developed an evolutionary biosocial/biocultural theory of the impact of pathogens on the social life of humans as well as other animal species that merits consideration. Termed the *parasite-stress theory of sociality,* it posits a variable adoption of in-group and out-group sociocultural tactics in response to the degree of local threat of infectious disease agents. In other words, these researchers argue that in reaction to the degree of risk of infectious diseases, which varies considerably by location, social groups develop patterns of interaction, including variation in intense versus less intense in-group contact and out-group avoidance (called *assortative sociality or homophily*). Moreover, they explain language diversity among neighboring peoples as emerging in the same way as an adaptation to the disease, protecting benefits of separating the in-group from others (Fincher and Thornhill 2008). Critical to this theory is the view that infectious diseases were major sources of morbidity and mortality and, thus, key forces of natural selection in human evolutionary history.

One of the issues parasite-stress theory raises is the fact that societies vary in the degree to which they emphasis strong family ties and durable extended family relations and, somewhat similarly, exhibit variable levels of religious group commitment. At issue here is the strength within a society of preferring to interact—including interact exclusively—with people who are perceived as being similar (i.e., relatives and those who share one's religion). Moreover, as part of this pattern are the multitude of ways—such as clothing patterns, tattooing and scarification, food preferences, and language and dialect—that people around the world use to mark in-group similarity and draw social boundaries around themselves. Also involved are behaviors designed to mark and adversely treat others as dissimilar, as people deemed to be different and beyond the borders of the in-group, including expressions of ethnocentrism, stigmatization, racism, and xenophobia. In accounting for the development of these sociocultural patterns, Fincher and Thornhill (2012:2) assert that they reflect "varying levels of parasite-stress experienced by people, both within a region and across geographic space." In other words, this theory posits that diverse patterns of social interaction and related behaviors have emerged in local and regional contexts over the course of human history as defensive strategies that respond to the level of infectious disease threat from surrounding peoples. As part of this theory, a parallel is drawn between the biological immune system and what is termed the *behavioral immune system*. The latter refers to culturally constituted behaviors and psychological orientations that both provide social groups protection from infectious disease agents and guide the social management of infectious diseases when they occur. Assert Fincher and Thornhill (2012:2):

> The behavioral immune system is comprised of ancestrally adaptive feelings, attitudes, and values about and behaviors toward out-group and in-group members, caution about or unwillingness to interact with out-group people, and prejudice against people perceived as unhealthy, contaminated, or unclean. . . . The behavioral immune system also includes the same types of bias against contact with nonhuman animals that pose human infectious disease threats.

A core component of this theory is its emphasis on local biologies, based on the assumption that immune responses, biologically and behaviorally, are most effective against local strains and species of pathogens to which a social group has been co-evolving with for some time and less effective against those pathogens that have been evolving in nearby host groups. As a result, out-groups may be infected with novel pathogenic varieties that in-group members cannot efficiently defend against. According to parasite-stress theory, the various group behavior strategies discussed above evolved to protect groups from their neighboring groups' diseases and are expressions of the significant impact of infectious diseases on sociocultural patterns.

The findings of various studies have been cited in support of this theory. Research by Jason Faulkner and colleagues (2004) and Carlos Navarrete and Daniel Fessler (2006), for example, shows that the numerical scores individuals receive on psychological tests that measure their level of xenophobia and ethnocentrism reflect their perceived vulnerability to infectious disease. People who believe that they are at high risk for infectious disease thus have greater levels of xenophobic and ethnocentric attitudes than those who perceive low infectious disease threat. Using World Health Organization data on *DALYs* (disability adjusted life years lost, which combines sickness and death measures) attributed to twenty-eight infectious diseases that are transmitted through human-to-human transmission (i.e., nonzoonotic diseases) and various behavioral datasets (e.g., the World Values Survey, the American Religious Identification Survey), Corey Fincher and Randy Thornhill (2012) hypothesized that (1) individuals who value strong family ties will be found predominantly in areas with greater parasite stress, (2) people facing higher levels of parasite stress will be more likely to adhere to local religious systems than those living in low parasite stress locations, and (3) the level of time and effort dedicated to participation in religious practice and the value people place on religious practice and ideals will be positively correlated with local parasite stress. Analyses confirmed all of their hypotheses for strong family ties and heightened religiosity, which they conclude provides strong support for the parasite-stress theory of sociality.

Not surprisingly this theory has its critics. Mícheál de Barra and Val Curtis (2012) question the key assertion that the pathogens of social out-groups are more dangerous than those found among in-group members. The existing literature, they argue, shows that the pressure of natural selection on pathogens favors traits that enable them to spread within their current host populations, not those that help them spread to neighboring groups. Also, the theory does not address the importance of ease of transmission between people (e.g., hepatitis C is much more easily transmitted sexually than HIV infection) on the virulence of a pathogenic agent, an issue discussed in Chapter 5. To cite one infectious disease case that raises serious questions about this theory, Chapter 2 discusses the condition that came to be known as kuru among the South Foré of New Guinea. As detailed there, it was in-group-affirming ritual behavior that was responsible for spreading this lethal disease among members of the in-group, and the lack of participation in these ritual behaviors protected out-groups from infection. Without doubt, the parasite-stress theory of sociality is intriguing; its ability to account for human or pathogen behavior, however, remains in dispute.

GLOBALIZATION OF INFECTIOUS DISEASE: DRIVERS OF DISEASE FLOW

Over time and at an ever-quickening pace, contact, exchange, and communication has been occurring across societies and regions of the planet. In the contemporary era people, products (including medicines), technologies, and infectious agents as well as ideas and other cultural components are moving rapidly around the world. This process of advancing cross-border social connectivity, known as *globalization*, has significantly diminished the spatial and temporal barriers between species and ecosystems and profoundly changed infectious disease ecology. Existing evidence suggests that there have been important alterations in the prevalence, spread, geographic range, and control of many infectious diseases because of globalization (Crowl et al. 2008). In the words of Gro Harlem Brundtland (2001), former director of the World Health Organization, "In a modern world, bacteria and viruses travel almost as fast as money. With globalization, a single microbial sea washes over all humankind." Indeed, as stressed in this book, the metaphorical sea to which Brundtland refers washes over far more humankind; it washes over animals as well, necessitating a more-than-human lens in the study of human health.

One of the reasons globalization promotes the spread of disease is modern human mobility (Tatem, Rogers, and Hay 2006). A glimpse at the role of human travel in infection can be seen in a recent study in New York City of identified cases of three infectious diseases, *hepatitis A, malaria,* and *typhoid*. Among individuals diagnosed with these diseases, 61 percent of hepatitis A cases, 100 percent of malaria cases, and 78 percent of typhoid cases were related to travel outside the United States (Adamson et al. 2010). Similarly, the rapid movement of people around the world was the key factor in the rapid spread of SARS from China to North America and elsewhere.

Another example of the mobility of infectious disease in a changing world can be seen in the case of *dengue*, a painful and debilitating viral infection. Dengue, a disease spread by a mosquito vector (primarily *Aedes aegypti*), became widely spread throughout tropical areas of the planet with the development of commercial shipping during the eighteenth century; in essence, the disease was "shipped" around the world (see Figure 1.2).

In the case of Southeast Asia, World War II pushed the spread of dengue as the movement of troops facilitated the dispersion of the various strains of dengue viruses across the region. The consequence was a situation known as *hyperendemicity*, which involves the simultaneous and overlapping circulation of multiple dengue serotypes. Co-infection with more than one strain produced the emergence of severe dengue hemorrhagic fever in the Philippines and Thailand during the 1950s. By the 1970s regular dengue epidemics were common throughout Southeast Asia as well as in Latin America, and *hemorrhagic fever* had become a leading cause of the hospitalization and death of children.

Research on shipping shows that the large metal shipping containers now used to move products around the world play a role in spreading other disease vectors and the diseases they transmit. This is one explanation for the diffusion of the West Nile virus to the United States around 1999. Cruise ships create another opportunity for the global movement of infectious agents. In 2010, for

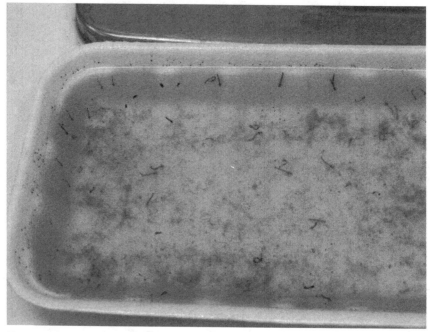

Figure 1.2 Aedes aegypti mosquito larvae. (Photo by Merrill Singer)

example, Cruise Line Association member companies recorded that 14.8 million people traveled by cruise ships, with an average travel time of seven days. Visiting various ports of call, cruises increase social connectivity worldwide, whereas cruise ships, as contained spaces, provide ideal conditions for the rapid spread of infectious agents (Garely 2012).

Food importation provides another pathway for infectious disease movement. The dramatic rise in the globalization of seafood along with the heavy demand in the comparatively wealthy US market has led to the rapid increase in the importation of marine food sources from around the world. The United States now imports more than 80 percent of its seafood supply, including both wild-caught and farm-raised fish and shellfish. This seafood is processed by thousands of suppliers based in over 150 countries, with China being one of the largest exporters of seafood to the United States. In 2007 the US Food and Drug Administration (FDA) reported that there were almost nine hundred thousand entries of imported seafood into the country; however, the FDA inspected only fourteen thousand, or just about 2 percent. One consequence has been outbreaks of fish poisoning caused by infectious agents, such as infected tuna steaks imported from Indonesia and Vietnam in 2006. A likely source of such outbreaks was inadequate temperature control between the time the fish were caught and the time they were consumed. Direct testing yields evidence of significant rates of the infection of imported seafood (Heinitz et al. 2000). In the contemporary globalized world, with shrinking government regulation, there is a significant potential for infection of imported seafood, a trend that global warming may exacerbate.

Health impacts are not the only consequences of the flow of infectious diseases. As a result of the skyrocketing increase in the movement of people and commodities around the planet, "the traditional 'drawbridge' strategy of disease control and quarantine [is] increasingly irrelevant" (Tatem, Rogers, and Hay 2006:16). This fact, however, has not stopped governments from attempting to use such methods in an epidemic, often combined with equally futile finger pointing at other nations as well as boycotts of their products without evidence supporting the health benefits of such action.

These examples affirm the importance of *microbial traffic*—the flow of pathogens to new host populations—for human health in a world where political and geographic boundaries no longer construct isolated microbial environments (Mayer 2000). Microbial traffic involves movement of pathogens from animals to people, people to other animals, and between human populations. Part of microbial traffic involves *genetic mixing*, the movement of genetic information across pathogen strains and species. Many of the emergent conditions that promote microbial traffic have their origin in human activities, reflecting constant changes in the relationship between humans and their environments. As Stephen Morse (1992:1327) observes, "people are creating much (although by no means all) of the traffic, even if we are doing it inadvertently." Morse views changes like deforestation, dam building, and the extension or technological transformation of agricultural production and other changes in land use as "traffic signals for microbial traffic" but argues that "we should see them [as well] as warning signals" (1992:1327). Further, these *anthropocentric* changes have helped to create "a remarkable new milieu referred to as 'the *global mixing bowl*' in which microbes have many new opportunities to create new niches, cross species boundaries, travel worldwide very quickly and establish new beachheads in the populations of people and animals" (American Veterinary Medical Association 2008:10, emphasis added).

As part of globalization processes, not only do infectious agents travel rapidly, but so do ideas about them. As political correspondent Declan McCullagh observed,

> SARS is the first epidemic of the Internet age, preying on the fact that as information becomes more communicable, rumors become more

communicable too. A teenager's Web hoax claiming Hong Kong borders would be closed prompted runs on canned food and toilet paper. A super market owner in Sacramento spent two weeks arguing that contrary to rumors, neither he nor his family was infected with SARS, and his stores were entirely safe. (quoted in Scott and Duncan 2004:2)

Pathogens, ideas and worries about them, and broader societal responses to them are in flux in the contemporary world, and increasing understanding of what is going on in these fast-paced times is a core item on the agenda of the anthropology of infectious diseases.

THE ANTHROPOLOGICAL DIFFERENCE: WHAT ANTHROPOLOGY ADDS

Why is there a need for an anthropology of infectious disease? Vitalizing the modern anthropological approach is a broad vision that incorporates a holistic understanding of human societies populated by people experiencing their world, including their health, through webs of meaning that are encoded in complex symbolic and semiotic systems; a recognition that humans are at once cognitive and emotional beings that bring a dynamic package of local and wider knowledges as well as feelings to their life experiences; an appreciation of the fundamental importance of human/environment interaction in shaping human activities and health; and an awareness of the role of structures of often unequal social relationship in the creation of threats to human well-being. In the specific domain of infectious disease research, anthropology is distinguished by a number of attributes, including an approach to research that examines interconnections and intersections among social, cultural, environmental, and biological factors, bringing to light vital linkages that might otherwise be over-looked. Anthropological studies tend to take place "in context" in the physical and social worlds in which people's lives unfold over time and in which they are infected and either suffer disease progression or improve. It was focused anthropological research, for example, that revealed that the specific culturally constituted ways and contexts in which drug users share drugs and not just the immediate sharing or multiperson use of syringes that was contributing to the spread of HIV infection in injecting populations (Koester and Hoffer 1994; Needle et al. 1998; Page et al. 1990). The anthropological emphasis on culture and context as factors that matter helps explain why people do what they do, an issue of considerable importance if what they do facilitates infection or protects them from it. Moreover, studying up and down, anthropologists are in a position to see how social structures and structural inequalities and not just personal decisions and individual actions create infectious risk and *risk environments* and link individual risk to social vulnerability. Consequently, anthropologists frequently suggest solutions to health problems that are informed by awareness of both the actual immediate and ultimate causes of disease. In a discussion of HIV transmission through sexual behavior, for example, anthropologist Richard Parker stresses the importance of refocusing understanding on sexual desire, which is often condemned in moralistic discussions of HIV risk, "from an individual to a collective phenomenon" (Parker 2009:xiv). Culture provides a frame of reference "through which sexual meanings are organized—and in relationship to which conflicting and contrasting sexual scripts are produced and reproduced" (Parker 2009:xiv). These, in turn, are shaped by other factors like social hierarchies and structural inequalities.

APPLYING THE ANTHROPOLOGY OF INFECTIOUS DISEASE

As practitioners concerned with addressing public health issues, anthropologists play diverse roles in infectious disease prevention and intervention. Such roles might range from identifying and addressing the reasons people may reject vaccination initiatives to designing and testing new models for deterring the transmission of sexually transmitted disease or even working to change unhealthy health policies and institutional practices. This work often confronts the special challenges of planned behavior change. A starting point in this kind of work is examining how public health officials conceive of how to best prevent or respond to infectious diseases (Nichter 2008) (see Figure 1.3). Traditionally most prevention research projects were vertically focused on one disease at a time, be it malaria, dengue, HIV, TB, or an array of other infectious threats to human health.

Instead, anthropologist Marc Nichter has pushed for examining common research issues that horizontally cross-cut diseases. This approach allows researchers to gain insights into how intervention messages about one disease affect thinking and practices involving other diseases. It also promotes consideration of how prevention messages can be bundled together to encourage universally beneficial prevention practices. It allows us to address the kind of problem Jen Pylpa described in northeastern Thailand (2004), where people were given disease-specific prevention messages about avoiding water-borne infections, diarrheal diseases, dengue, and malaria. As villagers integrated the various health and hygienic messages, many people came to believe—falsely— that drinking water containing mosquito eggs was the cause of dengue and malaria. They misapplied the message that, to avoid diarrheal disease, they should either not drink or treat pathogenically contaminated water.

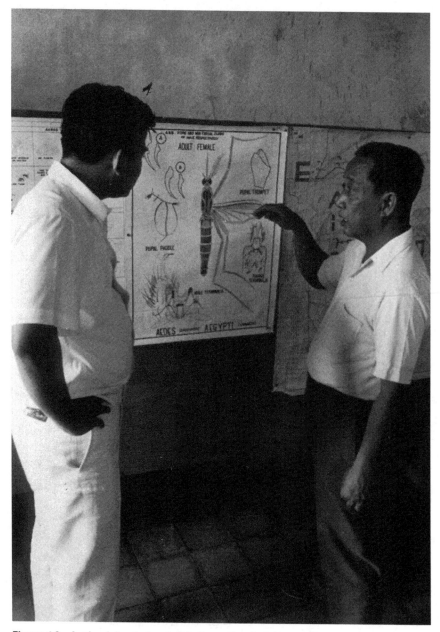

Figure 1.3 A physician being briefed on the Aedes eagypti.

What actual information could anthropologists generate to address this kind of problem? Lenore Manderson points out that anthropologists have adapted the methods of their discipline to collect data that can serve as "the informational basis for the development of [sound] policy, programmes or specific interventions" (1998:1021). Such data are based on observations of actual behavior, on-the-spot interviews about particular behavior practices, and assessments of the social and physical contexts in which disease transmission occurs and in which interventions will be implemented. For example, introducing effective hygienic practices may seem at first like a straightforward process, but in resource-poor settings, Manderson lists specific cultural and structural complexities that confront such a task:

> In poor communities, individual household latrines may not be affordable, and communal latrines may cease to be used because they are poorly maintained, smell and are surrounded by flies; insufficient [water] taps may be provided, taps may be placed in inconvenient locations, or people may maintain a strong preference for flowing river water over tap water; notions of hand washing vary and the action is not always sufficient to reduce bacteria; household animals and children may continue to pollute the environment and themselves; . . . householders may lack sufficient time to adhere to the wide range of actions required to ensure hygiene; and so on. (1998:1022–1023)

Targeted disease interventions require information on local knowledge and practices. Recognizing this, the National Institutes of Mental Health HIV/STD Prevention Trial Group (2007) adopted anthropological methods for identifying culturally appropriate local intervention approaches in five countries—Russia, Peru, Zimbabwe, China, and India. The group's researchers produced similar yet culturally distinctive findings that facilitated the local adaptation of the project's evidence-based, community-level sexual behavior–change intervention model. Anthropological methods were also used to implement the process evaluation that monitored the implementation of the intervention in all sites to assure that there was good adherence to the project model. The interactive nature of anthropological approaches allows for their "application in process evaluation to develop culturally appropriate, sustainable and effective interventions" (Hong et al. 2005:9).

What, exactly, are these special attributes of anthropological methods that generate such useful insights? These are discussed below.

ANTHROPOLOGICAL METHODS IN INFECTIOUS DISEASE RESEARCH

The methodological backbone of the anthropology of infectious disease is *ethnography*—the long-term observational and participatory field study of people and issues in social and environmental context. Within this framework anthropologists incorporate a diverse array of specialized methods.

At its core ethnography involves the prolonged immersion of the researcher or team of researchers into the social space and lifeways of the people under study. During their time in the field, anthropologists seek to participate (as conditions allow) in peoples' normal, everyday social lives and routine activities. This might entail attending healing ceremonies, accompanying someone to visit a loved one in the hospital, or simply joining families as they clean dirt from their harvested rice grains. During their daily involvement, anthropologists are systematically observing behaviors and relationships, listening to and participating in group conversations, and asking questions about the activities underway or other issues of concern. In addition to casual interviewing, anthropologists also use more focused and structured interviewing about specific issues, such as life history interviews. Although not all research in medical anthropology is ethnographic, there is a generally shared sense that ethnography offers valuable insights about health and behavior that are not easily acquired through other means.

Rather than a highly controlled and narrowly focused approach to data collection, ethnography provides a lens on issues of interest within their natural social context and in terms of how group members see, understand, and experience them. In her comparative study of the conception of contagion among various ethnic groups in Côte d'Ivoire in Western Africa and among Afro-Brazilian people in Bahia, Brazil, for example, anthropologist Andrea Caprara learned that in both settings "disease transmission is considered within a framework of relationships between analogical thinking and empirical experience, symbolic classifications and social organization and individuals and body conceptions" (Caprara 1998:998). In these settings people use cultural concepts of purity and impurity to define how diseases can be transmitted. People told her that saliva is an impure body fluid capable of transmitting disease not because it contains pathogens but because it is inherently unclean and polluting. By remaining in a local setting for some time, often for a year or more, anthropologists are able to glimpse behind the public masks and front-stage performances of social actors into backstage and often hidden arenas of experience and social interaction. As a result, they develop understandings of behaviors that might otherwise appear irrational, meaningless, or inscrutable or might go unnoticed and unknown to nongroup members.

Faced with various practical constraints, medical anthropologists also have developed methods for more tightly focused and short-term ethnographic assessment of pressing health issues. Rapid ethnographic assessment strategies are designed to shorten the time lag between the availability of findings and the implementation of research, which may be critical in an infectious disease epidemic. Rapid assessments carried out over a period of a few months now have a documented history of successful implementation in public health programs. To produce robust results in a condensed time frame, this approach builds on existing information, uses researchers who are already familiar with the local social and cultural contexts, seeks to develop a high level of community involvement, and is organized around a restricted set of research questions (Needle et al. 2003; Trotter and Singer 2005).

Specific methodological tools anthropologists use in the study of infectious diseases include *free listing* and *card sorting*, approaches designed to investigate people's underlying beliefs about the kinds and relationships among diseases, disease causes, and symptoms (Bernard 1995); *cultural consensus analysis*, which is used for assessing agreement among study participants about issues of concern (e.g., perceived nature of a specific disease) and for discerning the patterning of differences in cultural knowledge within and across social groups (Romney, Batchelder, and Weller 1987); and *narrative analysis*, such as having participants create fictional stories about responding to an infectious disease event in a family, which facilitates the identification of common themes shared among study participants (Winskell et al. 2013).

Anthropologists also have developed methods for linking local behaviors and issues to broader social factors, such as government policy structures, changing economic conditions, and cross-cutting forces like the work of international banking and lending institutions as well as nongovernment organizations headquartered in other countries. Sometimes called multisited ethnography, these approaches recognize that in the modern world we are all affected by far more than local-level events, information, and relationships. In their study of the South American cholera epidemic of 1994–1995, for example, Charles Briggs and Mariusa Mantini-Briggs recognized that, in addition to conducting local ethnography for their study of eastern Venezuela, they had to travel to Caracas; Washington, DC, Atlanta, Georgia; Geneva; Dhaka, Bangladesh; and elsewhere to interview public health officials about the Latin American epidemic. Work on the global stage allowed these researchers to "grasp how people and institutions located in very different sites are tied together" (Briggs and Mantini-Briggs 2004:xvi–xvii).

These strategies constitute only a short list of the numerous methods anthropologists use in their study of infectious disease but suggest the multiple avenues anthropologists traverse to make sense of the human health condition.

CONCLUSION: AFFIRMING BIOCULTURAL/ BIOSOCIAL UNDERSTANDING

The anthropology of infectious disease begins with the understanding that these conditions are at once pathological reality and social construction. Although there may be analytic utility in separating biology from culture and society and cultural from society as well, in the world outside of our investigative endeavors these phenomena are inseparable. Narrow "concentration on one to the exclusion of the other . . . has sometimes made a neater story, but an incomplete one" (Hays 2009:1).

With the rise of "germ theory" in the late nineteenth century, infectious disease in the purview of biomedicine came to seem like an unassailable biological reality, the investigation and medical response to which did not require much in the way of social or cultural inquiry. But although infectious diseases have necessary immediate causes in pathogenic infections, there are more distal causes of these causes that also must be understood to comprehend infectious disease fully as an aspect of and threat to human life and existence. Not only have humans and pathogens co-evolved, affecting and shaping each other over time in the ongoing transformatory dance of species with the challenges and opportunities presented by other species within and around them, but our languages, cultural traditions, and social organizations also reflect the long history of swimming in the microbial sea around us. The anthropology of infectious disease is a scholarly and applied discipline that, unlike many others, developed subdisciplines focused on both the physical and sociocultural aspects of our species and, as such, is keenly attentive to the avenues, mechanisms, and consequences of the human biosocial/biocultural interface in health.

DISCUSSION QUESTIONS

1. If it were possible to eliminate infectious disease by eradicating all microorganisms on Earth, would this be a good strategy?
2. How do you simultaneously study biological, cultural, and social structures and process?
3. What are useful questions to ask about quantitative accounts of an infectious disease epidemic?
4. How are processes of globalization changing infectious diseases?
5. Why is a narrowly biological understanding of infectious disease inadequate?
6. How has our species been shaped—physically, culturally, and socially—through our encounters with infectious disease?

7. What kind of infectious disease might a very poor, rural community be *more* likely to suffer? What infectious diseases might a poor, rural community be *less* likely to catch?

8. Make two lists with the headings "clean" and "dirty." Put each of the ten items below in one list or the other. Then reflect: Why did you categorize each item as clean or dirty? What do the words "dirty" and "clean" mean to you?

> Cockroach
> Sponge
> Saliva
> Kissing
> Bathtub
> Beer
> Ear wax
> Mailbox
> Mold
> Blood

CHAPTER TWO

Denizens of the Microbial World

> You are bound to get infections from time to time, and you are better off knowing something about what is going on.
>
> *John Playfair (2004:3)*

We live in extraordinary intimacy with microbes. They are in us, on us, and all around us. They "flow through our veins, lie in our eyes, and colonize our digestive and respiratory system" (Swerdlow and Johnson 2002:43). And they significantly affect our welfare: "Looking at the human body alone reveals distinct microbiomes in every orifice and a complex web of microbial interactions and metabolic products influencing every part of our lives" (Dove 2013). Microbes affect our digestion processes and produce vitamins and other elements that we need (Albenberg and Wu 2014). Gut-dwelling microbes like bifidobacterium and lactic acid bacteria feast on dark chocolate. When you eat chocolate, these organisms produce antinflamatory compounds that reduce the long-term risk of stroke (Moore, Goita, and Finley 2014). Some neuroscientists even suggest that certain bacteria may be necessary for the normal development of the human brain. Understanding microbes is thus crucial for anthropology, a field that seeks to comprehend humans in their full biosocial/biocultural complexity. This chapter presents an introduction and overview of microbes, both in general and especially as sources of infectious diseases.

KNOWING MICROBES

Microbes play many different roles in human society, and our perspectives of them vary:

> Different people see microorganisms from different perspectives. To evolutionary and molecular biologists, microbes are relatives, with whom we set up correspondence. To biotechnologists, they are workers, to be employed and perhaps, exploited. To environmental microbiologists, they may be merely scenery, or analogous to canaries in coal mines, but they are generally viewed as good neighbors if we have good fences. To clinical, food, and sanitation microbiologists, and to the defense establishment, microorganisms

are enemies to be tracked, contained, and killed, and to leaders of rogue states and terrorist organizations, they are useful tools which are much easier to get through airports than are firearms and explosives (Shapiro 2000:3).

The diversity of human perspectives on microbes, however, pales by comparison with the actual degree of heterogeneity found among microorganisms themselves. They come in numerous forms in a multitude of varieties with assorted capacities and an array of genetic patterns. Since the first complete microbial genome was sequenced in 1995—the pathogenic bacteria *Haemophilus influenzae,* which is linked to both ear and respiratory infections as well as *meningitis* in children—hundreds of microbial genomes have been sequenced and archived for public research in GenBank, a National Center for Biotechnology Information database.

This chapter explores the features of microbes, including their possible origins, varying and surprising lifestyles, impacts on human evolution and history, distribution, epigenetic features, roles as agents of human disease, and place in the epidemiological transitions that have occurred through time. It also reviews key features of the human immune system because of its importance in coordinating our response to pathogenic microbes. Finally, it presents a case study of one very mysterious microbe that caused a disease known as kuru in order to illustrate how human cultural behavior can be critical to disease transmission and shows one way anthropology has helped solve riddles of transmission.

MICROBES ON EARTH

Microbes have been present on earth longer than any other organisms and have evolved the ability to thrive in almost any environment that meets their minimal survival needs. Where did they come from? Presumably they evolved at different times and places on Earth in somewhat different ways. For the first 150 billion years or so of the 360 billion years that life has existed on Earth, bacteria were the only living inhabitants of the planet. Evidence suggests that bacteria originated in the ocean: land bacteria are more closely related to each other genetically than they are to ocean bacteria. Fossils of cyanobacteria (adapted to low-oxygen environments) from western Australia are the oldest evidence we have of life on Earth. Their remains are found as stromatolites, which look like tuber-shaped stone formations composed of layer after layer of bacteria remains (see Figure 2.1).

Since then microbes have played an important role in the course of life on Earth, including species extinction. Since life first appeared there have been several periods of mass extinctions, with the demise of almost all of the

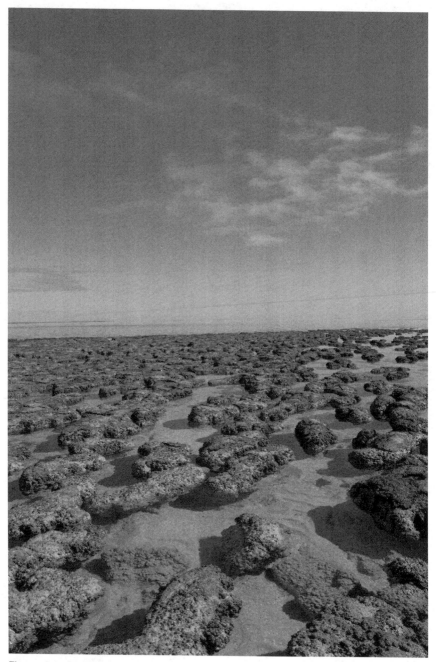

Figure 2.1 Stromatolites in Australia. (Photo by Robert Bayer)

dinosaurs some 65 million years ago being one of the best known of these jar-ring life events. Prior to the loss of dinosaurs there was an extinction event that has come to be known as the Great Dying, and until now it stands as the most dramatic of the five mass extinctions that have occurred. During the cataclysmic event 70 percent of vertebrate land species and 96 percent of marine species disappeared. A mass extinction of insects also occurred, with 83 percent of all genera ceasing to exist. What caused this great elimination of life forms that is well documented in the fossil record? For many years researchers believed that massive volcanic eruptions and raging natural coal fires filled the atmosphere with carbon, creating a greenhouse blanket that produced a significant, fateful rise in planet temperatures. More recently, however, researchers at MIT have suggested another culprit: methane-producing archaea called Methanosarcina (Rothman et al. 2014). In this scenario erupting volcanoes in what is now Siberia blew massive quantities of nickel into the world's oceans. This metal provided a metabolic fuel for an unparalleled explosion in the ocean-dwelling archaea population, facilitated by a genetic microbial innovation. These microorgan-isms, in turn, began to release ever-growing quantities of their natural discard: methane. Released methane emerged from the ocean and was transferred to the atmosphere, where it served as a far more effective greenhouse gas than CO_2. In addition, as it degraded and broke down into water and CO_2, it also produced a greenhouse gas with far greater capacity to remain in the atmosphere than methane itself. The combined effect of this microorganism's "methane bomb" and the resulting heat-retaining CO_2 blanketing of the atmosphere is the cause, according to MIT researchers, of both the massive scale of the Great Dying and the fact that it took 30 million years for life on Earth to recover with a broad reemergence of biodiversity and new life forms.

Today all surfaces on the planet are covered with bacteria. A single drop of ocean water (as far down as a hundred meters deep) contains on the order of a million bacteria, whereas an average gram of top soil has ten times that number, with representatives of six thousand to thirty-eight thousand different species (Curtis, Sloan, and Scannell 2002), including two hundred species of fungi (Leake et al. 2004). Researchers have even coined the term *plastisphere* to refer to the dense and diverse microbial communities living on the vast quantities of anthropogenic plastic debris that exists in open ocean ecosystems, includ-ing some opportunistic pathogens (Zettler, Mincler, and Amal-Zettler 2013). Overall the number of bacteria on Earth is estimated to be a figure containing thirty digits—numbering more than the amount of stars we believe exist in the universe (Wassenaar 2012).

We are uncertain about the origin of other microbes, such as viruses. It is clear that they are quite varied; some, such as poliovirus, have RNA-based genomes, whereas others, such as herpes virus, have DNA-based genomes. Some viruses, such as influenza and HIV, have single-stranded genomes, whereas others, including smallpox, have double-stranded genomes. Their physical makeup and strategies of replication are equally varied. Poliovirus has a diameter of only 30 nanometers, whereas *mimiviruses,* one of the giants of the group, has a diameter of 750 nanometers. Moreover, as Wessner (2010) points out, "According to a stringent definition of life, they are nonliving." This assertion is based on the fact that viruses lack cells, cannot turn food into energy, and, left without the components and structures they steal from their hosts, they are simply inert packages of specific biochemicals. But definitions, of course, are cultural constructions, and virologists disagree about whether to include viruses on the tree of life. Certainly, like living organisms, viruses have genes, are capable of reproducing themselves (with help from a host), and evolve in response to natural selection.

Even beyond its remarkable size, the giant mimivirus is unusual in another way. Its' genome, which is twice as large as any other virus and bigger even than many bacteria, contains more than a thousand genes that encode for proteins, something other viruses cannot do. In fact, since discovering mimiviruses, researchers have found an even larger virus, which they named, accordingly, the *mamavirus.* Like the mimivirus, the mamavirus was isolated from an amoeba living in a cooling tower. Mamaviruses are actually parasitized by another, smaller virus, dubbed the Sputnik virophage. These viruses cannot replicate unless a mamavirus is present, as they infect and hijack part of the mamavirus to replicate their own genome. Such is the complex, almost surreal world of viruses. More astonishing still, if all of the 1×10^{31} viruses on Earth were laid end to end, the line would go on for 100 million light years (Editor 2011).

Viruses have never been detected as fossils, probably because they are too small and too fragile to support the fossilization processes. Even in fossilized biological materials, such as plant leaves or insects in amber, preserved nucleic acid sequences of viruses never have been found. Researchers have devised at least three theories to explain the origin or viruses:

- Theory of "regressive evolution": viruses descended from free-living and more complex parasites that over time developed a growing dependence on host-cell intracellular "machinery" to replicate.
- Theory of "cellular origin": viruses had their origin as host cell DNA and/ or messenger RNA, but acquired the ability to exist separate from host cells.
- Theory of "parallel" evolution: viruses appeared with the most primitive organisms.

Some scientists even suggest that microbes constitute the smallest astronauts—that Earth was seeded with microbes cocooned in protective meteorite rocks from outer space. The Russian Federal Space Agency has been testing this idea by sending various microbes to Mars and back to see if they can survive the trip.

Over the course of their evolution microbes have developed some remarkable qualities. With brief life spans—some species can produce three generations within an hour—and high mutation rates, microbes have significant adaptive potential, including the ability to become genetically resistant to our antibiotic arsenal. Because their waste is oxygen, microbes, specifically bacteria, played the fundamental role in the initial oxygenation of Earth, making life on the planet possible. Moreover, researchers have begun to recognize the many fundamental impacts of microorganisms on the entire *biosphere*—the world of all living things (McFall-Ngai et al. 2013). They estimated that about 37 percent of the twenty-three thousand human genes have homologs with microbes, meaning that they are related evolutionarily to the genes of microorganisms. There is even speculation that because the internal temperature of mammals is the ideal environment for bacteria, microbes may have played a co-evolutionary part in the development of mammalian *endothermy,* internal heat generation.

BENEFICIAL MICROBES AND MICROBIAL SERVANTS

This book primarily is about microbes and disease, but it is important to remember that microbes play critical roles in human well-being and are useful for many things. Beneficial microbes exist throughout our bodies. On our outer surface staphylococcus bacteria secrete a substance that keeps our skin moist and flexible while at the same time producing a shield that diminishes the entry of infectious pathogens. In our nasal cavities *Lactobacillus sakei* bacteria provide protection from sinusitis by crowding out potential microbial intruders. Onset of sinusitis, it is believed, is linked to the loss of normal sinus microbial diversity due to an infection and the subsequent colonization of the sinuses by the bacterium *Corynebacterium tuberculostearicum,* which triggers painful swelling of the sinuses. In our colons bacteria help synthesize vitamins B and K, the latter of which is a vital component in blood clotting and maintaining healthy bones.

An example of a survival advantage a virus confers on us involves a gene sequence installed by members of a group known as human endogenous retroviruses that allows us to produce comparatively high levels of amylase in our saliva (six to eight times that of our closest mammalian relatives, the chimpanzees). This enzyme enables us to us to eat foods like rice, cassava, and potatoes by turning their high-starch content into sugar (Ting et al. 1992). Amylase is believed to have been critical to human evolution because it opened up an additional food source, one that was a game changer in some tropical and subtropical environments. Some anthropologists have even argued that the ability to cook and consume high-starch foods promoted the evolution of large brains, smaller teeth, modern limb proportions, and even male-female bonding (Wrangham et al. 1999).

Even microbes that have adverse effects—such as H. pylori, known for its role in acute and chronic gastritis, peptic ulcers, high correlation with gastrointestinal cancers—may also have benefits. There is now evidence that H. pylori may be active in preventing allergic diseases such as hay fever, eczema, and asthma; auto-immune diseases like multiple sclerosis and type I diabetes; and chronic inflammatory conditions such as inflammatory bowel disease. This recognition has led researchers to consider whether the microbe can be adapted for asthma and other prevention and treatment applications (Oertli and Müller 2012). Because H. pylori influences hormones that affect weight and body mass, researchers are also exploring the relationships between decreasing levels of H. pylori in children and growing rates of obesity:

> [...] chronic exposures to low-residue antimicrobial drugs in food could disrupt the equilibrium state of intestinal microbiota and cause dysbiosis [or microbial imbalance] that can contribute to changes in body physiology. The obesity epidemic in the United States may be partly driven by the mass exposure of Americans to food containing low-residue antimicrobial agents. (Riley, Raphael, and Faerstein 2013)

Other research has found that infection with one virus interferes with the functions of other more pathogenic viruses, a process known as a countersyndemic (Singer 2009c; see also Chapter 6 in this book). Progression of HIV disease, for example, occurs more slowly in individuals who are also infected with the hepatitis G virus (HGV) (Roossinck 2011). Unlike hepatitis A, B and C, HGV is nonpathogenic, leading researchers to prefer the name GBV-C. An important difference between GBV-C and the hepatitis-linked HCV virus is that most people with healthy immune systems who are infected with GBV-C are able clear it from their bodies, whereas fewer than 25 percent of those infected with HCV are able to do so. Because GBV-C and HIV are transmitted in the same way, the rate of GBV-C infection among HIV-positive people is particularly high (Williams et al. 2004). An important study that tracked HIV positive men for five years found that men without GBV-C were 2.78 times more likely to die than co-infected men with persistent GBV-C. In other words, GBV-C infection was associated with prolonged survival in individuals infected with HIV. Why? Research suggests that GBV-C induces cellular changes and cytokine concentrations that inhibit HIV replication (Stapleton, Williams, and Xiang 2004). One interpretation of human/microbe relationship in GBV-C infection is that it constitutes an example of *interspecies mutualistic symbiosis*: both species, virus and human, benefit from the interaction. Some microbes perform useful or even necessary biochemical functions for us, and in turn, by infecting us, they receive a nutrient-rich and warm home in which to live and reproduce.

Humans are an inventive species, so it is hardly surprising that we also consciously put microbes to work on our behalf. Bacteria, for example are used in making cheese, yogurt, and sourdough bread. Dead, weakened, or modified bacteria are employed in developing vaccines and medicines. A compound secreted by the soil-dwelling bacterium *Streptomyces griseus* is the source of the antibiotic drug streptomycin, the first drug to treat tuberculosis successfully. Another soil bacterium called *Mycobacterium vaccae* is being studied currently as a source of medicines to improve learning and treat depression. *Saccharomyces boulardii*, a tropical strain of yeast found in fruit, including lychee and mangosteen, is used clinically to treat gastroenteritis and diarrhea in children, antibiotic-associated diarrhea, and other intestinal infections. Bacteria also are used to clean water in sewage plants and oil spills. Bacteria were deployed after the massive BP spill in the Gulf of Mexico because of their capacity to digest oil. Penicillin, an antibiotic, is made from a fungus. Other fungi are used in the creation of synthetic insulin, a medicine in increasing need because of growing global rates of diabetes. Fungi also are of use to humans as food (mushrooms, truffles, tempeh), to make beer and bread (yeast), and to kill pests on farms. The colored veins in blue cheeses and the white rind on Brie and Camembert cheeses are fungi as well.

An even more intriguing use has been found for *Ophiocordyceps sinensis*, a fungus that parasitizes the caterpillars of a group of insects called ghost moths. The fungus germinates inside the caterpillar, kills and mummifies it, and sends out a stalk-like growth that bursts through the body of the larval moth. The fungus is highly valued as an herbal remedy in Tibet and China, and in the West it has come to be referred to colloquially as "Himalayan Viagra." So intense is the hunt for this fungus that people are doing extensive ecological damage digging up the ground in areas where ghost moths are found.

Viruses too have been harnessed in the service of humankind. Baculoviruses, probably the largest and most diverse group of DNA-based viruses, are insect pathogens that are deployed as biological controls in forestry and agriculture (Caraco and Wang 2008). Researchers currently are investigating the use of herpes viruses in the treatment of cancer by genetically reprogramming the virus to destroy cancer cells and eliminate cancerous tumors. Even the high-tech cyber industry is looking to the microbial world: biocryptography is a method for storing data inside microbes, using them as minuscule storage vessels.

HUMAN PATHOGENS AND THEIR IMPACTS

The WHO catalogs about two hundred different human pathogens linked to over twelve thousand recognized diseases, including the following six major groupings (see Table 2.1):

- Bacteria—one-celled nucleated bio-agents
- Fungus—entities with rigid cellulose—or chitin-base—cell walls that reproduce primarily by forming spores; most are multicellular except yeasts
- Virus—unnucleated entities composed of genetic material covered by a protein and lipid cover; an entity on the edge of life
- Protozoa—unicellular entities, including amoeba and paramecium, that are capable of self-propelled movement
- Prions—a term derived from protein + infection; they are unnucleated proteins in misfolded form
- Helminths—simple, invertebrate animals, such as intestinal worms

In addition to these, recent research on animals suggests a pathogenic role for what have been termed *retrotransposable elements,* which are parasitic strands of DNA that are capable of copying themselves and spreading throughout the genome. These entities may play a role in both cancer and aging (Sedivy et al. 2013). In considering these groups, we must always remember that nature is never neat and clear; at the edges categories blur. For example, the Rickettsia (the proximal cause of typhus) are different from other bacteria because they have the virus-like trait of lacking biological independence: they must rely on their host for several enzymes. There are other intermediate pathogenic forms as well, suggesting the complexities of this arena of work.

The impact of any particular infectious disease on humans is not uniform around the world or even around the block: the exact same pathogen might

Table 2.1 Pathogenic Sources of Various Diseases

Disease	Virus	Bacteria	Fungus	Protozoa	Helminthes	Prions
Heart disease	x	x	x	x	x	
Respiratory disease	x	x		x	x	
Pneumonia	x	x	x	x	x	
Cerebrovascular disease	x	x	x	x	x	
Eye infections			x	x	x	
Cancer	x	x				
Liver disease	x	x				
Blood diseases		x		x		
Kuru					x	x

have a very different effect on you from the person sitting next to you in the bus or a person living in another country. Researchers have identified a number of reasons for this variation. Historically the region of the world in which someone lives has been a primary factor in the likelihood that a particular pathogen will infect any particular person. For example, HIV infection is of far greater importance in sub-Saharan African than in Central America. Similarly many helminths are especially common in tropical zones, whereas malaria exists across countries in the warm belt circling the world at the equator.

A *virgin population* is a population being exposed to a spreading infectious disease for the first time. In no small part, the history of the European colonization of the so-called New World was a consequence of the fact that "relatively trifling endemic afflictions of the Old World regularly became death-dealing epidemics among New World populations that were totally lacking in acquired resistances" (McNeil 1976:185). The wealth of a country or region compared to other nations in the world is another significant factor; not surprisingly, many infections have higher impacts in poor countries, and what we think of as the *diseases of poverty* tend to be infectious conditions. To test the relationship between country status and infection, Matthew Bonds, Andrew Dobson, and Donald Keenan (2012) developed a computer model to estimate the relative effects of vector-borne and parasitic diseases on income, while controlling for other factors. They found that vector-borne and parasitic diseases have systematically affected economic development, as expressed in contemporary levels of per capita income. According to these researchers,

> The economic conditions of the extremely poor are, indeed, largely due to biological processes, which are manifest in health status. . . . Infectious and parasitic diseases effectively "steal" host resources for their own survival and transmission. . . . These [occurring] within-host processes at the individual level scale up to global patterns of poverty and disease. (Bond, Dobson, and Keenan 2012)

Sex (biology) also plays a role in patterns of infection. Tuberculosis, for example, tends to affect males more than females. Some infectious diseases, like pelvic inflammatory infection in women, are specifically tied to sex-related anatomy. Changes in the female body during pregnancy and lactation also can affect the infectious disease process. Some infectious diseases are more intense and threatening during pregnancy, whereas others affect the unborn child.

Gender—the culturally constructed social roles based on sex—is also a factor. In most societies, for example, women are more likely than men to be daily caregivers for the sick in both health care and home settings. As a result, women are more exposed than men to various infectious agents. Women also may bear a heavier burden than men if they are sufferers of infectious diseases such as *onchocerciasis* that cause body disfigurement. Marriage prospects for women with such diseases are more sharply curtailed than they are for male sufferers. Men, meanwhile, expressed more concern about the economic impact of infection as well as effects on sexual performance (Vlassoff et al. 2000).

Infectious diseases interact differently with people of different ages. Notes William McNeil (1976:116), an "infectious disease which immunizes those who survive, and which returns to a given community at intervals of five to ten years, automatically becomes a childhood disease." Children also may be particularly vulnerable because their immune systems are still developing. Infectious diarrheal diseases have the most impact on small children and, along with respiratory disease, significantly contribute to global childhood mortality from disease. The elderly, whose immune systems may be compromised by the breakdowns associated with aging, such as a reduction in macrophage production, also may be particularly susceptible to infection. Among healthy adults, for example, West Nile virus infection typically causes only mild flu-like symptoms; by contrast, among the elderly it is more likely to cause serious neurological diseases like encephalitis or meningitis.

We have already established that disease affects poor countries more heavily, as it does poor individuals or families. Infectious diseases are disproportionately common among the poor, and it is well established that poverty diminishes an individual's ability to cope with infectious disease. There are many reasons for this, including the fact that poor people are more likely to live and work in unsafe conditions. In the coal mining areas of central Appalachia, for example, where poverty is particularly severe, various helminth infections have been identified that are less of a problem elsewhere in the country. Of note is *Strongyloidiasis stercoralis,* or *threadworm.* Research has shown that a high percentage of patients in the region who suffer from *strongyloidiasis* infection are older white males, most of whom have underlying chronic illnesses such as chronic obstructive pulmonary disease. Researchers believe these men may have acquired strongyloidiasis infections while working in coal mines (Hotez 2008).

Previous exposure to a pathogen will also affect its impact on an individual. *Bacterial déjà vu* or *viral déjà vu* are terms coined by Nobel Prize Laureate Rolf Zinkernagel (Merkler et al. 2006) to explain why some people appear to be particularly susceptible to specific pathogens. In the context of chronic Lyme disease, an infection that is unresponsive to simple antibiotic treatment, and other diseases thought to be caused by insect bites, déjà vu refers to exposure to a pathogen at a formative life stage (e.g., childhood) that predisposes the individual to more intensive response if exposed to the same pathogen again later in life. Whereas people without previous exposure might experience only simple, treatable conditions, the déjà vu sufferer develops an infection that is resistant to short-course antibiotic treatment. This illustrates how pathogens can lie in a dormant state in human tissue only to be reactivated upon re-exposure, at which point they may be especially difficult to treat.

Only six deadly diseases—HIV disease, malaria, diarrhea, measles, pneumonia, and tuberculosis—cause some 90 percent of all infection-related deaths in the world. Children and young adults suffer the most: diarrheal diseases such as cholera, dysentery, or typhoid fever, for example, kill about 2 million children under age five, year after year. Infectious diseases disable millions more people every year. Measles, for example, can result in blindness, deafness, or brain damage (see Figure 2.2). *Lymphatic filariasis*, a parasitic worm disease, affects about 120 million people worldwide, and some 40 million people are disabled and disfigured by it. Acute respiratory infections, such as those caused by respiratory syncytial virus or Streptococcus pneumonia, are an additional source of childhood mortality and are often associated with other life-threatening diseases like measles. Low-income countries bear the biggest health burden of these infectious diseases, and poorer people suffer a greater health burden from infectious diseases than richer people in wealthier countries.

Despite global health programs targeted to improve the health of the poor of the world, three of the top five proximal causes of mortality in children ages

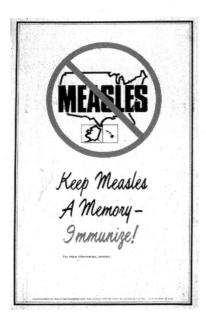

Figure 2.2 Centers for Disease Control Measles Immunization Poster. (Images from the History of Medicine)

one to four years are infectious diseases: pneumonia, diarrheas, gastroenteritis, and measles. Infectious agents associated with conditions like pneumonia, diarrhea, bronchitis, influenza, respiratory TB, dengue fever, malaria, and chicken pox are also the primary proximal causes of childhood morbidity.

COMPLEXITIES OF THE IMMUNE SYSTEM

Infectious disease is not directly determined by the presence or absence of pathogens. Over the course of human prehistory and history our ancestors evolved a multilayered immune system of structures and processes that provide constant protection from infectious agents. We now know that some of the genes and capacities of our modern immune system can even be traced to the Neanderthals. One example is as a small set of genes on chromosome 6 known as the human leukocyte antigen (HLA) class I genes, which carry genetic instructions for making HLA protein, used in identifying problems in cells such as cancer. These genes, apparently a product of the interbreeding of Neanderthals with direct human ancestors migrating out of Africa into Europe, may have conferred adaptive advantage in responding to the new pathogens our ancestors encountered in European and Asian environments (Abi-Rached et al. 2011). Once assumed to be an evolutionarily dead-end branch of the hominid family, Neanderthals may in fact be an important part of our engagement with the microbial world around us (Tishkoff and Verrelli 2003).

The modern human immune system has two primary components. The *innate immune system* is the body's first line of response to pathogens. Various features are present at birth, including skin, mucous membranes, and the vernix (a fatty substance covering the fetus that has antifungal properties) as well as internally dwelling macrophages (which, as we have seen, indiscriminately consume foreign entities in the body). The *adaptive immune system* is a complex, multicomponent system involved in creating an immunological memory after initial exposure to a pathogen. Special white blood cells that are part of this system help produce specific antibodies targeted to specific pathogens. Examples of cells in the adaptive immune system include T Helper Cells, or "CD4+ T Cells," which coordinate immune response to a detected infection; CD8 cells, called T killer/suppressor cells, which are involved in directly eliminating viral infected body cells and, sometimes, parasites; and B cells, which produce antibodies in response to foreign proteins, like bacteria and viruses. Another part of the adaptive immune system, memory T cells, protect the body from re-infection with a previously encountered pathogen. When a known pathogen is detected, a process called *immune reactivity*, memory T cells rapidly reproduce, hastening a quick immune response. Memory T cells also can trigger *autoimmune disease* when they cross-react with self-antigens, antigens that would normally be ignored, a response that sometimes is activated by infection or by environmental triggers. In autoimmune diseases the immune system attacks its body's own cells. More than eighty autoimmune diseases have been identified, including Type 1 diabetes, rheumatoid arthritis, pernicious anemia, psoriasis, and inflammatory bowel disease.

The immune system interacts regularly with other systems and tissues in the body. Critical and frequent interactions occur, for example, with the body's bone structure, particularly in the development of immune cells in bone marrow. The bone cavity in which marrow is found contains important stem cells that play a role in maintaining the immune system. Also within this space are *cytokines*, produced by immune cells to help maintain bone stability. Researchers refer to this vital interface as the "osteo-immune system" (Walsh et al. 2004). Aberrant activity in the immune system can lead a derangement of bone structure, as occurs in the disease osteoporosis, a progressive loss of bone mass and density.

Another complexity of the immune system involves so-called *gut flora*. During the birth process human babies must pass through the birth canal, which is a lactic acid bacteria–rich environment, and this experience helps educate the child's immune system about "friendly microbes"—those we need to survive. Researchers have long believed that during birth a baby's gastrointestinal tract is sterile and incapable of digesting food, but that within a few hours bacteria ingested during the birthing journey rapidly colonize the intestines. Recent studies suggest, however, that bacteria begin colonizing our guts while we are still in the womb (Funkhouser and Bordenstein 2013). This research shows that half of the fetal gut microbes are bacteria that produce lactic acid, such as lactobacillus, whereas the other half mostly consist of a family of friendly enteric bacteria like *Escherichia coli*. Copious doses of microbes are then added to a baby's gut during birth and through breastfeeding. Before long, the gastrointestinal tract contains about ten times as many bacteria cells as there are human cells in the body (Ley, Petereson, and Gordon 2006).

From birth on, our diet influences which bacteria come to reside in our guts, and this, in turn, determines which food breakdown products and metabolites are made available to our bodies. The composition of individuals' gut microbiota significantly influences the amount of energy available to them from the food they consume (Backhed et al. 2004). For example, strains of *Bacteroides plebeius* found in Japanese but not North American guts possess genes that aid in the breakdown and digestion of polysaccharies, found in seaweed. These genes appear to have been transferred to the gut bacterial genome from bacteria living outside of the gut, on marine red algae. The source of this transference appears to be tied to the historical centrality of seaweeds, especially Porphyra spp. (nori), in the daily diet in Japan, estimated to be on the order of 14.2 grams per person per day (Hehemann et al. 2010). By contrast, the gut species of most Americans is optimized for digesting a high-fat, high-protein diet, whereas people living Amazonia have gut microbes that are better suited for breaking down complex carbohydrates like cassava. Dietary increases in simple sugars and fat can change the relative frequencies of various gut microbes, affecting energy utilization and the development of metabolic disorders such as obesity (Walker et al. 2011). Decreased dietary diversity, in turn, may lead to a reduction in gut species diversity or atypical species composition, which may be linked to inflammatory bowel disease and vaginal infections like vaginosis (Fredricks, Fiedler, and Marrazzo 2005, Turnbaugh et al. 2006).

Because of microorganisms living in our intestines, each of us constitutes a community of hundreds of species—five hundred or more—many of which are as yet uncultivable and remain unidentified to science. Gut flora—although this common term is somewhat misleading, as it is comprised of fauna, that is, bacteria, not plants—includes 100 trillion bacteria representing one thousand different species and weighing some three pounds in people living in developed countries, about the size of a large guinea pig, and five in underdeveloped regions, because of the amount of "worm weight" or helminths.

Nobel Prize Laureate Joshua Lederberg proposed the term *microbiome* to describe the single biological unit composed of humans and the many microbes that dwell within them. Some researchers have even referred to the microbial cells inside the human body as a "newly discovered organ" in the sense that awareness of its presence, integration with the body, and considerable impact on human health is relatively recent. This growing insight supports the observation by Michael Hadfield, professor of biology at the University of Hawaii, that "it is hard to summarize a single 'most important conclusion' [about the fundamental importance of microbes] other than the admonition to biologists studying animals [including people], from behavior to physiology and ecology to molecular biology, that no matter what process you think you are studying, you must look for and consider a major role for bacteria" (quoted in Zyga 2013). Investigation of the health-related effects of microorganisms is supported by the National Institutes of Health's Human Microbiome Project, the ultimate objective of which is to assess the relationship of changes in the human microbiome to health and disease, a topic that currently is not well understood (Turnbaugh et al. 2007).

Recent research has shown that a high percentage of the microbes dwelling in the human body are not actually bacteria but are representatives of ancient, non-nucleated, single-celled organisms that have been termed Archaea, first discovered in the 1970s. These were previously called Archaebacteria but now are seen as having an independent evolutionary history from bacteria. They are, in fact, as different from bacteria as people are from bacteria. At first it was thought that Archaea only inhabited extreme environments such as hot springs and salt lakes, but it is now recognized that they live in multiple environments, from marshlands to the human colon and navel. In ponds, for example, Archaea help to breakdown leaves that fall into the water and sink to the bottom. In 1783 George Washington pondered the source of bubbles that rose from the bottom of pond water when he poked at it with his walking stick. He called the resulting bubbles flammable air because they could be lit by a torch. Unbeknownst to Washington, the bubbles were composed of methane, a byproduct of complex processes of leaf litter breakdown involving two stages of bacterial action and a final effort by Archaea.

In recent years researchers have discovered that the average human belly button hosts at least fifty microbial species; across a population of belly buttons researchers have identified thousands of species of microbial dwellers, some of which were previously unknown to science (Dunn 2012). Archaea also live in termites and play a key role in their consumption of cellulose. *Methanobrevibacter smithii* is by far the most common Archaean species in the human flora. No links have been established to date between Archaea and any human disease (Eckburg, Lepp, and Relman 2003).

The indigenous microbes in our bodies are of ancient origin; no doubt many of them have been with us throughout our evolutionary pathway to our current form as Homo sapiens. Specific kinds of indigenous microbes tend to colonize specific areas of our bodies: staph bacteria, for example, tend to colonize the skin; E. coli colonize the colon; and lactobacilli inhabit the vagina. As human ecology changes, so does our internal microbiota. In the past century the human condition, especially in developed countries, has undergone dramatic changes that affect the transmission and maintenance of indigenous microbes. Caesarean section, for example, limits the perinatal transfer of the maternal flora in the vagina to newborns. Replacing breast milk with formula changes the selection for gastric lactobacilli. Cleaner water diminishes our exposure to fecal organisms. Demographic developments in whole human populations, including the trend toward smaller families with fewer children, lowers intrafamilial transmission of microbes. In short, our relationship with microbes, internal and external, pathogenic and nonpathogenic, is dynamic; it is constantly changing and, in the process, changing us.

Notably, gut flora are important for the maturation of the immune system, the development of normal intestinal morphology, and the maintenance of a continued and immunologically balanced inflammatory response. The gut flora reinforce the barrier function of the intestinal mucosa, helping it to prevent the attachment of pathogenic microorganisms and the entry of allergens. Some members of the gut flora may contribute to meeting the body's requirements for certain vitamins, including biotin, B-complex vitamin, and vitamin B12. Anthropogenic alteration of the gut flora of the intestine, such as occurs with antibiotic use, but also with disease and aging, can reduce its beneficial role in human health.

Working alongside gut flora are *mitochondriam,* which are tiny, rod-like structures found in most of our cells. These entities help us break down glucose into usable energy to power the work of our bodies. Because of their genetic makeup, we believe that mitochondriam evolved from bacteria and represent the remaining vestiges of a relationship that was sufficiently beneficial to host and microbes alike that the bacterial ancestors of mitochondriam lost their independent identities and became an integral component of animal cells. This process occurred among predecessors of the human species long before the evolution of Homo sapiens (Gray, Burger, and Lange 1999).

Although various microbes are beneficial for human health, even so-called good microbes can, under certain circumstances, go bad—that is, become pathogenic. This occurs primarily for four reasons:

1. A microbe common to one location in the body winds up in another location in the body.
2. The body's immune system is compromised.
3. There are disease interactions (i.e., syndemics).
4. There are unusual exposures.

A case of a microbe going bad because of being "out of place" is the cause of a frightening disease called *necrotizing fasciitis,* popularly called "flesh-eating disease." This is a fast-moving condition, spreading at a rate of three centimeters an hour and leading to death in about 25 percent of cases. The disease is caused by a bacterium called *Streptococcus pyogenes,* or Group A Streptococcus (GAS), which is the source of various skin and throat diseases, including strep throat. Sometimes GAS travels to parts of the body where bacteria usually are not found, like the blood and muscles. Resulting infections are referred to as "invasive GAS disease," one expression of which is necrotizing fasciitis.

Often pathogens do not merely infect and cause disease; they may also change the internal biochemical environment in the human body in ways that make the human host a more hospitable place for their growth and reproduction. This is achieved by secreting substances like sulfonolipid capnine, which controls the human innate immune response. Over time pathogens may succeed in suppressing the immune response through a gradual process of initial and subsequent infection that is known as *successive infection*. Without treatment, successive infection can contribute to the development of common symptoms of aging (e.g., memory loss). Even long after a pathogen is cleared from the body, the alterations in our internal environment may persist and affect our health. In the case of invasive GAS disease, some researchers believe that it is a consequence of S. pyogenes evolving to produce proteins that trigger the body's immune system to destroy body's tissues. By trying to fight the bacteria, the body instead destroys itself, a type of autoimmune disease (Didierlaurent, Goulding, and Hussell 2007).

Pathogen research is increasingly recognizing host manipulation of this sort. We now know, for example, that Anopheles gambiae mosquitoes infected by malaria are more attracted to human odor than mosquitoes that are not infected, increasing the rate of transmission of malaria to humans (Smallegange et al. 2013). This occurs because the *Plasmodium falciparum* parasite that is the immediate cause of malaria changes the olfactory systems of infected mosquitoes in ways that increase the allure of human odors. This change enhances the mosquito's ability to find a human blood meal to feed their eggs. Additionally, infected mosquitoes feed more often and withdraw more blood from human hosts, increasing the opportunities for the parasite's transmission.

A less commonly mentioned component of the body's defenses against pathogens are the array of powerful acids found in the stomach. Gastric acid, which is composed of hydrochloric acid, potassium chloride, and sodium chloride, assists digestion by breaking down proteins in food. In addition, it helps to control ingested pathogens. This function was confirmed by a study carried out by Rosemary Morrison and coworkers (2011) of the effects of pharmaceutical therapies like Prilosec, Prevacid, and Zantac that are designed to suppress stomach acid and are among the most widely sold drugs in the world. These researchers found that patients who receive acid suppression therapy are at heightened risk for *Clostridium difficile infection* (CDI), which causes more deaths in the United States than all other intestinal infections combined. Intense CDI commonly results in the need for surgery within a few days after onset and has mortality rates as high as 50 percent in some populations.

THE SOCIAL LIVES OF MICROBES

Given their comparatively simple structures as self-replicating, unicellular entities, until recently we assumed that microbes lead solitary lives without much in the way of social interaction, communication, or cooperation. We now realize that microbes "exhibit a stunning array of social behaviors" (West et al. 2007:53). Here are five fascinating examples of their social diversity.

First, some microbes produce materials that are directly beneficial to other microbes. For example, iron is a critical element in bacterial growth; however, it is hard to for bacteria to obtain iron because most environmental iron is in an insoluble form or actively sequestered by host species as a protective measure to withhold it from pathogens (Skaar 2010). To meet this challenge, the human pathogenic bacterium *Pseudomonas aeruginosa* (associated with cystic fibrosis) has evolved the capacity to produce and release *siderophore pyoverdine,* an iron-scavenging substance that is advantageous in low-iron contexts. Notably, siderophores provide iron-access survival benefits both for the bacteria that produce them as well as their geographic neighbors who do not. Similarly, microbial collaboration enables the production of compounds that break down antibiotics, such as the enzymes that destroy penicillin.

Second, bacteria appear to have an ability to assess the number other bacteria nearby, called *quorum sensing,* that allows a coordinated response in a population of bacteria. Examples of such responses are the use of cell-to-cell signaling molecules to improve group access to nutrients, collective defense against competitors, and pathogenic virulence in interaction with hosts (Williams et al. 2007). Quorum sensing underlines the truly interactive nature of microbes and suggests the need for terms like "microbial society."

Third, bacteria form multicellular communities known as *biofilms* (e.g., dental plaques), which have various properties, including providing group protection from antibiotics and host immune system responses. Biofilms, which appear early in the fossil record—over 3 billion years ago—grow as accretions by gradually accumulating additional layers of microbes. They are not simply random assemblages of cells that adhere to surfaces but rather are structurally and dynamically complex biological systems. Various forms of cooperative behavior are involved in the construction of a biofilm, including the production of the chemicals that hold biofilm structures together or protect against protozoan predation. There is even speculation that within biofilms there is a division of labor among member bacteria, suggesting complex forms of social behavior (Boles, Thoendel, and Singh 2004).

Biofilm formation constitutes a protected mode of growth that allows microbes to survive even in hostile environments and also to diffuse to colonize new environmental niches. Biofilm formation confers protection from a range of environmental challenges, including UV rays, metal toxicity, acid, dehydration, antibiotics, and host defenses (Hall-Stoodley, Costerton, and Stoodley 2004). It is found in both nonpathogenic and pathogenic species (e.g., E. coli and V. cholera). This capacity presents a challenge for the surgical implantation of medical devices like heart valves, intravenous catheters, joint prostheses, peritoneal dialysis catheters, pacemakers, cerebrospinal fluid shunts, and endotracheal

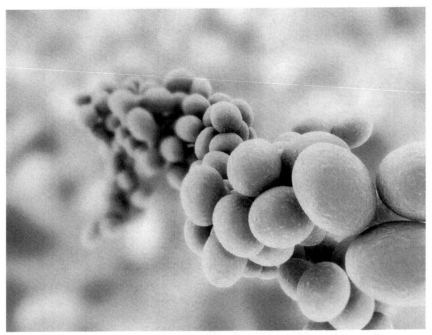

Figure 2.3 Staphylococcus. (Photo by Sebastian Kaulitzki)

tubes because biofilms, particularly those built by *S. epidermidis and S. aureus,* form on the surfaces of these devices and disrupt their effectiveness. Bacterial *endocarditis* occurs when microbes like streptococci and staphylococci (Figure 2.3), which generally live on people's skin or in the oral cavity, gain access to the body, enter the bloodstream, and colonize implanted devices.

Bacterial biofilms play an important role in urinary tract infection, which is the most common infection in women, the second most common bacterial infection across genders after respiratory infection, and the most common hospital-acquired infection. Specifically, biofilms may enable bacteria to withstand immune responses and antibiotic treatment. As a result, repeated urinary tract infections are not necessarily caused by the continual reintroduction of pathogens but rather are the consequence of the continuous presence of pathogens in biofilms attached to the urinary tract wall and the periodic release of some bacterial cells leading to active re-infection.

A fourth example of social behavior that has been discovered in microbe populations is that some cells do not develop and divide at the normal rate but instead remain in a quiescent or dormant state. Called *persister cells,* they are resistant to antibiotics. Persister cells can survive, phase into active development, and perpetuate a species after a deadly assault by pharmaceutical drugs. Persister cells play an important role in blocking the total eradication of infectious agents with antibiotic drugs and in the development of multidrug tolerance in bacteria, fungi, or other pathogens. Multidrug tolerance differs from multidrug resistance in that although it confers temporary protection from antibiotic activity, it is not a mutation-based genetically heritable quality (Lewis 2007), as discussed below. The discovery of persister cells and, indeed, many of the social aspects of microbes are affirmation of what has been called *Orgel's second rule*, after the late biochemist and theoretician Leslie Orgel: "Evolution is cleverer than you are." Orgel meant that the long-term trial-and-error course of evolution does not require invoking an "intelligent designer" or the hand of god (Dunitz and Joyce 2013).

Finally, cooperative behaviors among microorganisms are involved in pathogenic virulence and microbes' ability to cause harm. Virulence regulation in pathogens is based on various cooperative behaviors in gaining optimal use of a host's resources, including enhanced virulence in one lineage of a microbe to gain host resources ahead of competitor microbial lineages.

In sum, rather than leading independent lives, microbes, like many other life forms, are social beings with complex and consequential relationships that we are only beginning to understand. This knowledge is proving invaluable in our quest to comprehend how microbes cause disease and how we can respond to improve health.

PATHWAYS OF PATHOLOGY

Microbes are of most interest to medical anthropology, of course, because of their role in infections that are responsible for about 35 percent of the total mortality of humans each year and about 40 percent of lost DALYs (daily adjusted life years) a measure of the loss of "healthy life" that combines disability and mortality. Over the course of a lifetime an average person acquires approximately 90 trillion bacteria, some of which contribute to what epidemiologists refer to as an individual's *pathogenic burden* or *infectious burden*. A critically important trait of infectious diseases is that they are *communicable diseases* that pass from one person to another or from an animal to a person, either directly (e.g., by breathing in the water droplets exhaled by another) or indirectly (e.g., by touching an elevator button touched by an infected individual or through a vector species like a mosquito). Some researchers differentiate communicable diseases caused by microscopic infectious agents (e.g., bacteria, viruses) from those caused by often somewhat larger parasites such as *hookworms*. However, some microscopic infectious agents, such as HIV, roughly fit the definition of a *parasite*—an organism that feeds on and is sheltered on or in a different organism while contributing nothing to the survival of its host. Thus, a separation of communicable diseases on the basis of the size of the infectious agent is probably not particularly useful. What is useful is gaining a good understanding of the nature of pathogens, their strategies of survival and reproduction, and their interactions with human hosts.

The first critical development in understanding pathogens was the recognition that diseases can be induced by tiny organisms, which took centuries for humans to achieve. In fact, in some ways we are still achieving it. For example, in the HIV disease pandemic University of California molecular and cell biologist Peter Duesberg has continued to assert that HIV does not cause disease. This thoroughly discredited claim adversely influenced the policies of the administration of Thabo Mbeki of South Africa for a number of years and contributed to costly delays in the startup of HIV disease treatments. This tragic turn of events is best understood in light of past disease history in South Africa, like the earlier use of tuberculosis and syphilis to construction theories of black inferiority and sexuality during the era of apartheid (Fassin 2007). Recognition involves an ongoing process of investigation and learning about pathogens and pathogenic processes. One argument of those who denied that HIV was the immediate cause of AIDS was that viruses do not "park themselves" in the body and lie dormant for years before springing to life and causing infection. We now recognize that this is precisely what some pathogens do, and just how they do it is beginning to become clear. The virus involved in chicken pox (*Varicella zoster*), for instance, can lay dormant in dorsal root ganglions, which are sensory nerve cells found just outside the spinal cord. The virus reactivates as a person ages and their immune system weakens or as a result of stress or injury, causing painful outbreaks of shingles. The reactivated virus cannot cause chicken pox again, but it can lead to a blistering rash.

Four key concepts in our evolving understanding of pathogens and their relationships to humans are dynamism, virulence, anthropogenesis, and human development. With respect to pathogens, *dynamism* means that pathogens and the diseases they induce are not static; they change over time and place. For example, the Bubonic *plague* swept through Europe in the fourteenth century and killed 25 to 75 million people, perhaps half of the European population at the time, triggering changes that helped fuel European economic development. This was followed by a long period of only local breakouts, most recently in Peru in 2010 and, subsequently, a few small outbreaks in the United States and Madagascar. The disease has not disappeared or been controlled by biomedicine. Under the right set of conditions it could leap again to the front stage of major infectious disease threats. The ways in which pathogens change in response to the challenges they face, including those presented by immune systems and modifications in human sociocultural patterns, is an essential arena of biological knowledge, one that is far more complex than we realized until relatively recently.

Virulence—the harmfulness of a pathogen—is tied to the ease and facilitation of transmission as well as the route of transmission. Vector-borne pathogens tend to be more virulent if a person (host) becomes sick because sickness prevents the person from actively interfering with disease vector activity. The sufferer lies down and is more subject to vector bites, so the sickness facilitates transmission of other vector-borne pathogens. By contrast, rhinoviruses, the most common viral infective agents in humans and the primary immediate causes of the "common cold," are burdensome but tend not to keep people lying in bed for long periods. As a result, the viruses facilitate the likelihood of interaction with and—through sneezing and coughing—the transmission of the virus to others.

Anthropogenesis refers to the significant role of humans in shaping pathogen behavior and evolution and, as a result, the effects of pathogens on our and other species. Everything we do—for example, how we handle our garbage, including everything from what we consume, the kinds of packaging used by the producers of commodities, our cultural attitudes about handling waste, and the quality of municipal systems for garbage collection and deposit—can affect pathogens and their vectors. As Daniel Reidpath, Pascale Allotey, and Subhash Pokhre (2011) have shown for a mosquito vector of the dengue virus, the more litter that is created and discarded in the area around a home, the more abundant mosquito breeding sites are in proximity to the humans mosquitoes feed on, the greater the incidence of encounters with mosquitoes, and the higher the levels of infection. A particular interesting example of human effect on microbial evolution is seen in the case of convergence of the zoonotic pathogens *Campylobacter jejuni* and C. coli that is being driven by human activities. These two related but evolutionarily distinct bacteria are among the most common infectious agents responsible for human gastroenteritis worldwide. Intensive livestock breeding of chickens or other domesticated poultry as well as cattle, however, has brought these two species together and created conditions that provide opportunities for genetic exchange. As a result of the flow of genes, particularly from C. jejuni to C. coli, species boundaries are breaking down and the two bacteria are merging, or despeciating (Sheppard et al. 2008).

Through their behaviors, pathogens have impacted *human development*. They help shape humans biologically, socially, and experientially, influencing the pathways we have taken through evolution and history (Sabbanti, Manfredi, and Fiorino 2010). Pathogens have been active not only in the natural selection of human biology (e.g., in the co-evolutionary makeup of our immune systems) but also in the formation of human cultural forms and practices—the culturally compelling but ineffective urge to wear surgical masks in public borne of fear of infectious disease, the equally urgent but equally ineffective admonishment to "cough in your elbow," and the increasing ubiquity of antibiotic hand cleanser dispensers. Lawrence Sawchuk (2010:116), writing about cholera epidemics in Gibraltar, stresses, "The effects of an epidemic cannot be measured by the toll of the sick and dead alone" but must include an account of the impacts on ways of life, political structures, and people's understandings of and behaviors in the world.

One consequence of enduring human/microbe interaction is the emergence of a *mutual causation process,* stated simply: species A adopts a new behavior, which facilitates a responsive change in species B, which, in turn, provokes changes in species A, which again impacts and leads to new changes in species B, and so on (Kwa 2008). For example, the more people (species A) living in suburban settings who use backyard flower pots as a form of decoration, the greater the number of new breeding habitats for mosquitoes (species B), which brings them in closer proximity to an important food source for their developing eggs—human blood. In turn, people change their behavior by developing new methods for warding off mosquitoes and new antibiotics for treating malarial infections; in response, mosquitoes develop genetic alterations that enable them to be resistant to those antibiotics. Cormier (2010) has proposed an example of this process in the case of New World malaria. She believes the disease was transferred from Old World human populations to monkeys in the New World during the colonial era, when human cultural practices such as the hunting of monkeys for food and the raising of captured baby monkeys as pets set up intimate interactions during which diseases were transmitted between monkeys and people. Humans responded by developing new or adapted cultural practices—such as the bathing of infected individuals in aromic plants—to treat malarial fevers.

Internally, within an individual's own body, similar processes transpire. This progression, known as *host-pathogen coevolution,* is characterized by reciprocal adaptive changes between pathogens and host immune systems. Host immune systems put pressure on pathogens to develop adaptive responses, and researchers have identified many of these. Some pathogenic species, such as the viruses involved in causing measles and mumps, respond to host immune pressure by becoming (primarily) specialists in the infection of young and immunologically naïve hosts (e.g., children). Because of this strategy, they do not need to develop immune system evasion capacities. Infection caused by these viruses commonly leads to acute disease followed by the elimination of the pathogens by the host through adaptive immunity. Through this process the host gains lifelong protection against re-infection by these viruses. However, viral species continue to survive by being highly contagious and continuing to spread rapidly to new, immunologically naïve hosts, which is why we tend to think of the disease conditions they cause as childhood diseases. And so the co-evolutionary process goes. In developed countries and among wealthy populations mortality from these diseases is extremely low; in underdeveloped countries, however, where rates of malnutrition are high and health care systems are weak, the fatality rate of measles can be many times greater than in wealthy countries.

Other pathogens use an array of immune evasion strategies that are based on mutations. In other words, by continuously changing, pathogens may be able to avoid being detected by the immune system (Brunham, Plummer, and Stephens 1993). In the case of viruses, for example, DNA viruses, positive single strand RNA viruses, negative single strand RNA viruses, and retroviruses have all adopted their own genetic mechanisms to counter host immune responses. Not all of these mechanisms are the products of natural selection operating on random mutations that allow preservation of advantageous gene-link traits. We now know that some mutations are not completely random but are, in fact, built in, following a made-to-mutate capacity. These involve a set of highly mutable genes that Richard Moxon and colleagues (1994), who study the meningitis-linked bacteria *Haemophilus influenzae,* call *contingency genes.* These genes code for the biochemistry of the surface structures of these bacteria. H. influenaze evade immune responses because constant modifications of their contingency genes cause their surface molecules to change continually. Research by Moxon and coworkers shows that mutation in contingency genes occurs at a higher rate than in other areas of the genome. This allows the potential expression of millions of variants, some of which may confer survival benefits because they hinder recognition by immune cells.

Research by Barbara Wright with the bacterium E. coli found that rates of mutation go up in hard times when this bacterium is facing significant environmental challenge (e.g., lacking needed amino acids necessary for reproduction). Observes Wright,

> Within an hour following starvation, bacterial cells undergo major metabolic transitions . . . in which genes required for cell division are repressed while a number of other genes are derepressed. During this transition from exponential growth to stationary phase, events related to gene activation parallel a sharp increase in supercoiling, suggesting that transcriptional activation may drive supercoiling and the resulting DNA secondary structures that are precursors of mutation. (2000:2995)

In effect, Wright is arguing for the existence of a Lamarckian side to evolution involving a role for environmentally induced, acquired characteristics. Although long considered irrelevant to contemporary Darwinian biology, this line of understanding, which asserts that an organism can pass on to its offspring characteristics that it acquired during its lifetime, has gained new acceptance in recent years because of the discovery of epigenetics.

In short, not all of the biological aspects of infectious disease–related co-evolutionary biology involves genetic adaptations. Extremely complex *epigenetic* factors—influences that do not involve genes—also are at play. In response to a detected microbial attack, for example, the immune cells of hosts undergo dramatic changes that facilitate key defensive responses. Successful pathogens, however, commonly develop nongenetic mechanisms to deregulate host genes' protective activities involved in bodily defense. Host cell transcription structures, which are critical to the reproduction of cells in a body, are a common target of such epigenetic processes. *Listeria monocytogene,* the pathogenic agent of listeriosis and one of the best-studied bacterial pathogens, for instance, induces host cell signaling changes involving repression of host gene expression in ways that favor pathogen survival, progression, and virulence. Specifically, L. monocytogene secretes a toxin called listeriolysin that causes a down regulation of host genes that encode the production of proteins involved in defensive inflammatory response by the immune system. Listeriolysin also allows L. monocytogene to gain entry into mammalian cells and to live and reproduce inside them in a domain in which they are protected from antibodies in the blood stream (Hamon, Bierne, and Cossart 2006).

Epigenetic factors also are important in *pathogen latency.* The starting point for understanding this side of pathogenic activity involves a set of changes in the normal biochemical process known as *DNA methylation,* a biochemical progression that entails the addition of a methyl group of molecules to two of the four DNA nucleotides, namely cytosine or adenine. DNA methylation is significant because it alters the expression of genes in cells as they divide and differentiate from embryonic stem cells into very specific body tissues, such as liver, lung, or heart tissue. Liver and lung cells have the same genetic content, yet when liver cells divide they produce daughter liver cells, whereas lung cells produce daughter lung cells. As Eva Jablonka and Marion Lamb (2005:113) observe, even though "their DNA sequences remain unchanged during development, cells nevertheless acquire information that they pass on to their progeny." The information guiding cell production, in other words, is not programmed by genes but rather acquired through a nongenetic inheritance system.

DNA methylation appears to be essential for normal development, as experiments show that mice embryos whose methyltransferase genes have been destroyed die, usually around day nine of gestation. One line of thinking is that methylation is a component of an ancient genomic immune system that consists of the following two phases: bodily detection of foreign DNA sequences (e.g., those of a virus) and methylation, which entails silencing or turning off the foreign DNA before it can invade body cells, hijack their resources, and make new copies of itself that become integrated into transcribed components of the host's genome. DNA methylation also suppresses the expression of endogenous retroviral genes, which appear to be viral elements in the human genome that closely resemble and can be derived from retroviruses, and other potentially damaging sections of DNA that have been incorporated into the genome of the host over time. In bacteria, for example, DNA methylation appears to help protect them from infection by *bacteriophages* (from the Greek for "to devour bacteria"), which are viruses that can infect and replicate in bacteria.

In latent viral infection, however, production of aberrant DNA methylation occurs, which triggers the production of "turned off," or persister, pathogen cells. Because they are already "turned off" (but not destroyed), they remain available to be "turned on" at a later point in time and, thus, are reservoirs of recurrent infection. This process appears to reflect part of the ongoing evolution of pathogens in response to host defenses. As a result of epigenetic latency processes like this, pathogens are much harder to defeat than we recognized in the past.

Epigenetic factors also can be at work in cancers triggered by pathogens. As Hélène Bierne and colleagues (2012) report with reference to the pathogen *H. pylori,* an acquired risk factor for stomach *carcinogenesis*:

> it has been shown that eradication of H. pylori infection in human patients leads to a decrease but not to full disappearance ... of genes closely correlated with the risk of gastric cancer development. ... This is a strong indication that a bacterial infection may leave epigenetic imprints in a tissue enabling permanent changes in gene expression. Given the fact that cancer must arise from a cell that has the potential to divide, this bacterial reprogramming might be induced in long-living cells, such as stem cells or progenitors, thereby being propagated to daughter cells.

Epstein-Barr virus (EBV), a herpes virus that is the etiologic agent involved in causing infectious mononucleosis, is associated with tumor production. Atsushi Kaneda and colleagues (2012) suggest that EBV-infected cells acquire extensive methylation involved in the silencing of multiple tumor-suppressor genes and that, as a result, these cells become malignant. Epigenetic gene silencing, in short, promotes cancer because it inactivates genes that evolved as part of the body's defense against tumors. Epigenetic factors also are involved in prion-triggered diseases such as kuru, as examined later in this chapter. Manipulation of gene expression by nongenetic or epigenetic factors can play an essential part in the biological drama of infectious diseases and must be assessed in understanding these conditions. More broadly, recognition of the importance of epigenetics is leading to a fundamental rewriting of what has been called the Modern Synthesis (Mayr 1982) that links genetics, random mutation, and natural selection as the primary pillars of biological evolution.

PATHOGENIC INFLUENCE ON HUMAN BIOLOGICAL EVOLUTION

Changes in human ecology, including our relationship to the environment and the intentional and unintentional pattern of alterations we make in the environment, lead to modifications in the microbes that populate our bodies and our infectious disease–related health. During much of our evolutionary prehistory hominid ancestors of modern humans foraged the African savanna in small, nomadic bands. Early hominid populations probably were too small and dispersed to support many of the acute communicable pathogens that subsequently came to haunt human communities. A nomadic lifestyle involved a continual pattern of breaking camp and relocating to a new area as local food sources were depleted or went out of season. This pattern also made pathogens less prevalent in general. However, the fact that viruses, such as chicken pox and herpes simplex, may survive in isolated family units suggests that they could have been sustained in dispersed and nomadic populations of early prehumans and humans. Parasitic worms also may have been important pathogens during this phase of human prehistory (Perlman 2013). The current distribution of parasite species common to human and nonhuman primates provides evidence for longstanding hominid-parasite relationships that predate the divergence of the hominid lineage.

As humans have evolved, so too have their infectious diseases. Some diseases that once were rare have become common. Others have disappeared completely, and new infectious agents have emerged over time. Each has had its effects on human health and well-being as well as on our evolution as a species. Ancient human ancestors, for example, were covered with thick, long hair, so why did (most of us) become comparatively hairless, or at least develop very short hairs over most of our bodies? Hairiness has its evolutionary benefits, after all—warmth most notably, and hair confers the ability to be active on cool nights, a behavior impossible for hairless reptilians. One theory, first suggested in the 1800s, is that our evolutionary transition toward hairlessness confers advantage in dealing with ectoparasites, such as lice, ticks, flies, fleas, and the infectious diseases they transmit as vectors. Research has shown, for example, an association between body waxing and a drop in ectoparasites (Armstrong and Wilson 2006).

Of course, all of our closest primate relatives, such as the bonobos, chimpanzees, and gorillas, still are furry—what about them? Are ectoparasites and the diseases they spread a problem for them? These primates are, in fact, quite covered with ectoparasites, but they may control them in three ways. First, they move their resting places every night, as fleas can go through their life cycle only if their host animal lives in a fixed den, lair, or house. Second, they engage in regular social grooming to remove ectoparasites. Finally, they have developed long-term biological relationships with their pathogens, allowing the development of natural immunities (Rantala 1999). From an evolutionary standpoint the problem is not biting ectoparasites per se—this is an irritant but probably not decisive from an evolutionary perspective. Rather, the problem is the many infectious, debilitating, and potentially lethal diseases these ectoparasites transmit as vectors, which may well have been a factor in our own evolutionary movement toward hairlessness in a time of transition to less-than-nightly geographic mobility and temporary shelter construction in response to ecological conditions.

Other impacts of infectious disease on our evolutionary course have been identified. In perhaps the most well-known case, during the 1940s several physicians in Africa noticed that patients who suffered from sickle cell anemia, a serious hereditary blood disease, were more likely to survive malaria, a disease that infects one in every twelve people on the planet and kills over a million people every year, mostly children. Sickle cell is a mutation in the DNA code of the gene that tells the body how to make a form of hemoglobin (Hb), the oxygen-carrying molecule in our blood.

Studies of the geographic distribution of what came to be called the "sickle cell gene" found that it was most concentrated "in a large and rather continuous region of the Old World and in populations which have recently emigrated from this region, while it is almost completely absent from an even larger region of the Old World which stretches from Northern Europe to Australia" (Livingstone 1958:533). In sub-Saharan Africa, where the ancestors of humans first evolved, it is unlikely that malaria was a major threat at the stage when all people lived in small mobile bands and had foraging economies based on hunting and the collection of wild edible plant foods. These conditions did not favor the occurrence of human malaria, although the disease no doubt was present at the time in other mammalian herd species. Anopheles mosquitoes (see Figure 2.4), the vector that spreads malaria, tends to breed in warm, sunlit pools of water and not in heavily forested environments, whereas sustaining malaria infection requires a sufficiently large host population to ensure that infected individuals will be bitten by mosquitoes, take up the malarial parasite during a blood meal, and transmit parasites to other individuals. With the development of horticulture,

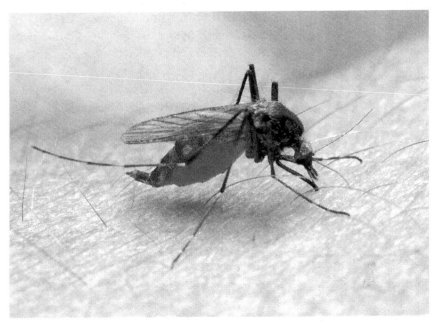

Figure 2.4 Sucking Anopheles mosquito. (Photo by Vladvitek)

the ecology of malaria changed. Clearing of forested areas for the planting of crops allowed both the entry of sunlight to ground level, where it could reach cultigens, and the development of pooled water following rains. This technological transition, which was facilitated by the development of iron tools, promoted a more sedentarized way of life while also creating concentrated populations of readily available human hosts in local residence. The conditions were created, unintentionally through the course of human cultural evolution, that allowed the targeting of humans as a source of blood meals for mosquitoes and the jump of malaria from other mammals to our species. This evolutionary pathway also led to the adaptive occurrence of sickle cell disease.

Two factors provided clues for unraveling the sickle cell mystery: the particular pattern of geographic distribution of the sickle cell gene and recognition that it achieved high frequency in some populations despite the fact that, historically, individuals who received the gene from both parents rarely survived long enough to reproduce. Both suggested to researchers that there may be some biological benefit conferred on individuals who receive the gene from only one parent. Ultimately researchers established that the sickle cell allele HbS carriers have been naturally selected because the trait provides some degree of resistance to malaria. The red blood cells of these individuals, containing some abnormal hemoglobin, tend to adopt a sickle shape when the malaria parasite infects them. These infected cells flow through the spleen, which culls them out because of their damaged sickle shape, eliminating the parasite along with them. The disadvantage of this adaptation is that receiving this sickling trait from both parents causes sickle cell disease. In the 1990s, even as treatments, which are directed at managing symptoms, have improved the longevity of sufferers of this disease, in the United States sufferers' median age at death was only forty-two for males and forty-eight for females, who died of anemia and multi-organ dysfunction (Platt et al. 1994).

The introduction in 2000 of a vaccine that protects against invasive pneumococcal disease, an infection triggered by colonization with the bacterium *Streptococcus pneumonia,* has contributed to the survival of children with sickle cell disease (Yanni et al. 2009). Research in Jamaica found median survival rates of 53 years for men and 58.5 for women (Wierenga, Hambleton, and Lewis 2001). Before the introduction of the vaccine children with sickle cell disease had a six hundred times greater risk than their healthy peers of acquiring invasive pneumococcal disease. In children, interaction of sickle cell disease and pneumococcal disease constitutes a deadly syndemic that unites the consequences of an adaptive response to an infectious parasite with an infectious bacteria. Risk of fatal infection with pneumococcal disease among sickle cell sufferers has increased with the appearance of drug-resistant pneucococci, as penicillin-resistant pneumococci are consistently more common in children with sickle cell disease than otherwise healthy children (Steele et al. 1996).

As this case suggests, most biological adaptations are less than fully optimal; they are compromises that have their benefits as well as their costs. The evolutionary advantages of limiting the lethal impact of malaria, however, appears to have outweighed the evolutionary cost of sickle cell disease, resulting in the survival of the HbS allele in the human genome. As noted in Chapter 1, parallel cases that affirm the centrality of genetics in infectious disease course have proved to be elusive, very likely because of the multidimensional shaping of infectious disease—the complex interplay of biology, environment, culture, and society. What is clear is that microbes have been significant in the processes of becoming human (Fuentes 2013).

INFECTIOUS DISEASES AND
EPIDEMIOLOGICAL TRANSITIONS

Three far-reaching transitions in the configuration of infectious and other diseases have occurred over the sweep of human history (Armelagos and Harper 2005). Beginning about ten thousand years ago a major shift occurred in many human populations: the transition from a nomadic hunting-and-gathering lifestyle to sedentarism and primary food production. This shift, involving major changes in human social organization, diet, demographics, and behavior, created conditions favorable for disease agents among animals to transition to human hosts and for preexisting human pathogens to evolve to more virulent forms. The increase in infectious disease mortality that arose in the context of these changes is known as the first *epidemiological transition*. The human adoption of permanent settlements created larger aggregates of potential human hosts, as described for malaria, as well as increased contact with animal vectors such as rats that live on the human food supply. The frequency of interpersonal contact within and between communities also increased. These changes likely fostered the spread and evolution of more acute infectious diseases. Humans became susceptible to measles, plague, tuberculosis, and other *zoonoses*—infectious disease agents that successfully transfer from an animal population host to a human population host. Subsequent urbanization, which in Europe began in the Middle Ages, was one of the main factors facilitating the devastating spread of *Yersinia pestis*, the Black Death, through the crowded cities of Europe.

Improved sanitation systems implemented by European governments, enhanced nutrition during the nineteenth century, and, eventually, the introduction of antibiotics ultimately reduced the prevalence of plague along with cholera, tuberculosis, typhoid, scarlet fever, dysentery, childhood infections, and other ancient diseases proximally caused by microbial foes, primarily in wealthier and technologically more developed nations (Hardy 1993). This change constitutes the second epidemiological transition. (Unfortunately it has been accompanied by the rise of noninfectious chronic and degenerative diseases among longer-lived people.) A significant moment in the history of human infectious diseases began at the tail end of the Middle Ages with the beginning of the Colonial Era and the economic and political extension of European cultural and social forms to all corners of the world. Alfred Crosby (2004) termed the global spread of Europeans, European animals, European plants, and European infectious diseases *ecological imperialism*. This centuries-long event significantly exacerbated health problems in colonized areas of the world and helped to create the contemporary global health profile.

We are living in the third epidemiological transition, which is characterized by the resurgence of infectious diseases, including the reappearance of diseases that previously were somewhat controlled (e.g., tuberculosis) and the emergence of new infectious diseases in human populations (e.g., HIV infection). Moreover, as Ron Barrett (2010:84) notes, "Humankind is rapidly developing a global disease ecology, one that involves the [international] convergence of disease patterns as well as the diffusion of pathogens across populations and national boundaries." This third epidemiological transition also involves the evolution of pathogens' resistance to antibiotics and an increased impact of syndemic interaction among diseases, both infectious and noninfectious.

PATHOGENIC INFLUENCES ON HISTORY

Across these three epidemiological transitions infectious diseases have helped to shape the course of human history. Commenting on the effect on human history of bubonic plague, or the Black Death, as it was known, Shirley Lindenbaum (2001:363) argues that it contributed to "the emergence of nation states, the rise of mercantile economies, and the religious movements that led to the Reformation." Additionally the epidemic may have "brought about new ways of understanding God, the meaning of death, and the role of authority in religious and social life" (Lindenbaum 2001:363).

In the same vein, in *Twelve Diseases That Changed Our World,* Irwin Sherman (2007) describes the various ways pathogens have transformed human societies through time. For example, *yellow fever* influenced the building of the Panama Canal, the Louisiana Purchase, and, in fact, the pre–World War II development of the southern United States. Although malaria hampered the economic development of some countries, one of the reasons Europeans were able to colonize Africa was that they were used quinine, derived from the bark of the cinchona tree, which was reasonably effective as an antimalarial drug. Why did Europeans have quinine? They acquired it when they colonized South America; the Quechua Indians of Peru and Bolivia originally discovered the medicinal properties of the cinchona tree, and Jesuit missionaries learned about the drug from indigenous peoples and began shipping it to Europe, providing an important weapon in the Europe's ever-expanding colonial onslaught.

In the 1500s, European travelers introduced exotic diseases into the Americas that, by some estimates, killed over 50 percent of the population of Mexico, enabling a very small European army to conquer a sophisticated warrior society. As Francisco de Aguilar (1993:121) wrote at the time of the sacking of the Aztecs—in a tone that clearly reflects the Spanish cultural view of disease among the indigenous people—"When the Christians were exhausted from war, God saw fit to send the Indians smallpox, and there was great pestilence in the city." Similarly Bernadino Vazquez de Tapia (quoted in McCaa 1995:423), who accompanied Hernán Cortés, wrote,

> The pestilence of measles and smallpox was so severe and cruel that more than one-fourth of the Indian people in all the land died—and this loss had the effect of hastening the end of the fighting because there died a great quantity of men and warriors and many lords and captains and valiant men

against whom we would have had to fight and deal with as enemies, and miraculously Our Lord killed them and removed them before us.

As these accounts suggest, the devastating spread of Europe infectious disease among New World indigenous people affirmed to Europeans their physical superiority as well as God's blessing of their imperial conquest.

Based on a reexamination of diverse original sources on the 1520 small pox epidemic in Mexico, Robert McCaa (1995) concluded that in some provinces half the population died, whereas in others the rate was somewhat lower. The same pattern prevailed throughout the Americas: from the Caribbean to coastal Brazil and northward to New England and New France (e.g., Louisiana), no indigenous group was spared the harsh impact of European pathogens. It is fair to say that Native American susceptibility to immunologically unfamiliar European epidemic diseases, and not a technological or cultural advantage—and certainly not any innate biological superiority—was the key factor allowing Europeans to conquer the so-called New World, subjugate its peoples, and reap the bounty of its resources. The impact of these European infectious diseases was "in all likelihood the most severe single loss of aboriginal population that ever occurred" in human history (Dobyns 1963).

In a single stroke Europeans constructed both a new social world and, at the microscopic level, a new world of infectious disease ecology. Infectious disease, in other words, was an enabler of the entire colonial era and helped bring into being the postcolonial period, which we now inhabit. The Irish famine also had a major influence on the history of the United States. An infectious disease of potatoes in Ireland in part brought on the famine, but social factors—including unequal access to food, large food exports to England, land acquisitions and exploitation by absentee landlords, and other inequities—were central factors contributing to the death of around a million people. Another million Irish immigrated to the United States, where they played a major role in expanding the Democratic Party, developing labor unions, and molding the nation's character in numerous other ways.

Malnutrition and infectious disease are closely related in the context of inequality, and all the more so in the context of violent conflict. Influenza very likely influenced the course of World War I by sickening and killing soldiers and straining military health care. Some historians believe that the influenza infection President Woodrow Wilson was suffering with at the time affected negotiations during the Treaty of Versailles (Tice 1997). More broadly, of the astounding 62 million civilian and 45 million war-related deaths in the twentieth century alone, a large percentage were due to infectious disease rather than battlefield injuries (Levy and Sidel 2008). In the *Global Burden of Armed Violence* the Geneva Declaration Secretariat (2008) reports that for each of the more than half a million people who died violently in a war between 2004 and 2007, another four died from infectious diseases and malnutrition brought on by war.

During the civil war in Somalia in 1992 blocking access to food was used as a weapon against civilians, leading to famine, a breakdown of public health programs, mass migration, and, then, further exposure to food insecurity in refugee camps due to the contamination of food and water supplies under war conditions. One consequence was a high rate of infection-caused diarrheal disease among both children and adults. Approximately 74 percent of children under five years of age living in the refugee camps died from diarrheal disease acquired from infected water. This grim pattern has become common in contemporary armed conflicts, and it is exacerbated when health care infrastructures and providers are targets of attack.

Trypanosoma, a family of parasitic protozoa, also have influenced the course of human history. Its name is derived from the Greek words for "body" and "borer." In humans trypanosomes proximally cause the fatal disease in Africa that we call sleeping sickness. In the New World a trypanosome is the proximal cause of Chagas disease. Sleeping sickness has been identified in thirty-six sub-Saharan countries, mostly in rural areas, where it is spread by the tsetse fly vector. In 2009 about ten thousand cases of sleeping sickness were reported to the World Health Organization (2013c). Once an infected tsetse fly bites and infects a human, the protozoa drills through the skin layers and causes a skin lesion, triggering fever, headaches, and joint pains. In a second stage of development the parasite crosses the blood-brain barrier and infects the central nervous system, resulting in the symptoms that give it the name "sleeping sickness." Untreated, it commonly leads to death. As a result of sleeping sickness, areas of African savanna became uninhabitable by humans. Some of these areas hold Africa's great ungulate herds—gazelle, gnu, wildebeest, zebra—which are bitten by tsetse flies but only suffer mild illness. The tsetse fly limited human predation, so today the African savanna ecosystem supports a higher diversity of ungulate species than is found in any other ecosystem or continent on Earth. In the comparable prairielands of North America, by contrast, lack of an equivalent disease and vector meant that there was little to stop the near extermination of what had once been vast herds of another ungulate, bison.

There is far more to the human encounter with trypanosomiasis in Africa. One aspect of note has been its historic relationship with European colonialism on the continent. Colonial powers viewed trypanosomiasis as a peculiarly African condition, a cultural construction that intermingled growing medical awareness of an infectious disease spread by the tsetse vector with a stereotypical portrayal of Africans as innately lethargic. For some period of time the colonial medical community even debated whether Europeans in Africa could be infected with this African disease, though eventually it was accepted that they could (Bloom

2008:104). Missing from colonial understandings of sleeping sickness was the role of colonialism itself in spreading the disease. Systems of colonial labor were at fault, for example, when they forced African men to work clearing brush and woody vegetation along riverbanks or to perform similar toil in risky settings where tsetse flies congregate. Social disruptions caused directly and indirectly by colonialism, including population migrations, invasive expeditions, and wars, further contributed to the spread of the disease, despite colonial efforts to implement disease control measures. In one of the "telling ironies of history, [colonial regimes] likely contributed to both cause and cure as they regulated outbreaks in part induced by the larger disruptions of imperial expansion" (Redfield 2013:184–185).

THE HYGIENE HYPOTHESIS

The changing relationship between humans and their environment has given rise to a phenomenon that has been called the *Hygiene Hypothesis*. This proposition is based on an important principle of organisms, including infectious disease agents, namely that *organisms reflect their evolutionary history*. An interesting nonmicroscopic example of this is the case of the pronghorn "antelope" that inhabits western and central North America, first brought to scientific awareness by the Lewis and Clark Expedition of 1804–1806. Pronghorn are distinguished by their speed as runners; indeed, they are the fastest land mammal in the Western Hemisphere. Their bodies evolved in response to being chased by a very fast predator that no longer exists (the American cheetah), resulting in the production, under contemporary conditions, of "overspeed." The result is energy waste while in flight from contemporary but much slower predators.

As this example shows, when the species that are critical to the evolution of another species are removed—whether as a result of human overhunting, habitat change, or other cause—their specialized adaptive features become anachronistic as well as potential sources of illness. In applying this idea to humans, Rob Dunn (2011:ix), in his book *The Wild Life of Our Bodies: Predators, Parasites, and Patterns that Shape Who We Are Today*, argues that although as a species we evolved in a world of microbes, including pathogens, parasites, and beneficial organisms, "We no longer see ourselves as part of nature." In the name of progress and sanitary living we scrub much of nature off of our bodies and our kitchen counters, hoping to "get rid of germs." Nature, in the new world we have created, is the frozen landscape outside the bubble of our built environments, a kind of living painting that is pleasant to view and contemplate but one we are glad to have escaped. Yet something appears to have gone wrong. Just as we seem to be on the verge of "ridding ourselves of the old threats, a set of 'new' diseases—including Crohn's, inflammatory bowel disease, rheumatoid arthritis, lupus, diabetes, multiple sclerosis, schizophrenia, and autism, among others—has become more and more common" and a new threat to our existence (Dunn 2011:18).

In explaining the rise of many of the new noninfectious diseases, the Hygiene Hypothesis asserts that a lack of early childhood exposure to infectious agents and parasites resulting from our sanitizing cultural practices increases susceptibility to allergic diseases in children by suppressing natural immune system exposure to pathogens. The rise of autoimmune diseases and acute lymphoblastic leukemia in young people in the developed world has been explained in terms of the Hygiene Hypothesis.

In the late 1980s David Strachan (1989) proposed that hay fever and eczema, both allergic diseases, are less frequent in children from large families, a situation that, he theorized, creates multiple opportunities for early childhood exposure to infectious agents that further our immune system development and diminish autoimmune allergic responses. In recent times the emergence of multiple hygienic practices, elimination of childhood diseases, widespread use of antibiotics, extensive availability of antibacterial soaps, and the relative availability of effective medical care have further diminished exposure to many "traditional" diseases of early childhood development. As a result, some argue, we are supersensitive to allergens (see Figure 2.5).

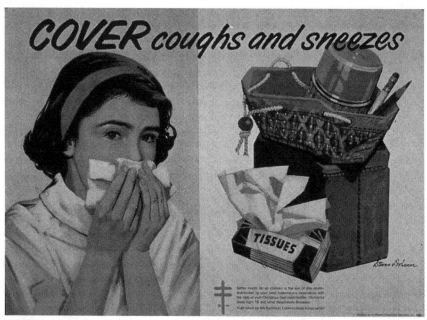

Figure 2.5 1960s Public health message. (Poster by Stevan Dohanos, National Tuberculosis Association)

Various studies have provided supportive evidence for the Hygiene Hypothesis. Research by Markus Ege and colleagues (2011), for example, compared school-age children in Bavaria, Germany, who lived on farms with those who did not live on farms. Farm children were found both to have lower prevalence of asthma and allergies and to be exposed to a greater variety of environmental microorganisms. Moreover, the diversity of microbial exposure, including fungal and bacterial species, was found to be inversely related to the risk of asthma. Although the Hygiene Hypothesis remains somewhat controversial, it reveals the complexities of our evolutionary relationship with the multiple microorganisms with which we share the planet. One implication of the Hygiene Hypothesis is that no less than the beneficial microbes in our gut or on our skin, there are ways in which, having adapted to their presence, we also need pathogens. Our interaction with them promotes survival, just as it exacts a cost.

CASE STUDY: KURU

Early in the twentieth century, health scientists became aware of a new disease that appeared to exist primarily among the South Foré people of New Guinea. The disease was known to the South Foré as *kuru,* a word that, in their language, means "to shake." The disease also is called "trembling sickness" or "laughing sickness" because of the sufferer's symptoms, namely palsy, contracted face muscles, and the loss of motor control, resulting in the inability to walk and, eventually, even to eat. Kuru victims become progressively emaciated and inevitably die. The disease was responsible for around 2,500 deaths before it was curtailed.

Epidemiological studies found that kuru was increasing in prevalence at the time it came to the attention of health officials, a pattern that continued through the 1950s. At its peak it primarily afflicted women in their twenties and thirties—in other words, during their most fertile reproductive years. In a group the size of the South Foré, kuru presented a significant threat to survival. In the 1950s and 1960s the kuru epidemic may have killed 25 percent of the female population among the South Foré; as a result, in some villages there were few female survivors of marriageable age. Historically, South Foré men had several wives, but because of kuru, men who had lost wives were left with child care duties. Men were resentful and confused by this situation as, growing up and learning South Foré culture, they were accustomed to a clear-cut, gendered division of labor.

Because the South Foré have a personalistic explanation for illness—namely, they believe spiritual beings or magical manipulation cause illness—they came to accept that kuru was the work of sorcerers who used contagious magic. The basic principle of contagious magic in various ethnomedical traditions is that "once two things have been in contact, they remain in contact spiritually forever." Hence, all of your fingernail or hair clippings are still connected to you, and magic performed on them will affect you. Sorcerers were believed to be people who had occult knowledge that they could use to harm their enemies through contagious magic. The South Foré became very focused on cleaning up their house sites to make sure sorcerers could not obtain and magically manipulate any of their hair, fingernail clippings, feces, or personal belongings. Additionally, the South Foré organized sorcerer hunts, and identified sorcerers were forced to "confess" and then join antisorcerer cults. This strategy, though unquestioningly meaningful culturally, failed to produce the desired result and did not slow the increasing number of kuru victims.

In the early 1950s a team of Australian doctors began working to discover the cause of kuru in hopes of finding a cure. Some researchers traced cases of the disease in family lines to see whether it was hereditary; it wasn't. Other researchers collected water, soil, plant, and animal specimens to test for environmental toxins that could be causing the disease; none were found. Eventually kuru was discovered to be an infectious disease of the brain and nervous system. Researchers thought initially a virus with a prolonged incubation period caused kuru, but the implicated virus could not be found.

In the late 1950s an American pediatrician named Carleton Gajdusek came to Papua New Guinea to try to identify the infectious agent that caused kuru. Through the microscopic examination of tissue from people who died of the kuru, he discovered that the disease organism was carried in the blood and was concentrated in brain tissue. Meanwhile Shirley Lindenbaum, an Australian anthropologist working with her husband, Robert Glasse, carried out an ethnography of kuru to help clarify what was going on (Lindenbaum 1978). They found that kuru was of relatively recent origin, that it had spread from place to place since its emergence, and that mortuary cannibalism might transmit it (Mathews, Glasse, and Lindenbaum 1968). Their research showed that the South Foré ate parts of their deceased relatives' bodies as a component of their funerary practices. Foré believe that the living have a responsibility to ensure that the dead are transformed into spiritual ancestors: "By eating the dead, the female affines [relative by marriages] of the deceased person confined the dangerous ghost [of a deceased individual] inside themselves, thus protecting the family from ghostly attack and the pollution from a decomposing body" (Lindenbaum 2013:178). Ritual cannibalism freed the ghost to journey to the land of the progenitors and be reborn there as a living ancestor. In these rituals women butchered the corpses and were the main cannibals. They also gave portions to their small children to eat. Men generally thought this practice was unmanly.

They had pigs to eat, whereas the diet of women and children was normally poor in animal protein. In his Nobel Prize lecture on kuru, Gajdusek (1976) also noted that the disease could be spread to individuals who participated in cannibal rituals but did not consume ancestor body parts as a consequence of pathogen exposure through cuts and abrasions or through the intentional rubbing of brain tissues on the bodies of the living. Lindenbaum (2013) comments that although transmission through cuts is possible, the South Foré deny that rubbing brain tissue on their bodies was ever a cultural practice.

Ultimately evidence mounted that a prion was the immediate cause of kuru. The word prion is derived from the words "protein" and "infection." Prions are pathogenic variants of proteins that are naturally produced in nerve cells and certain other cells. Their structure contrasts with all other known infectious agents, which contain nucleic acids (either DNA, RNA, or both) along with protein components. When a prion encounters a normal protein cell it is able to convert it into a prion, leading to a buildup of prions clumped together and empty spaces or holes in the brain. In the case of kuru the eating of body parts of individuals who had been infected spread the prion.

In the early 1960s cannibalism was outlawed in Papua New Guinea, and government patrols enforced the ban. Since the practice ended, no new kuru infections have been identified, and the last kuru death occurred in 2007. The disease is now considered to be eradicated. Kuru is not unique, however, and is closely related to *Creutzfeldt-Jakob disease*. The latter disease is now popularly referred to as "mad cow disease" because it is a variant of the disease in cattle (bovine spongiform encephalopathy). There is a similar disease called scrapie that afflicts sheep and causes them to have tremors, stagger, lose their eye sight, and die. One of the complications of prion diseases is the long incubation period, as much as fifty years, between infection and symptom onset.

The case of kuru affirms the biocultural/biosocial patterns of infectious diseases: the spread of the disease occurred because of human cultural beliefs and practices involving mortuary cannibalism. Similarly, industrial patterns of animal husbandry and feeding have facilitated the spread of prions among animal species. Although cattle are herbivores, they are being fed the remains of other cattle in the form of meat and bone meal, allowing infectious agents in slaughtered animals to spread. Various other livestock handling practices of industrial food production, from keeping massive numbers of animals in crowded conditions and heavily using antibiotics to promote rapid growth, have also been identified as sources of risk for human infectious disease (Davis 2005).

Another lesson of prions is that they represent a case of cell replication that does not involve genes. Prions can become self-propagating (and infectious), but they lack nucleic acid (RNA or DNA). They are a nongenetic, or epigenetic, entity (Krimsky and Gruber 2013). Expanding research on such phenomena is reshaping existing biological thinking and narrow, gene-based biological determinism while opening the conceptual space for considering the importance of nongenetic factors, including culture and society, in accounting for infectious disease.

CONCLUSION: LIVING WITH MICROBES

This chapter delved into many of the complexities of human/pathogen interaction through time and place. A take-home message of the chapter is that you cannot fully understand humans as a species, the course of our history, the natures of our societies and cultures, or our relationship to the world around us without considering pathogens. Developing such understanding is the raison d'être of anthropology and the bedrock of its mission as a scholarly discipline and as an applied field concerned with improving the human condition, we must pay close attention to the big effects of tiny organisms.

Discussion Questions

1. What are some of the key interactions between pathogens and our immune systems' components that shape health and disease?
2. Why was there such a dramatic increase in concern about "germs" in the Western world during the twentieth century?
3. What are the lessons of sickle cell disease for human evolution?
4. Why was anthropology of value in figuring out the transmission of kuru?
5. What are the pros and cons of labeling gut flora as a human organ?
6. In light of the Hygiene Hypothesis, should we change our child-rearing practices?

CHAPTER THREE

More Than Human

> Life thwarts full definition, even comprehensive theorization, not
> because it is mysterious but because it is impossible to separate fully
> forms of explanation from the apparition of living things themselves,
> forms of life from life forms.
>
> *Stefan Helmreich (2009:9)*

THE WIDER COMMUNITIES OF HUMANS

Our bodies contain many nonhuman cells, making each one of us, in a sense, a kind of biological community of diverse species. Previous chapters showed that we are more than just human in our composition. The title of this chapter explores the theme "more than human" in the study of microbes in another sense; namely, it covers the relationships between our species and other microbe-bearing animals and plants in the world. An important consequence of these relationships is that, although microbes adapt biologically and behaviorally to the bodily conditions inside the species they inhabit, they also migrate, jumping to new species and adapting to somewhat different conditions within their new hosts. In the process microbes that were not particularly harmful to their original hosts may become pathogenic in their new biological environments, even severely so.

Our relations with other species and their microbes have had their effect in making us who we are and in shaping human health. These relationships have an immediate bearing on the field of anthropology. Animals, plants, fungi, virus, and bacteria—combined these constitute somewhere between 2 million and perhaps as many as 15 million species, yet they were once confined to the margins of anthropological research. Today they have begun to appear alongside humans in the way anthropologists think about the world. Increasingly we have come to recognize that species, including our own, co-evolve in close interaction with and in continuing response to other species. In this sense we have helped to make each other (Singer 2014). This fact is readily apparent in considering our long history with canines. Their roles as hunters, watch dogs, companions, bed warmers, and more have left imprints on us just as our selective breeding practices have shaped them, turning predator wolves that howl into friendly dogs that bark with wagging tails and floppy ears. Today even the smallest organisms and those seemingly least like us, such as microbes, are being rethought in anthropological texts. As our knowledge expands "about microbial genetics, structure, and function, the more we marvel at the sophistication of the survival strategies of microbes" (Smolinski, Hamburg, and Lederberg 2003:57). The more we understand our world, the greater we realize the powerful role of microbes, beneficial and otherwise, in the making of the human condition.

This chapter engages this second meaning of "more than human." It examines the spread of diseases across species and the fundamental role of zoonotic pathogens, such as HIV and Lyme disease, in the continued production of human health. The chapter ends with a consideration of a migrating disease called Nipah and the role of bats as vectors of this multispecies infectious disease. This case illustrates how the ways we change the environment can come back to harm us in the form of new zoonotic diseases.

EMERGENT AND ESTABLISHED ZOONOTICS AND HUMAN HEALTH

In general, pathogens are host specific, surviving only within one or a narrow range of life forms, and are unable easily to transfer to or live within other organisms. The bacteria *Shigella flexneri*, for example, which causes dysentery in parts of the world lacking clean drinking water, only infects humans and other primates. Similarly, Chytridiomycosis is an infectious disease only found among amphibians. It is caused by a fungus that has been linked to a dramatic drop in amphibian populations around the globe and possibly the extinction of some species (Daszak et al. 2003). It is not, however, at least directly, a threat to humans, as it has not made the rather considerable jump from amphibian to mammalian bodies. But it may affect us nonetheless. We are learning that amphibian bodies contain chemicals such as peptides that are useful in treating some human diseases—and there are numerous other reasons why their extinction is of no small importance to our species. The red-eyed treefrog, *Litoria chloris*, which dwells in Australia, has the highest levels of peptides that kill HIV, possibly by penetrating the virus's outer membrane envelope and creating damage that causes the virus to fragment. The loss of such a species has potential ramifications for human health. Anthropogenic global warming may facilitate the spread of Chytridiomycosis, as frog immune systems appear to lose effectiveness during erratic shifts in temperature (Pounds, Fogden, and Campbell 1999). In other words, our actions may be endangering species of value to us in dealing with our own infectious diseases.

Sometimes, as it turns out, microbes do successfully adapt to new host species. The term zoonoses refers to infectious disease agents that successfully transfer from an animal population host to a human population host. It is estimated that 60 percent of newly identified emerging infectious diseases in humans have their origin in other animals (Jones et al. 2008). So-called *avian influenza* (bird flu) is one such disease that potentially threatens millions of people. This pathogen has broken through the *species barrier,* mutating in a way that has allowed it to live in the internal body and cellular environment of a new species. Breaking through this barrier involves a process of reproduction, mutation, and natural selection. When it occurs it means that, as a consequence of continuous errors in the reproduction of a pathogen, by chance the right genetic combination that enables infection of the new species occurs and the altered pathogen survives and infects the new host.

There are two risks to humans from the cross-species transfer of zoonotic diseases:

1. Direct transfer from animals to humans. For example, bovine tuberculosis, seen in people who work around cattle or drink untreated cow's milk, is caused by the pathogen M. bovis.
2. Human-to-human transmission of a disease that began as a zoonotic disease infection, such as HIV.

HIV appears to have evolved from a simian immunodeficiency virus (SIV) found among chimpanzees, more specifically *Pan troglodytes troglodytes* living in southern Cameroon (Gao et al. 1998). After initial transfer to human hosts, SIV adapted and evolved genetically to become HIV, which became an explosive immediate cause of human disease.

Pathogens also pass from humans to other animals, with repercussions for species that are important to us as sources of food or that play other vital roles in complex ecosystems. An example of this transfer is the case of respiratory syncytial virus (RSV), the leading cause of lower respiratory tract infections in infants and young children as well as a risk to health among those over sixty-five years of age (Thompson et al. 2003). Ecotourism programs that bring people into chimpanzees' habitats appear to be triggering outbreaks of respiratory disease caused by this virus among our primate relatives. In the first confirmed case of a virus transmitted directly from humans to great apes in the wild, this virus jumped from human tourists to several groups of chimpanzees in West Africa during the period 1999 to 2004, with devastating consequences for an already endangered species. Cases like these create a serious challenge to efforts to sustain ape populations because they show that "the close approach of humans to apes, which is central to both research and tourism programs, represents a serious threat to wild apes. This represents a dilemma because both activities have clear benefits for ape conservation" (Köndgen et al. 2008:262).

The breaking of species barriers has emerged as a critical part of the chain of events causing a global rise in infectious diseases, and as a result, the fundamental importance of animal diseases as a threat to humans has escalated. Researchers like anthropologist Melanie Rock (2013) stress that human health cannot be understood adequately without reference to animals. Epidemiologists, social scientists, physicians, veterinarians, and others concerned with preventing emergent human infections by monitoring and controlling animal diseases, including those of companion species (e.g., dogs), have formed the One Health Movement (Rock et al. 2009). From the perspective of scientists and practitioners involved in this effort, the "convergence of people, animals, and our environment has created a new dynamic in which the health of each group is inextricably interconnected" (American Veterinary Medical Association 2008:3).

Although animal pathogens can affect human health when they jump species, this is not the only way they affect our well-being. Disease among food animals, for example, threatens the human food supply, a not insignificant issue in a world in which food insecurity is a major global health concern. Exemplary is the disease known as porcine reproductive and respiratory syndrome (PRRS), which only affects pigs. By suppressing the swine immune system, PRRS allows persistent infections to become established, leading to respiratory disease, abortion in pregnant sows, and the death of piglets. The virus that causes PRRS has the ability to evolve rapidly, which makes developing vaccines and treatments difficult. Because of the enormous number of swine deaths caused by PRRS outbreaks, this animal disease has had major consequences for the food supply chain and on economies and livelihoods in swine-producing countries and regions (Muirhead and Alexander 1997). In the United States alone the total annual economic impact of PPRS is estimated to be about $560 million (Neuman et al. 2005).

Another infectious animal disease of concern is the highly contagious viral condition of cloven-hoofed livestock known as foot and mouth disease (FMD). It too has caused considerable losses to the US economy, totaling almost $40 billion. Along with yet another animal disease, bovine spongiform encephalopathy, which has infected humans as well, FMD has generated widespread food safety fears and emotional distress among livestock producers. FMD is considered to be one of the worst animal plague endemics in many parts of the world (Tully and Fares 2008).

Infectious disease of food plants presents one more way pathogens threaten human health and well-being. Currently the United States and Brazil, for example, the two global leaders in the production of citrus crops, are facing devastation from a bacterial disease known as citrus greening or yellow dragon. The bacteria, *Candidatus liberibacter,* is spread from citrus tree to tree by a pin-pointsized insect called a *psyllid,* which feeds on citrus trees and serves as vector of the bacteria. As a result of the rapid spread of the disease, which causes the fruit to become bitter and drop to the ground and eventually kills the tree, the entire orange juice industry in the United States is at risk (Alvarez 2013).

Infectious disease also threatens bananas. Known as Panama disease, it is linked to a fungus called *Fusarium oxysporum.* The danger is significant, as this pathogen wiped out much of the world's banana crop in the first half of the twentieth century. At the time the dominant species of banana consumed around the world was known as the Gros Michels variety. The type of banana now dominant on the world market is the Cavendish banana, and growers selected it to replace the Gros Michels specifically because of its apparent resistance to the fungus. But Panama disease is now spreading across the world and poses a devastating threat to the Cavendish banana industry (Ploetz 2005).

An additional aspect of the role of other species in human health involves the complex developmental stages in the life cycles of many pathogens. *Cysticercosis* and *taeniasis,* for example, are the names of two diseases caused by the helminth *Taenia solium,* more commonly known as the pork tapeworm. Pigs become infected with T. solium when they ingest food or water contaminated with the tapeworm's eggs. Following ingestion, the eggs develop in pig muscles. Humans become infected when they ingest raw or undercooked infected pork—infection is tied to cultural practice. Cysticercos develops in humans when T. solium infects the brain or muscle tissue, whereas taeniasis involves intestinal infection. Neurocysticercosis, infection of the brain, is particularly menacing and causes seizures.

These examples of infectious diseases among livestock and crop species affirm the importance of maintaining an eye on the big disease picture rather than adopting a narrow, anthropocentric focus on immediately known human diseases.

CLASSIFYING ZOONOTICS

The World Health Organization (Battershell 2011) has developed the following classification system of zoonoses based on the nature of the pathogen's life cycle:

- Direct zoonoses—these zoonoses are transmitted from an infected verte-brate host to another host through direct contact by way of an inanimate object or anthropod vector. During transmission these pathogens do not undergo developmental change or propagation. An example of this kind of zoonosis is rabies, a disease that kills over fifty thousand people a year worldwide and is transmitted directly from animals to people.

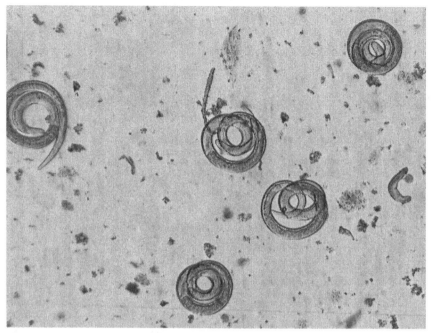

Figure 3.1 Trichinella spiralis, a parasitic worm. (Photo by Olga Rudneva)

- Cyclozoonoses—these zoonoses require more than one vertebrate host but no invertebrate host is needed. Examples of cyclozoonoses are *hydatid disease* (linked to the larval form of the pathogen *Echinococcus granulosus*) and trichinosis (linked to *Trichinella spiralis*) (see Figure 3.1).
- Metazoonoses—these zoonoses require an invertebrate host, where the pathogen multiplies or develops before it can infect a vertebrate host. An example of a metazoonotic disease is bubonic plague.
- Saprozoonoses—these zoonoses are transferred through a nonanimal reservoir, such as a plant, or through the abiotic environment, such as through water or soil. Tetanus is an example of a saprozoonotic.

Nathan Wolfe and colleagues (2007) have proposed a staged pathway of evolutionary development of zoonotic diseases. In the first stage the triggering pathogen is found only in nonhuman animal species. Stage two is characterized by species jump, and new infections of humans are the result of animal exposures rather than human-to-human transmission. In the next stage animal pathogens are transmitted to humans and are able to undergo several cycles of human-to-human transmission before an outbreak dies out, a pattern seen in sudden outbursts of ebola that end within a confined period of time. This pattern may have also characterized the early history of HIV, with multiple short-lived transfers from animals to humans over time before the virus fully adapted to the human biological environment (Karesh and Noble 2009). Stage four is a mixed cyclical stage involving infections associated with animal exposure combined with long sequences of human-to-human transmission without new animal transmission. This pattern is seen, for example, in Chagas disease. In the final stage the pathogen has become fully adapted to the human host and is genetically differentiated from its ancestral species found in animals (e.g., HIV). In this stage human-to-human transmission is the only route of new infections.

Zoonotics, in short, come in diverse forms with varying life histories and stages of adaptation to human hosts. Their significance as a factor in health is tied not only to these biological characteristics but also to their interface with human social and cultural systems as well as demographics. As the total human population on the planet continues to grow, more bodies are made available as reservoirs for disease. A larger overall population also means that there are greater numbers of older people and people with existing health conditions that degrade their immune systems. Moreover, in some regions of the world economic instability is causing breakdowns in public health systems, including prevention education programs. Because of expanded food production to meet the food needs of a growing population, some animal populations also are expanding. The movement of people, which has dramatically increased, also facilitates the movement of zoonotics to new places. Infectious agents can be unknowingly transported through the shipment of infected animals or carried on clothes or the flesh of people who have come in contact with animals.

In other words, human behavior is critical to the spread of zoonotics as well as to their control. Wildlife biologists use the term *pathogen pollution* to accentuate the continued and disruptive anthropogenic movement of infectious agents outside their natural geographic or host species range as well as to draw parallels to other ways in which human activity is adversely affecting the environment (Cunningham, Daszak, and Rodriguez 2003). As Chapter 4 will emphasize, pathogen pollution is accentuated by its interaction with other forms of anthropogenic pollution and ecosystem degradation.

PETS IN THE BEDROOM AND MICROBES IN THE OFFICE

To begin to examine the role of cultural practices and social structures in human exposure to zoonotic disease, it is useful to examine microbes living close to home in the spaces of human occupation, such as homes, offices, or related settings. Domesticated pets that live in human homes, for example, represent a routine means of animal/human interaction. In the United States, where over

60 percent of households have pets, there are around 60 million domestic dogs and 75 million cats, and 56 percent of dog owners (especially those with small dogs) and 62 percent of cat owners allow their pets to sleep with them in bed (Chromel and Sun 2011). This widespread cultural practice—one that is not limited to the United States—which usually involves a view of pets as members of the family or as friends, has been found to be a factor in several bubonic plague outbreaks, such as in New Mexico in 1974, a result of infected flea bites. In Argentina, where Chagas disease is found, domestic transmission is significantly higher when infected dogs sleep with their owners (Gürtler et al. 1991).

Additionally, *cat-scratch disease* is a zoonotic condition named for its route of transmission. Its immediate cause is *Bartonella henselae,* a *proteobacterium,* which is a phylum of bacteria that includes a wide variety of pathogens. Research shows that sufferers of this disease are more likely than matched controls to have been scratched or bitten by a kitten, licked on the face by a kitten, slept with a kitten, or combed a kitten (Zangwill et al. 1993). Kissing family pets on the nose and mouth or allowing a pet to lick your face are also routes of pet-to-human disease transmission. Being licked by pets as well as being bitten is also a common source of human infection with *Pasteurella multocida,* a *coccobacillus* that causes soft tissue inflammation but also can lead to serious conditions like *osteomyelitis,* endocarditis, and meningitis. *Capnocytophaga canimorsus* infections in humans also have been associated with being licked by or sleeping with a dog or cat. Although virulence is low in healthy individuals, in people with preexisting conditions, including alcoholism and compromised immune systems, this bacteria can cause severe disease.

In a study of people's homes in Raleigh-Durham, North Carolina, Rob Dunn and colleagues (2013), aided by a large group of "citizen biologist" volunteers, took swabs of pillow cases, the insides of refrigerators, toilet seats, TV screens, door jams, and other household surfaces. Based on a genetic analysis of these swabs, they found that each of the household locations they sampled was home to bacterial communities that were distinct from those found on other surfaces. They also examined whether the variability in bacterial diversity across homes could be attributed to outdoor environmental factors, indoor habitat structure, or the occupants of the home. What they found was that the presence of dogs had a significant effect on bacterial community composition in multiple locations in indoor environments. Homes occupied by dogs harbored more diverse communities and higher relative numbers of dog-associated bacterial species. The finding showed that when "you bring a dog into your house, you are not just bringing a dog, you are also introducing a suite of dog-associated taxa directly into your home environment, some of which may have direct or indirect effects on human health" (Dunn et al. 2013). Not all of these effects, they stress, involve infectious disease, as several studies suggest that pregnant women who live in houses with dogs are less likely to give birth to children who develop allergies or *atopic dermatitis* (e.g., Aichbhaumik et al. 2008). One product of recent research on pathogens in the home, although not reflective of zoonotic transmission, involves the frequent presence of the fungal pathogens *Exophiala dermatitidis* and *Exophiala phaeomuriformis* living on rubber molding in dishwashers, despite the high temperatures, high moisture, and alkaline pH values found therein (Zalar et al. 2011). Both of these fungi are linked to serious systemic disease in humans.

In the United States the most common parasitic zoonotic infections of humans associated with dogs are caused by *hookworms* (*Ancylostoma spp.*) and *roundworms* (*Toxocara canis*). A CDC study found that about 14 percent of the US population is infected with roundworms, leading to a zoonotic infection called *toxocariasis* (Won et al. 2008). This condition is most common among African American children as well as in people in lower socioeconomic groups. The mode of transmission occurs when humans come into contact with sand or soil that is contaminated with infected roundworm eggs and larvae from dog or cat waste. In most individuals who are infected, symptoms are minimal, but in some people who develop a high number of roundworm larva or have repeated infections, symptoms can include fever, coughing, enlarged liver, and pneumonia. Although it rarely occurs, human roundworm infections can cause blindness.

Overall, more than one hundred known zoonotic diseases have been identified as coming from domesticated pets. At the same time there is little doubt that relationships with pets often improve human health and a sense of well-being, and the therapeutic aspects of such relationships are well established (an issue also of concern to the One Health initiative). Some dogs, for example, have been found to be able to anticipate and alert family members to seizure onset in epileptic children (Kirton et al. 2004).

Beyond the bedroom, offices, where millions of people around the world now spend long hours of their day, are another site of pathogen contact. Bringing pets to the office or transporting pathogens picked up from pets at home are the primary ways zoonotics wind up in offices. Employees working in crowded office buildings commonly share workstations, computers, chairs, restrooms, tables and countertops, and public areas that have been found to contain a wide spectrum of microbes. In a study carried out in thirty different offices in three US cities (Tucson, New York, and San Francisco) of five shared surface areas, Krissi Hewitt and coworkers (2012) found significant differences in the abundance of bacteria between offices most populated by men and women, among the various surface types that were tested, and among the three test cities. More than five hundred different bacterial genera were identified. Most abundant were bacteria that are common inhabitants of human skin and nasal, oral, or intestinal cavities. Other commonly occurring genera in their samples appeared to have environmental origins, such as soils. The bacterial array of the Tucson samples was distinct from those from New York and San Francisco, which were indistinguishable. Overall, these researchers' analysis affirms that "humans move through a sea of microbial life that is seldom perceived except in the context of potential disease and decay" (Feazel et al. 2009).

In addition to surface-dwelling species *air-borne pathogens* are well adapted for spreading in indoor environments like offices. Conditions that are maintained in offices to increase human comfort—protection from sunlight, controlled temperature, regulated humidity levels—can foster pathogen survival during their exposed and vulnerable transmission from one person to the next. Most air-borne pathogens die in outdoor air, but indoors they can rely on help from humans to create an environment that fosters propagation. It is estimated, for example, that one-third of so-called common colds—infections of the upper respiratory tract caused by over two hundred different viruses—are contracted in office settings. Many infectious diseases, such as those caused by norovirus and influenza viruses, frequently spread person-to-person in indoor environments. *Norovirus,* a major cause of gastroenteritis in hospitals around the world, can lead to short-term ward closures and staffing shortages. Air-borne routes also spread tuberculosis. The infectious agent is invisible to the naked eye, being just one to five microns in size (a micron is about one-hundredth the width of a human hair). Exhaled by an infected individual, the pathogen can remain air-borne in room air for a long period of time. Computer simulation models have shown that placing an individual with a highly infectious case of tuberculosis on the first floor of an average ten-story building will, over an eight-hour period, cause a person on the tenth floor to have accumulated enough exposure to have a 33 percent risk of contracting tuberculosis (Department of Aerobiological Engineering 1998).

Many other human cultural practices facilitate the zoonotic transmission of infectious diseases from animals to humans. One notable illustration involves the dog-keeping practices of the Turkana people of northwest Kenya and neighboring Dassanetch and Nyangatom peoples in southwestern Ethiopia. In these societies, which inhabit an arid environment in which water is scarce, women use nurse dogs to lick and clean the rear ends of small children who have defecated. Dogs also are encouraged to lick clean cooking- and serving-ware in households. As a result of this cultural hygienic practice, hydatid disease, a potentially lethal parasitic infection immediately caused by the larval stages of several different tapeworm species, is spread from dogs to humans (Fuller and Fuller 1981). Dogs, in turn, are infected by their contact with herd animals like sheep and camels, including the ingestion of infected animals that have died. Having gained access to human hosts by way of infected dogs, the pathogen that immediately causes hydatid disease breaks free of its protective outer shell, penetrates through the intestinal wall, and makes its way to a body organ. The Turkana and neighboring peoples are highly infected with hydatid—7 to 10 percent of people and as many as 65 percent of their dogs test positive—but culturally they do not associate infection with associated symptoms, including cysts of the liver (abdominal pain), lungs (causing coughing and shortness of breath), and other body systems, with an infectious disease spread by dogs or the hydatid cysts they witness in their livestock (Magambo, Njoroge, and Zeyhle 2006). Like modern office workers who do not think that the built environment of the office is a place of risk, or people in the United States and Europe who bring their dogs and cats to bed with them, the Turkana do not view their socially quite useful dogs as vectors of disease.

THE ORIGIN OF AIDS AS A ZOONOTIC DISEASE

Following many years of debate about the origin of HIV infection as a human disease, the historic facts are now becoming clear. The evidence supports the importance of a biosocial/bicultural understanding of this major infectious disease. Genetic and other research indicates that although HIV first came to human attention in the late twentieth century, the disease is far older and can be traced back at least to the early 1900s. The disease began when SIV (simian immunodeficiency virus), a viral ancestor of HIV found in chimpanzees (*SIVcpz*), made the zoonotic jump to humans. Researchers believe that ancestors of this virus had an earlier origin in monkey species and then spread to chimpanzees, most notably the chimpanzee subspecies *P. t. troglodytes,* through predation on monkey species like red-capped mangabeys. Based on the development of an innovative, noninvasive screening technique for testing fecal samples of wild chimpanzees for SIV antibodies, researchers were able to establish "that chimpanzees are indeed the natural reservoir of SIVcpz and the source of HIV-1" (Sharp and Hahn 2010:2490).

The number of different SIVs that have been identified has expanded rapidly over the past twenty years and are now known to infect approximately forty primate species from sub-Saharan Africa. Although many of these SIV species are nonpathogenic in their primary host, extensive research with two communities of chimpanzees in Gombe National Park in Tanzania found that SIV infection was associated with a ten- to sixteen-fold increase in risk of chimpanzee death. The studies also revealed that fertility was significantly reduced in SIV-positive chimpanzee females, including both lowered birth rates and reduced survival of their young (Santiago et al. 2003). In light of the discussion of the stages of zoonotic transition, this research suggests a movement of the viral line that developed into HIV-1 as follows: monkey species SIV (nonpathogenic to host) →chimpanzee infection and adaptation of the virus to replicate efficiently in the new host (pathogenic)→human infection and further adaptation to the human host (pathogenic) and human-to-human transmission. Notably, because of the genetic similarities of chimpanzees and humans, adaptation of SIV to the chimpanzee body environment may have facilitated a subsequent jump to humans. In this multistage, multispecies adaptive history, as Sharp and Hahn (2010:2492) suggest, "It will be of particular interest to understand the extent to which co-infection with other viruses, bacteria, protozoa (such as Plasmodium) or multicellular eukaryotes (e.g., worms) influence[d] the course of SIVcpz infection and pathogenesis." As discussed in Chapter 6, this kind of syndemic interaction among pathogens is increasingly proving to play a critical role in the evolutionary history of infectious diseases.

Available evidence supports the conclusion that the disease that many years later would come to be known as AIDS moved from chimpanzee to human populations sometime between 1884 and 1924, at about the same time that urbanization was expanding in west central Africa (Worobey et al. 2008). Urbanization of colonial Africa created the conditions that allowed HIV-1, the form of the virus that sparked a global pandemic, to spread rapidly among humans; namely, the development of densely settled populations composed of high percentages of sexually active young adults (see Figure 3.2). This location for the origin of HIV-1 is supported by findings showing that it is the only region where all three of the subgroups of HIV-1 (known as M, N, and O) are found. HIV-2, a less pathogenic variety than HIV-1, very likely jumped to humans from Sooty Mangabey monkeys early in the twentieth century. More recently a new type of HIV was discovered in Cameroon, and it appears to have evolved from *SIVgorilla*.

One model of interspecies pathogen transmission has been labeled the *Hunter Theory*. In this model SIVcpz was transferred to humans when humans stalked, killed, butchered, and ate chimps (a food source called "bush meat") or when chimp blood got into cuts or wounds on the hunter. Hunting of monkeys and apes for human food is common in most areas where nonhuman primate species are found. Normally the hunter's immune system would have successfully eliminated SIV, but mutations appear to have enabled SIV to transition to the new human host and became the new species HIV-1. Given the high mutation rate of this RNA virus and growing human penetration of forested areas in Africa facilitated by extensive logging, this transition is not surprising. In research in rural Cameroon Wolfe and colleagues (2004a) found that, although the Cameroon government forbids the hunting of wild animals, it is widely accepted and permitted for personal

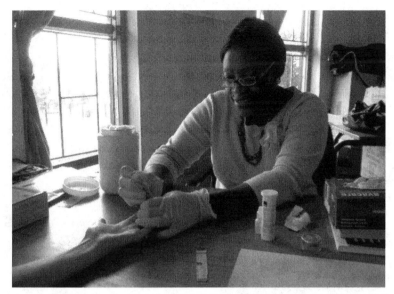

Figure 3.2   HIV testing in Lesotho in Southern Africa. (Photo by Nicola Bulled)

consumption. They demonstrated that retroviral transfer from primates to hunters is continuing (Wolfe et al. 2004b). In a sample of about a thousand people in Cameroon they found that 1 percent were infected with *Simian Foamy virus* (SFV), a disease that previously was thought to only infect primates but now appears to have made an initial jump to humans.

In addition to the sociocultural factors implicated in the origin of HIV, including hunting, urbanization, and sexual practices, a set of political economic forces was also important. During the late nineteenth and early twentieth centuries European colonial regimes ruled much of Africa. In some areas, such as French Equatorial Africa and the Belgian Congo, colonial domination was particularly severe, and many Africans were forced into labor camps where sanitation was poor, food scarce, and physical demands punishing. These conditions were sufficient to lower the efficacy of people's immune systems, facilitating the ability of SIV to penetrate the human immune system and human biochemistry and evolve into HIV (see Figure 3.3). In their heated race for wealth and power, the colonialists cut trails into dense forests that previously had few human intruders. To achieve this feat, thousands of Africans were forced into service clearing roads and as porters carrying extracted resources like elephant tusks. One of these colonial roads led directly to the area researchers have identified as the likely place humans were first exposed to SIV. The near-slavery condition African workers faced may have contributed to the search for wild sources of food, including bush meat, to

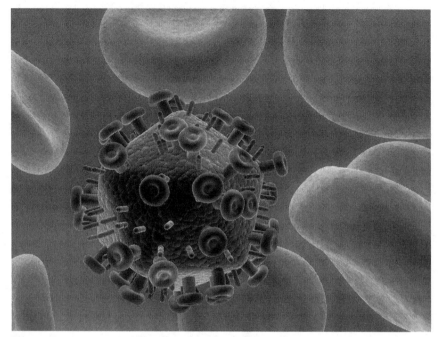

Figure 3.3 Human Immunodeficiency Virus. (Photo by Sebastian Kaulitzki)

supplement what meager food colonial bosses offered. In short, although HIV had its origin in Africa, its emergence as a global pandemic would not have occurred without the colonial restructuring of human/environmental relations European colonists in Africa initiated (Timberg and Halperin 2012).

Other social forces have more recently expanded the hunt for bush meat, including expanding populations and the demand for food, logging, and mining activities that also have increased access to deeper forest areas as well as the depletion of Atlantic fish stocks off the coast of West Africa by European super-trawling ships that has forced people to find other sources of protein. These developments are significant from the standpoint of infectious diseases because there are other primate viruses that can and have begun to make the jump to humans.

THE BIOSOCIAL/BIOCULTURAL HISTORY OF LYME DISEASE AND THE INTRICACIES OF LYME DISEASE ECOLOGY

The origin of *Lyme disease* as a specific, named infectious threat to human health dates to the mid-1970s, when several American researchers recognized a cluster of cases of arthritis in and around Lyme, Connecticut. Subsequent researchers determined that these cases were a symptomatic expression of an infection by a new pathogenic agent transmitted by tick bites. Contrary to our image of how medical science works, social science investigation of the discovery and description of the cause and nature of this new infectious disease shows that it was not achieved through the direct and systematic unveiling through rigorous biomedical research of a given set of biological and epidemiological facts; rather, it involved the social construction of a categorically new disease involving a number of interacting factors.

The first cases of what would eventually be called Lyme disease in the United States and, ultimately, worldwide attracted medical attention because of the actions of two people from the Lyme, Connecticut, area. One, a woman named Polly Murray, had been sick since the 1960s with intermittent symptoms, including rashes, swollen knees, stiff joints, and sore throat. She reported in her book *The Widening Circle* (Murray 1996) that she had consulted over twenty-five physicians without getting a satisfactory explanation or relief from her symptoms. Alarmed by the appearance of similar symptoms in her sons and neighbors, Murray called a state public health official in the fall of 1975 and was referred to Allen Steere, a Yale rheumatologist-in-training. That Steere was already studying diseases like arthritis was probably critical to the subsequent turn of events.

At about the same time another women, Judith Mensch, contacted state health authorities and the CDC seeking an explanation for why her daughter as well as other children in her neighborhood were being diagnosed with juvenile rheumatoid arthritis, a rare and sporadic affliction. She too was referred to Allen Steere. Intrigued by these cases, Steere, other Yale researchers, and a Connecticut public health official conducted a survey with parents, physicians, and school nurses in and around the town of Lyme and identified a group of about fifty children and a few adults who suffered from inflammatory joint disease. About one-fourth of these individuals also reported having an unusual skin rash. Given epidemiological experience, the high prevalence within the same time and geographic zone and within certain families suggested the possibility of an infectious disease.

Steere discussed these cases with a Yale dermatologist who had treated a number of rash cases the previous summer in nearby Groton, Connecticut. The following year a patient with the same kind of rash presented with the tick that bit him. Because of an explosion in the number of ticks that were being reported in and around the town of Lyme over the previous decade, Yale entomologists initiated a tick survey. They found a dramatically greater number of ticks in the area of the identified cases compared to a nearby area without cases. Ticks, in fact, transmit numerous human diseases (see Table 3.1). One such disease

Table 3.1 Tickborne Diseases of the U.S.

Tick vectors	Diseases transmitted to human
Blacklegged tick (*Ixodes scapularis*)	Anaplasmosis
Blacklegged tick (*Ixodes scapularis*)	Babesiosis
Lone star tick (*Ambylomma americanum*)	Ehrlichiosis
Blacklegged tick (*Ixodes scapularis*)	Lyme disease
Gulf Coast tick (*Amblyomma maculatum*)	Ricketsiosis
American dog tick (*Dermacentor variabilis*), Rocky Mountain wood tick (*Dermacentor andersoni*), and Brown dog tick (*Rhipicephalus sangunineus*)	Rocky Mountain Spotted Fever
Lone star tick (Ambylomma americanum)	Southern Tick-Associated Rash Illness
Relapsing fever tick	Tickborne Relapsing Fever
American dog tick (*Dermacentor variabilis*), Wood tick (*Dermacentor andersoni*), and Lone star tick (*Amblyomma americanum*)	Tularemia

even disables the body's ability to tolerate consumption of red meat and pork. Exposure to tick saliva—which contains proteins that enable the tick to prolong attachment to a host and successfully feed—appears to cause an allergic reaction to a carbohydrate called alpha-gal found in meat. This reaction, which may have evolved as part of the body's effort to reduce tick attachment, includes the release of histamine and resulting symptoms, such as swelling, hives, and breathing problems. There are a growing number of individuals with this allergy around the world (Commins and Platts-Mills 2013).

The identification of the Lyme spirochete pathogen was made by Willy Burgdorfer, a zoologist and microbiologist, and collaborators who were studying a different tick pathogen. Unexpectedly, they noticed microfilaria (small worms) in two ticks and decided to dissect the ticks' digestive tracts to find additional specimens. Instead, they found spirochetes living there. Subsequently, the same spirochete was found in patients reporting the symptoms that would eventually be termed Lyme disease. In their first scholarly report, however, the Yale investigators named the "new" disease Lyme arthritis and asserted that it was a "previously unrecognized condition" (Steere et al. 1977). Ultimately these US cases were linked to European cases that had been identified as much as six decades earlier (Farmer 1996) and named after the now widely known characteristic "bull's eye" skin rash. It was also recognized that arthritis was only one of several symptoms and one that did not occur in all patients. Given the standards of scientific labeling, at this point, the name of the disease should have been changed to reflect the infectious agent or the earlier European label of neuroborreliosis. Instead, Lyme arthritis was changed to Lyme disease as the enduring name of the condition, fixing the importance of the US/Yale investigators' contributions and emphasizing the newness of the disease. Thus, a typical scholarly publication on Lyme disease in the United States today begins, "Lyme disease, first described in 1976." As the physician-anthropologist Paul Farmer (1996:259) notes, however, "Neuroborreliosis was studied long before the moniker Lyme disease [was] coined, and before suburban reforestation and golf courses complicated the equation by creating an environment agreeable to both ticks and affluent humans." In fact, at a 1909 research conference Swedish dermatologist Arvid Afzelius presented a study of an expanding, ring-like rash, which he named erythema migrans, that he observed in an older woman after a tick bite.

What occurred in the mid-1970s in Connecticut was a clustering of infections in a localized area in a population that was socially empowered to motivate state and researcher attention. What US research "discovered" appears to have been a disease that was already known with somewhat different symptoms in Europe. It came to attention in the United States for social as much as for biological or medical reasons. Robert Aronowitz (1991) has argued that recognition of the mid-1970s cases along the Connecticut shoreline was in no small part a consequence of the fact that a symptom like arthritis, associated with older people, was being seen in children. Among adults, in whom inflammatory arthritis is much less unusual, cases did not stand out as representing a new disease. An additional reason the historical recognition of Lyme disease unfolded as it did is that there was skepticism among US researchers about the European evidence and of the findings of researchers from a different discipline (nonrheumatoid researchers).

Nonetheless, genetic research at the University of Bath in the United Kingdom by a team headed by Klaus Kutenbach (Margos et al. 2008) suggests that the Borrelia bacterium evolved initially in Europe and spread to North America aboard ticks on migrating mammals prior to the arrival of humans in the New World. There are early historic accounts of ticks annoying explorers and colonists in forests in the Northeast, suggesting that the conditions ripe for *B. burgdorferi* transmission in this region developed hundreds of years ago. Other social factors and changing socioeconomic patterns also were important, including the process by which preferred middle-class housing led to the conversion of rural farmland into a suburban landscape, increasing woodland and populations of deer that carry ticks. These changes pushed Lyme along the path to becoming the most frequent vector-borne disease in North America. Of historic note, Native Americans living in the Northeast forests prior to European arrival had already recognized that by using fire to control forest growth and creating meadows, deer populations increased and were easier to hunt. Deer very likely passed along tick infections to Native American communities prior to the arrival of European invaders.

The presence of ticks in the Northeast was confirmed in the mid-eighteenth century by Pehr Kalm (1773), a Swedish botanist who was sent to America by Carl Linnaeus, the Swedish botanist, physician, and zoologist who began the development of the binomial nomenclature now common in scientific naming (e.g., *Escherichia coli*). Kalm found that New York forests "abound" with ticks when he visited in 1749. After the arrival of Europeans there was considerable deforestation of much of the Northeast as farms were created during the eighteenth and nineteenth centuries, resulting in the near elimination of white-tailed deer (and forest-dwelling white-footed mice) and presumably also of ticks such as the black-legged tick. With the industrial revolution, however, farms were abandoned, forests grew back over farmed land, and the deer and mice returned—and so too did the ticks. Notably the *erythema migrans* rash, the hallmark of B. burgdorferi infection, was already being described in midwestern and Pacific states at the time Lyme disease was first "described" in Connecticut.

"If an acorn falls in the forest, will you contract Lyme disease?" This curious query appeared in a story reporting the findings of a study by Richard Ostfeld of the Cary Institute of Ecosystem Studies showing a statistical relationship between the bountifulness of forest acorn production in autumn and rates of nearby human Lyme disease. As it happens, oak trees drop few or no acorns in most years. This is thought to be an adaptation that makes acorns an unreliable food source and thus prevents mice and chipmunks populations from concentrating around oaks. As a result, not all of an oak's acorns are eaten, and thus, some can germinate when they do fall. This process is called predator satiation, safety in numbers. Mice especially like acorns because they are so big, offering plenty of food. Acorns, in turn, are so big because of an adaptation to forested areas with thick layers of leaf litter on top of the soil. Big acorns provide a lot of energy for a seedling, whose tap root must penetrate the hindering leaf litter to reach the soil below. The years that oak trees produce a bumper acorn crop in the autumn are known as mast years, from the Old English word for the nuts of forest trees that have accumulated on the ground. Ostfeld's study found that autumns in which forests produced a lot of acorns were followed the next summer by high mice populations.

High numbers of mice represent an increase in the number of hosts for ticks, including infected ticks; other research shows that 90 percent of ticks that feed on mice in some areas are infected with Lyme disease (Ostfeld 2011). Ticks are dormant for almost a year after feeding on mice and then resume feeding on new hosts, including on humans. As a result, there is more Lyme disease among nearby humans two years after a high acorn year. Notably, the size of deer populations in the area was not found to be predictive of more Lyme.

And then there is the issue of the role of Japanese Barberry. This hardy semideciduous shrub (specifically *Borrelia thunbergii*) was introduced into the United

States from Europe in 1875 because it was seen as attractive (a cultural value), required little care (a cultural preference), and was resistant to deer (a cultural ideal for the suburban gardener); moreover, it grows well in abandoned farm areas that have reverted to forest. The berries are edible and used in herbal medicines. By the 1980s, however, it has come to be seen as an invasive species because it pushes out native species. Barberry is important to the story of Lyme disease because it creates a perfect, humid environment on the ground for the growth of mice and tick populations. According to Jeffrey Ward of the Department of Forestry and Horticulture at the Connecticut Agricultural Experiment Station in New Haven, "When we measure the presence of ticks carrying the Lyme spirochete (*Borrelia burgdorferi*) we find 120 infected ticks where Barberry is not contained [i.e., not under control], 40 ticks per acre where Barberry is contained, and only 10 infected ticks where there is no Barberry" (quoted in Foran 2012). So humans' intentional introduction for cultural reasons of a now-invasive—if decorative—plant also is contributing to the prevalence of Lyme disease.

Another human impact that promotes Lyme disease is forest fragmentation. This occurs when large, continuous forests are divided into smaller patches, for example because of road construction, clearing for agriculture, urbanization, or other human development. White-footed mice are more abundant in forest fragments in some parts of the country, probably because fewer predators like coyotes and foxes and competitors like rabbits remain there. The mice are particularly abundant in land segments that are smaller than about five acres. Research by Ostfeld and coworkers found that forest patches smaller than three acres have an average of three times as many ticks as do larger fragments and seven times more infected ticks (Allan, Keesing, and Ostfeld 2003). As many as 80 percent of the ticks in the smallest patches are infected, the highest rate these scientists have seen.

In sum, Lyme disease was as much constructed through complex social and historic processes and behaviors as through scientific biomedical discovery of a previously unknown disease. This "discovery" of a disease that was both around for a long time and already known by a different name in Europe occurred because of changing social/residential conditions, environmental conditions, medical career issues, the politics of science, and professional disciplinary attitudes.

In fact, the oldest known case of Lyme disease was the Tyrolean Iceman, a 5,300-year-old Copper Age mummified individual, discovered in 1991 on the Tisenjoch Pass in the Italian part of the Ötztal Alps. Genetic sequencing of the Iceman identified 60 percent of the genome of *Borrelia burgdorferi*. Robert Aronowitz argues (1991:101), "Lyme disease embodies and reflects aspects of our current and past beliefs about sickness and how these beliefs, rather than being marginal influences on a fundamental biological reality, have shaped almost every aspect of medical practice and lay response."

The case of Lyme further affirms the degree to which infectious disease epidemics are as much cultural constructions and products of social structures as they are biological processes. This is further affirmed by looking at the Lyme disease controversy. Public health is rarely a strictly medical issue; it is, for multiple reasons, customarily a political issue as well. In the case of Lyme disease there has been considerable debate about what has been called "chronic Lyme disease," including whether such a thing exists and, if so, how prevalent it is, what are the criteria for diagnosing it, and what is the appropriate treatment. In chronic Lyme disease diverse symptoms are said to persist despite antibiotic treatment. The mainstream medical perspective, held by the CDC, the Infectious Diseases Society of America, the American Academy of Neurology, and the National Institutes of Health is that the existence of chronic Lyme disease is not supported by convincing scientific evidence. Others, especially those who believe they suffer from the disease, sharply and vocally disagree.

Debate continues over whether Lyme disease is an acute, treatable, minor disorder or a chronic, serious, widespread, poorly treated infectious threat to public health (Murray 1996). Caught in the controversy, Allen Steere (the Yale rheumatologist who investigated the Connecticut cases) at one point had to hire security guards for public appearances because he feared the wrath of angered individuals who claimed they had chronic Lyme disease that was not responsive to simple antibiotic treatment but were being shunned by biomedicine (Grann 2001). Left untreated, there is no debate that Lyme disease can cause significant problems in the joints, heart, and central nervous system. Still in dispute is the effectiveness of short-term antibiotic treatment.

Adding to this discussion, anthropologist Mark Macauda and colleagues (2011) stress the importance of doctor-patient communication in the treatment of Lyme disease, beginning with physician understanding of how patients perceive the disease. Using interviews and surveys with approximately four hundred participants in Rhode Island and Connecticut, where the disease is highly endemic, these researchers examined public perceptions of Lyme disease. They found people to be generally knowledgeable about the disease but tended, going against the dominant medical view, to believe both that Lyme disease symptoms and that the spirochete that is the immediate cause of the disease can persist after a patient has received antimicrobial treatment. When these researchers asked their study participants about the value of continuing antibiotic treatment for more than two months, about half of them thought that it was sometimes useful, whereas about a quarter believed that it was always useful. Notably, almost all reported that they had either been diagnosed themselves with Lyme disease (about 25 percent of participants) or that they knew someone who had experienced Lyme disease, and these personal experiences and interactions were more often referred to as a more important source of Lyme disease understanding than information from medical professionals. Macauda and colleagues also show that the concept of chronic Lyme disease entered into the public discourse by way of media reports, influenced the policy arena (several states passed legislation to legally protect doctors who provide long-term antibiotic treatment), and generated conflict in civil society. They assert that popular "opinion can alter how [a] disease is treated, both at the population level through legislation, and at the individual level in the doctor's office" (Macauda et al. 2011:861).

The case of Lyme disease clearly demonstrates the critical value of a "more than human" perspective that includes other mammalian species, ticks, pathogens, and even plant species in understanding human infectious disease.

CASE STUDY: NIPAH AND FLYING FOXES

During 1998–1999 a significant outbreak of encephalitis and respiratory illness occurred in Malaysia. Epidemiologic investigation identified the immediate cause to be a previously unknown virus. The new pathogen was given the name Nipah virus after the area in Malaysia in which it was first discovered. During the initial wave 265 people were diagnosed; 40 percent of them died. Almost all of the victims were found to be directly involved in the raising or butchering of pigs.

This finding sparked an effort to control the infection through a government-mandated slaughter of massive numbers of pigs, causing considerable economic loss for small farmers. Subsequently a small epidemic developed in Singapore in which eleven individuals who handled pigs imported from Malaysia fell ill, one of whom died. Outbreaks also have occurred in Bangladesh and neighboring parts of India. Ultimately, it was determined that the Nipah virus was related to another pathogen that caused several outbreaks in Australia, where it was at first called the equine morbillivirus and later labeled the Hendra virus after the town where it first appeared. Both the *Nipah and Hendra* were determined to be members of the Paramyxoviridae family of viruses, a name derived from the Greek words for "beyond slime." Other members of this family include the measles virus, mumps virus, and respiratory syncytial virus.

Researchers believe that certain species of "flying foxes" (pteropid fruit bats) are the natural hosts of both the Nipah and Hendra viruses. Bats and flying foxes, members of the order Chiroptera (which means "hand wing"), are among the most abundant, diverse, and geographically disperse vertebrates. A considerable number of viruses have been detected in bats, most of which are not known to be transmitted to humans; however, bats are reservoir hosts for a number of infectious agents found in humans, including the rabies virus and related *lyssaviruses* (Calisher et al. 2006).

Flying foxes are found across a wide area encompassing parts of Australia, Indonesia, Malaysia, the Philippines, and some of the Pacific Islands. Research by Kaw Bing Chua and colleagues (2003) found that industrial planation development and pulpwood extraction have caused decreases in the availability of flowering and fruiting forest trees that fruit bats use for foraging. In Malaysia the World Bank estimates that trees are being cut down at four times the sustainable rate. Bats also were driven from their traditional habitats by the dense smoke of fires set to clear forested areas for developing cash-crop plantations. In response, the bats began to encroach into cultivated fruit orchards, bringing with them the Nipah virus. At the same time, farmers were moving pigpens into orchards to take advantage of available space. Fruit bats, which are highly social animals that roost in family groups on branches, routinely dropped partially eaten fruit into the pig sties below and their excreta into feeding troughs, which pigs consumed, leading to their infection. Existing evidence "suggested that climatic and anthropogenic driven ecological changes coupled with the location of piggeries in orchards allowed the spill-over of this novel *paramyxovirus* from its reservoir host into the domestic pigs and ultimately to humans and other animals" (Chua et al. 2002:265). In Bangladesh, anthropological research revealed that other human behaviors, such as drinking fresh date palm sap from clay collector pots set in palm trees led to human infection because bats were visiting and drinking from the pots (Luby et al. 2006). Flying foxes also were identified as the source of transmission of Hendra to humans.

In the case of Hendra, in 1994 an outbreak of an acute respiratory illness in humans and horses took place in Australia in a suburb of Brisbane called Hendra. Small outbreaks over several subsequent years followed. By the end of 2012 a total of thirty-nine outbreaks of Hendra virus had occurred in Australia, all involving infection of horses. The virus found to be the infectious agent was scientifically placed in the same genus as Nipah.

As this description suggests, the encephalitis outbreak first seen in Malaysia toward the end of the twentieth century was dependent on complex interactions of multiple species, including humans, fruit bats, pigs, fruiting trees, and the Nipah virus. Similarly, fruit bats, horses, humans, and Hendra virus interactions produced acute respiratory disease in Australia. Just as our bodies contain more than human cells, our health is dependent on many other species, large and visible as well as microscopically small and outside of our unaided ability to see; yet all of these life forms are interacting and changing their patterns of interaction in consequential ways. These interactions are essential to the making of human health and disease. Moreover, as we have seen, crucial interactions occur not only at the biological level but also at biocultural and biosocial interfaces.

CONCLUSION: HEALTH AND THE CO-EVOLUTION OF SPECIES

This chapter locates human infectious diseases and infectious disease impacts on human communities within a holistic, nonanthropocentric, and co-evolutionary perspective. Although the ultimate concern of the anthropology of infectious diseases is human health, a traditionally narrow focus only on humans—divorced from an appreciation of humans as interlocked in a complex and dynamic web of species relations through time and place—considerably limits understanding and effective response to infectious diseases.

Why is it important to know the zoonotic origin of HIV disease, for example? In part, having an objective understanding of where the disease came from is useful in countering moralistic, nationalistic, sexist, homophobic, and other stigmatizing and blame-pointing cultural misinterpretations of the nature of this impactful disease. The origin of HIV appears to lie in the blameless search for food among people hard pressed by the disruptions and coercions of colonialism and its enduring legacy. Additionally, such understanding has led to the search for and successful discovery of other primate diseases in the process of transitioning to human diseases. Beatrice Hahn, who led the research team that discovered the chimpanzee origin of HIV, has commented, "The fact that it could be with us for quite a long time before we even realized it was there is kind of eye-opening.... I think it's something to keep us on our toes. It helps us understand that we can be surprised" (quoted in Carmichael 2006). Finally, knowledge of where the virus originated and how it evolved could be crucial in developing a broad-spectrum vaccine and more effective treatments against HIV disease with fewer side effects.

Beyond HIV and other human infectious diseases, it is evident that our lives are codetermined by animal and even plant pathogens as they influence our food supply or other environmental resources. The directionality of effect flows both ways; our diseases jump to animal species and our actions in the world contribute powerfully to the spread and virulence of infectious diseases.

DISCUSSION QUESTIONS

1. What are some of the ways in which our manipulation of the environment is coming back to harm us in the form of new zoonotic diseases?
2. What does the case of Lyme disease teach us about biosocial/biocultural understanding?
3. To protect ourselves from new viral infections, should we exterminate species like bats that are important vectors?

4. How did biology, culture, and social structure work together to create the global HIV pandemic?
5. Why does learning the evolutionary origin of a pathogen matter?

CHAPTER 4

Environmental Disruption, Pluralea Interactions, and Infectious Diseases

> Beginning with the invisible releases of radiation, and the toxic pollut-
> ants like DDT, and then the by-products of large-scale industrialization
> like acid rain ... we began to alter even those places where we were
> not. ... The by-products—the pollutants of one species have become
> the most powerful force for change on the planet.
>
> *Bill McKibben (2006:xix)*

AGENTS AND OBJECTS OF CHANGE

Changes in the broader relationships between humans and the physical environment are reconfiguring our relationships with pathogens. The ways we
are restructuring Earth are contributing to the appearance or diffusion of new
infectious diseases or the movement of older diseases to new areas. We are
reshaping the planet's surface in countless ways, from mountain-top removal
to deforestation; depleting ocean species; penetrating environmental zones
previously free of human presence; increasing pressure on local resources; creating diverse forms of environmental degradation and simplification; promoting
greater frequencies of novel interactions with animal species around us; and
inducing shifts in climate. As contrasted with a century ago, "The world is a different place—more chaotic, storm tossed, disease ridden" (McKibben 2006:xiv).

This chapter examines the issue of *environmentally mediated infectious disease*,
especially as a result of human activity in the world, with special emphasis on the
adverse interaction of multiple human-influenced environmental changes on pathogen pollution, the spread to new areas, and increased impact of infectious diseases.
The chapter stresses the lesson that, because of biosocial and biocultural dynamics,
human beings are "not simply agents of environmental change" but, by causing
the spread of infectious diseases, "are also objects of that change" (Nash 2006:7).

ENVIRONMENTAL SHAPING OF INFECTIOUS DISEASE

A growing body of research affirms that environmental change significantly
influences emerging and reemerging agents of infectious disease (McMichael

and Martens 2002). Joseph Eisenberg and coworkers (2007) have proposed a framework for tracking the relationship between environmental changes and infectious disease transmission. Their approach brings together three features of environment/infectious disease relationships, which will be discussed in turn:

1. Environmental change is manifest in a complex web of ecological and social factors that help to shape the landscape of infectious disease.
2. The transmission dynamics of pathogenic agents mediate the effects environmental changes have on infectious disease impact.
3. Infectious disease burden in a population—determined by the incidence and severity of infection—is a product of the interplay between environmental change—including changes wrought by human activity—and the transmission cycle or route of transmission of a pathogen.

First, Eisenberg and colleagues point out, "There has been a tendency to delineate environmental changes into those that are social, such as urbanization, and those that are ecologic, such as deforestation, but in actuality any process affecting human health has both social and ecologic components that are inextricably linked" (2007, 1220). In other words, it is impossible to fully disentangle the natural and the "unnatural" (or human-influenced) features and characteristics of the environment. Thus, "climate change may impact the characteristics of El Niño, roads may contribute to urbanization, deforestation may amplify climate change, and the impacts of natural disasters might be augmented by anthropogenic changes such as loss of wetlands" (Eisenberg et al. 2007, 1220). Similarly a new road can lead to shifts in population that affect the spread of sexually transmitted diseases, whereas deforestation and the building of a dam may affect the breeding habits of disease-bearing mosquitoes that leads to increased incidence of malaria.

Second, environmental factors can impact the rate of infectious disease transmission by modifying population levels of hosts, vectors, and pathogens (e.g., new roads and urbanization that result in increased human concentration) or by changing the life conditions of hosts, vectors, and pathogens (e.g., rising temperatures, drought, storms). The nature of these impacts, however, is different across the various *transmission dynamics* of pathogenic agents, namely direct human-to-human transmission (e.g., HIV infection), vector-borne transmission (e.g., Chagas disease), environmental contact transmission (e.g., food-borne infectious diseases like listeria), and zoonotic transmission in which human-to-human diffusion does not occur and infection is dependent on animal reservoirs (e.g., Lyme disease). Environmental changes that affect animal species that serve as reservoirs (e.g., the return of deer to now suburban areas of the US northeast) influence the spread of Lyme disease, for example, but have no impact on the spread of HIV infection or on food-borne infections. Similarly, rapid global travel that allows the movement of people around the planet facilitated the spread of HIV disease but had no comparable effect on the spread of malaria.

Finally, the infectious disease burden in a population is a product of interaction between environmental change and the transmission cycle of pathogens. A case in point is rotavirus, which is estimated to cause four hundred thousand to seven hundred thousand deaths in children around the world every year (Parashar et al. 2003). Rotavirus is transmitted from an infected person's body into the environment in feces. The virus spreads by what is known as "the fecal-oral route," which means that the virus must be shed by a person who is infected and then enter another person through their mouth. Often this occurs through the infection of drinking water sources. Rotavirus is a threat to children because it produces gastroenteritis and diarrheal disease, which cause dehydration. Although the virus is found worldwide, in both developed and developing countries alike, and by age five almost all children in the world will have at least one episode of retrovirus gastroenteritis, the health burden of this disease is not equally distributed socioeconomically. As Umesh Parashar and colleagues (2003:569) observe,

> The incidence of rotavirus disease is similar in children in both developed and developing nations. However, children in developing nations die more frequently, possibly because of several factors, including poorer access to hydration therapy and a greater prevalence of malnutrition. An estimated 1,205 children die from rotavirus disease each day, and 82 percent of these deaths occur in children in the poorest countries.

In developed countries, changes in the environment (improved sanitation, access to health care) have had far greater impact on lowering the burden of the disease associated with rotavirus infection than has occurred in developing nations. As this framework underlines, understanding infectious disease requires examining social, cultural, environmental, and biological factors in tandem.

GOING TO DISEASE: HUMAN PENETRATION OF INFECTED ZONES

We know that forests, especially tropical forests, constitute natural reservoirs of diverse species, including potentially pathogenic microbial species. The high temperatures and considerable rainfall in these lush environments promote this diversity of species and the existence of insect vectors that can transmit diseases. It is possible as well that warmer temperatures support the replication of pathogenic agents both inside and outside of other organisms. Human penetration of tropical rainforests, historically and more recently—including efforts aimed at logging and deforestation, extraction of other forest resources, clearing for settlement, clearing for corn fields for the production of biofuels, mining, and increased international tourism in tropical regions—has led to the leakage of tropic infectious zoonotics into nontropical human populations and, in cases such as HIV disease (see Chapter 3), even to lethal global pandemics (Wolfe et al. 2000).

Deforestation can also influence diseases carried by certain snails. As with mosquitoes, deforestation alters snail diversity in forests because few snail species are able to adapt to the new, deforested conditions. But the ones that do adapt to the more open, sunlit areas are generally also those better able to serve as intermediate hosts for the parasitic flatworms that cause the disease schistosomiasis in people. Also known as bilharzia, this disease can lead to chronic ill health, reducing peoples' capacity to work or even causing death. It adversely affects almost 240 million people worldwide, and it is estimated that over 700 million people live in endemic regions, especially in tropical and subtropical areas, and in poor communities without clean drinking water and adequate sanitation. In such areas a large proportion of women may suffer from female genital schistosomiasis, acquired while standing in infected water (e.g., washing clothes in an infected lake or stream). Disease is caused when the pathogenic worm enters the body and deposits its eggs in the blood vessels surrounding the bladder or intestines (see Figures 4.1 and 4.2).

Deforestation can lead to widespread ecosystem reconstitution that influences vector-borne disease transmission through altered vegetation, the introduction of livestock, and the development of human settlements in cleared areas. There are several examples of the direct effects of deforestation on vector-borne human diseases, such as malaria, as discussed in Chapter 1 and below. Deforestation and animal vectors' ability to adapt to human blood as an alternative source of food also affects other human vector-borne diseases (Walsh, Molyneux, and Birley 1993).

Savannah blackflies, for example, which transmit a more severe form of onchocerciasis than do forest-dwelling blackflies, increase in density as forest cover decreases and urban and savannah areas are created in previously forested regions (Wilson et al. 2002). Similarly, cutaneous leishmaniasis, transmitted by sandflies, is increasing in deforestation regions in places like Costa Rica. Forest clearing in Costa Rica is tied to the development of large-scale commercial agriculture and accelerated human population growth. These changes, in turn, are "associated with new inequities in land tenure . . . increased numbers

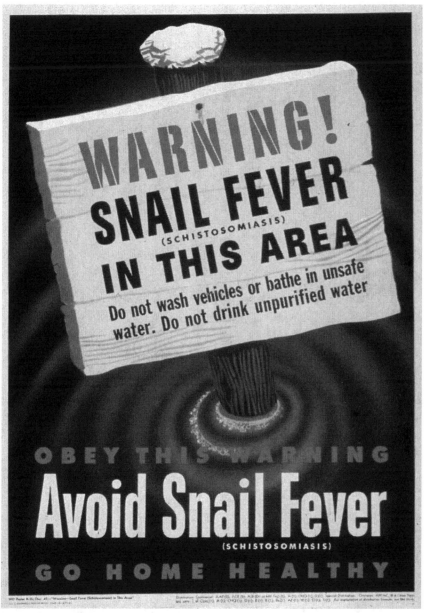

Figure 4.1   Schistosomiasis prevention poster. (Images from the History of Medicine)

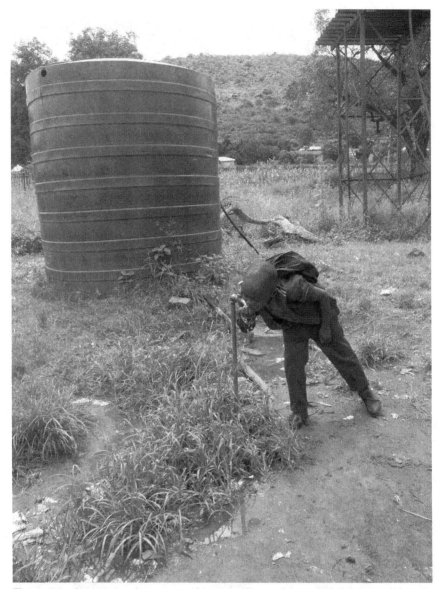

Figure 4.2 Access to clean water is a significant factor in infectious risk, Lesotho in Southern Africa. (Photo by Nicola Bulled)

of landless peasants, and hence further pressure to cut down forests for local subsistence agriculture . . . and extraction of other natural resources" (Chaves et al. 2008). Risk of leishmaniasis is highest in communities living inside or close to fragmented forests now intermixed with agricultural plots. Reservoirs

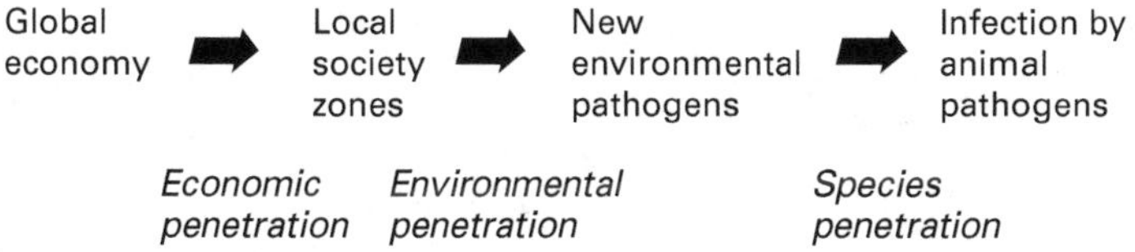

Global economy	Local society zones	New environmental pathogens	Infection by animal pathogens
	Economic penetration	*Environmental penetration*	*Species penetration*

Figure 4.3 Tripartite Model of Biosocial Penetration.

of leishmaniasis include small mammals, whose density increases in fragmented forests because of a loss of predators in such environments.

Deforestation also is linked to the spread of *buruli ulcer* (BU), a necrotizing and potentially disfiguring cutaneous infection caused by *Mycobacterium ulcerans*. After tuberculosis and leprosy, BU is the third most common and least understood of the major mycobacterial diseases, which include infections associated with tattooing. Unlike tuberculosis and leprosy, BU is related to environmental factors and is not transmissible between humans. M. ulcerans has been recovered from various insects, so researchers believe insect bites may be involved in the transmission of the mycobacterium (Williamson et al. 2012). The rapid surge in BU cases beginning in the early 1980s may be associated with forest clearing and other topographical changes, such as building dams and irrigation systems (Meyers 1995).

Figure 4.3 shows a *tripartite model of biosocial penetration,* which is one way to conceptualize the entwinement of biosocial factors active in the causes and evident in the consequences of environmental penetration. Like all models, this figure simplifies extremely complex and locally varied processes: (1) the global capitalist economy, with its built-in emphasis on the endless hunt for resources, routinely penetrates and reconfigures local societies; (2) which serve as vehicles for the penetration of new environments for resource extraction and production; and (3) which creates exposures to and opportunities for human penetration by novel infectious disease agents. In some cases, such as HIV, this penetration and adaptation by a simian infectious agent traveled all the way back up the "supply chain" and became the source of a global pandemic.

ANTHROPOGENIC GLOBAL WARMING AND THE SPREAD OF INFECTIOUS AGENTS

Scientists across many subfields are in very broad agreement that our planet is warming; that human activities such as the burning of fossil fuels, high-tech agriculture, and deforestation are primary drivers of this warming process; that the pace of warming is accelerating faster than anyone previously realized; and that the changes wrought by climate change will have far-reaching human health impacts. Many analysts believe that climate change and the socionatural crises it is creating is the number-one threat to human health in the twenty-first century (Baer and Singer 2009, 2014; Foster 2002; McMichael 2013). Included among the many health risks of climate change are enhancements of conditions that foster the spread of infectious diseases through various pathways, including vector-borne diseases, water-borne diseases, wind-blown pathogens, and moisture-related mold infections (see Figure 4.4).

The relationship linking climate, environment, and infectious diseases predates and is analytically independent of the issue of anthropogenic global warming. For example, rainfall and drought have always played a key role in the incidence of malaria in affected areas, the dry season contributes to

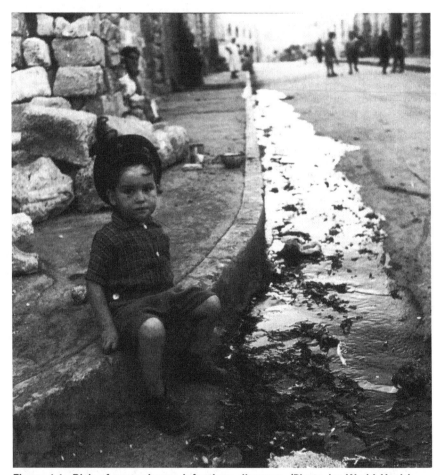

Figure 4.4 Risk of water-borne infectious diseases. (Photo by World Health Organization)

meningococcal disease in parts of sub-Saharan Africa, and warm ocean water spreads cholera in the Ganges River delta (Greer, Ng, and Fisman 2008). These examples all come from places in the developing world that lack the socioeconomic protections developed nations enjoy, including improved water systems, high-quality housing, and reduced exposure to disease vectors.

Influenza is another infectious disease global warming is affecting that is tied to considerable human morbidity, mortality, and economic burden across time and place, although certainly not evenly among nations or social groups. Influenza pandemics occur annually, with regular replacement of the dominant viral strains that circulate the globe. In temperate zones influenza events exhibit a seasonal pattern that appears to be driven by climate factors (Ebi et al. 2001). Research has focused on what is called the El Niño Southern Oscillation (ENSO), a cyclical interannual climate variation between warm and cold phases that affects global atmospheric and oceanic circulation patterns (Baer and Singer 2014). Several studies have linked the spread of infectious diseases like dengue, Rift Valley fever, malaria, cholera, and diarrheal diseases to the phases of this cycle (Checkley et al. 2000; Hales et al. 1999; Pascual et al. 2000). In revealing research with datasets covering ten seasons in France, Cécile Viboud and colleagues (2004) established a link between the impact of influenza on morbidity and mortality and global climate index factors. They found that the mortality impact of the dominant influenza strain was significantly higher during the ten seasons with colder ENSO conditions than during the sixteen seasons with warmer ENSO climates.

Anthropogenic global warming is creating pressing and mounting problems even beyond cyclical climate patterns that have always been with us. The magnitude of the changes that are occurring in our world led Nobel Prizing–winning atmospheric chemist Paul Crutzen and biologist Eugene Stoermer (2000) to suggest that the current geographic age of Earth should be renamed the Anthropocene (Age of People). Their argument is that for the last 150 years human activities, more so than natural forces, have had the most impact on shaping the biogeological environments of the planet and its climate. For Crutzen this realization began with research on the ecosystem of the Amazon Forest, including flows of matter, energy, and chemical components. Following these flows, he identified deforestation, which has resulted in a loss of one-fifth of forested land since 1970, as a transformation of organic matter into airborne smoke particles and chemical compounds (e.g., CO_2) that alter the atmosphere. Since Crutzen and Stoermer began pushing for recognition of the significant extent of human reshaping of climate, the world has experienced ever-higher levels of CO_2 and other gases in the atmosphere and the tumultuous effects of resulting climate change.

This climate trend already is influencing various human disease vectors that seasonal temperatures once restricted in their distribution. Vectors are spreading to new areas because insect and other arthropod (e.g., ticks) vectors of infectious diseases are ectothermic (cold-blooded) and, as a result, subject to the effects of temperature on their reproduction, development, behavior, and range. Temperature also affects the development of pathogens residing in vectors. A temperature rise of only 2°C (3.6°F) could expand malaria's domain of active infection from 42 percent to 60 percent of the planet. A temperature rise at this level, moreover, will more than double the metabolic rate of malarial mosquitoes, increasing their feeding on human blood to nourish their eggs (Gage et al. 2008). Research on densely populated areas in the traditionally cooler highlands of Colombia and Ethiopia shows that in warmer years malaria infection occurs at higher elevations (Siraj et al. 2014). In Ethiopia researchers estimate that just a 1°C (1.8°F) rise in temperature could lead to an additional 3 million cases per year in children under fifteen years old, a population particularly vulnerable because they have never been exposed to the disease.

Other infectious diseases also are expected to spread. Various studies suggest a climate connection to the last major outbreak of plague, which is spread by fleas harboring *Yersinia pestis*. Although this epidemic began in western China in the mid-nineteenth century, it was the Indian subcontinent that was most severely affected, particularly during the years between 1896 and the 1920s. The timing of plague outbreaks in this region was "heavily influenced by seasonally varying climatic factors, primarily rainfall and temperature" (Gage et al. 2008:443–444). Based on an examination of plague cases in New Mexico in recent years, Robert Parmenter and colleagues (1999) demonstrated that human cases occurred more frequently following periods of above average rainfall. Researchers believe that increased rainfall—an outcome of climate change in some regions—facilitates the availability of rodent food sources and increased rodent reproduction, increasing the likelihood of human contact with infected rodents. In addition to malaria and plague, vector-borne ailments whose geographic ranges are expanding because of global warming include West Nile virus, Rift Valley fever, yellow fever, Hantaan virus, Lyme disease, Dengue fever, cholera, and *aspergillosis* (see Table 4.1).

The environmental effects of global warming are diverse and include an increase in the frequency of extreme weather, including large storms and flooding. Fungal species, which grow best in damp environments, and the infectious diseases they cause are thus becoming more common. Fungi form a large group of organisms that includes mushrooms as well as microorganisms such as molds. Fungi only became important human pathogens in the twentieth century as a result of immune-system-damaging HIV infections and medical interventions

Table 4.1 Infectious Diseases That are Spreading Because of Global Warming

Malaria
West Nile disease
Rift Valley fever
Yellow Fever
Hantaan virus infection
Lyme disease
Plague
Dengue
Cholera
Aspergillosis

that diminish immune capacity. As a group, mammals, including humans, are quite resistant to fungal infection. Mammals maintain high internal body temperatures relative to environmental temperatures, creating conditions that restrict the growth of the majority of fungi. In recent years, however, the threat of fungus species to health has been spurred by:

- the global food crisis, as plants are the group worst hit by fungus infection, and the threat appears to be growing (e.g., potato blight, rice last, wheat stem rust, soybean rust, corn smut);
- animal species die-offs due to fungal disease (e.g., the disease current causing mass die-offs of mosquito-eating bat and frog species); and
- flooding and the spread of pathogenic house molds.

Invasive, opportunistic mold infections have become significant causes of death in immunocompromised individuals, such as bone marrow transplant recipients and HIV patients. Molds are also of special risk to individuals with asthma or other allergic sensitivities. *Aspergillus* is the most common of such molds, although *Fusarium* species are growing in frequency as factors in human health. Conditions caused by Aspergillus include allergic reactions, internal bleeding, jaundice, lung infections, and infections in other organs. Since 2011 a number of US states have experienced an increase in corn and other crop food contamination with Aspergillus. Because this mold is so toxic, truckloads of corn with more than twenty parts per billion, or about one hundred kernels in an average load, are not allowed to cross state lines. Aspergillus is very responsive to the drought conditions that have plagued parts of the United States because, unlike other molds that are adapted to moist environments, it prefers the hot, dry climates that global warming is exacerbating in some regions.

Some fungi produce poisonous substances known as *mycotoxins*. The fungus species *Stachybotrys chartarum*, for example, produces an especially damaging mycotoxin that causes mucosal bleeding, cognitive dysfunction, extreme rashes, vomiting and nausea, and cell death. Although the reason for fungi's mycotoxin production is not clear, we know that in infectious situations they weaken the host and improve the environment for further fungal proliferation. The mycotoxins fungi produce are considered active, and the US military developed them as potential biological weapons. Concerns about food-based mycotoxins provoked the US Food and Drug Administration to regulate and enforce limits on concentrations of mycotoxins in products of the food and feed industries beginning in the mid-1980s. The most well-known mycotoxin is the potent human liver carcinogen known as *aflatoxin*. It is produced by two related fungi species, *Aspergillus flavus* and *A. parasiticus,* that grow on various food crops. Aflatoxin contamination is now "a global food security issue, but it's especially a problem in developing countries, which are often largely populated by subsistence farmers who don't have the resources, technology or infrastructure needed for adequate grain testing" (Bloudoff-Indelicato 2012).

The case of Hurricane Katrina offers a window into the growing impact of global warming on human mold exposure. The extensive flooding this intense storm caused created conditions that supported widespread mold growth and had "likely significant impacts on respiratory morbidity" (Kinney 2008:465). Chris Mooney has described the New Orleans community of Lakeview in the months after Katrina struck and flooded much of the city. Houses were deserted, piles of debris sat on each curbside, vegetation everywhere was dead, and inside the hollow shells of homes there were "huge tapestries of mold on the walls" (Mooney 2007:1). A CDC survey found that 46 percent of homes in New Orleans had visible mold growth, and 17 percent had heavy mold coverage of indoor house surfaces (Ratard et al. 2006). Indoor air samples revealed that Aspergillus was the predominant mold present. The CDC investigation concluded that postremediation workers and residents involved in cleaning and restoring their homes were potentially put at risk for the negative health effects of mold exposure. Notably, numerous homes that were structurally sound after the storm still had to be gutted before they could be renovated because of dangerous mold growth (Government Accounting Office 2008).

A fungal infection spurred on by climate change appears to be the driving force in an increasingly important life-threatening disease known as coccidioimycosis (cocci for short), or Valley Fever (Irfan 2012). Labeled "a silent epidemic" by the Centers for Disease Control and Prevention, this airborne disease is striking more people each year, primarily in the Southwest, especially California, Texas, and Arizona, but also in arid areas of Central and South America. US cases rose from 850 in 1995 to over 20,000 in 2011 (CDC 2012). In part, the rising number of cases reflects population growth in the Southwest and California, areas that emerged in the US imagination as ideal "new start" settings away from crowded Eastern and mid-Western sectors of the country. It is estimated that 30 to 60 percent of people who dwell in an endemic region where coccidiodes fungi (including both *Coccidioides immitis* and *Coccidioides posadasii*) live in the soil are exposed to spores at some point during their lives. Although most people suffer limited consequences, others develop severe infections, including chronic pneumonia, and over 150 people die annually because of the disease. The disease has different manifestations, however, depending on where fungal spores nest in the body. Symptoms can include significant weight loss, cognitive impairments, heart problems, lung damage, and bone deterioration.

Fungal pathogens commonly are controlled by the presence of predatory bacteria and other organisms that feed on them. But these controls diminish— and acute infections rise—when rainfall is followed by a prolonged drought or a drying period, the kinds of shifting weather patterns produced by anthropogenic climate change. Hotter, drier climate, increasingly typical in the Southwest, is associated with an increase in the level of wind-blown dust that breaks off fungal spores and carries them into the lungs of unsuspecting hosts. Construction projects that disrupt the soil and release dust into the air also contribute to the spread of coccidiodes spores. As with other infectious diseases, it is evident that the interaction of biological (fungal spores in interaction with human bodies), environmental (changing climate, soil conditions), social (the production of greenhouse gases, the push for new construction), and cultural factors (beliefs about the "good life" that brought many migrants to the Southwest and California) is driving an increase in cases of Valley Fever.

Unmistakably, climate change is altering relations among microbes, insect vectors of disease, animal population reservoirs of potentially zoonotic infectious diseases, and humans. As humans continue to cause global warming, although trends will vary by geographic region and level of national wealth, we expect to continue to see a widespread increase in vector-borne infections, water-borne gastrointestinal diseases, airborne respiratory diseases, and the emergence of new zoonotic diseases in human populations.

INDUSTRIAL FOOD PRODUCTION AND PATHOGENS

On May 23 and 24, 2000, approximately 160 people living in the small rural community of Walkerton, Ontario, Canada, sought hospital treatment for a set of intense gastrointestinal symptoms, including bloody diarrhea, vomiting, severe stomach cramps, and fever. Another 500 people contacted local hospitals complaining of similar potent symptoms. Before the outbreak ended, over 2,300 became sick and 7 died (Ali 2004). Epidemiological investigation concluded that the cause was contamination of a drinking water well by cattle manure containing the potentially deadly strain of the E. coli bacteria known as O157:H7 (and to a lesser extent, *Campylobacter jejuni*). The health threat of this strain of E. coli was first recognized during the 1980s, when cases of foodborne transmission caused human illness, a development that coincided with the importation of cattle from Argentina, where rates of infection in humans were already comparatively high. Although E. coli is usually a harmless bacteria in the intestines of cattle, the virulent E. coli O157:H7 strain is believed to be a product of the transfer of a gene from the dangerous Shigella bacteria, a process known as *gene assortment* (Heymann and Rodier 1997). E .coli O157:H7 is especially dangerous to young children and the elderly.

This case raises the broader issue of the role of industrial food production, or what is sometimes called factory farming, on the spread of infectious diseases. In the United States, for example, the dramatic pace of the transformation of food production from family farming to agribusiness is striking. Since World War II the overall number of farms in the country has shrunk but the size of the remaining operations has grown; this is especially the case with livestock and poultry production. Since the 1950s the total production of meat has more than doubled, but the number of producing operations has decreased by 80 percent. There has been a sweeping shift in food animal production to much larger, more concentrated facilities, with animals often raised in close confinement in outdoor pens. Huge cattle operations produce enormous quantities of manure that must be managed to avoid contamination of water systems. In the United States in 2007 over 2 billion head of livestock and poultry produced approximately a billion tons of manure and associated contaminants (Environmental Protection Agency 2013). Often on cattle operations manure is stored in a building or stockpiled, whereas drainage ditches may flow through animal-occupied areas, discharging storm water, manure, feed, and other waste into collection ponds or lagoons. Global warming and associated increases in intensive storms can overwhelm these facilities and break down barriers between farms and waterways.

The contemporary food industry presents a significant potential infectious disease risk, combining an abundance of manure, the presence in cattle of numerous infectious agents that can lead to human disease, and the potential for contamination of groundwater. Manure can provide an advantageous environment for pathogen survival because of the availability of nutrients, protection from UV radiation, and control of temperature extremes. The degree of threat is influenced by the ability of microorganisms to survive under various environmental conditions and in diverse media (e.g., soils). Some pathogens of animal origin, like Cryptosporidium while in the oocyst stage, are notable because of their evolved capacity to persist in damp environments for months, resist our conventional techniques for disinfecting drinking water, and cause disease for which we lack treatments. Similarly, E. coli O157: H7 is particularly well adapted to a range of extreme environments because of its resistance to salt and chlorine. In the case of the Walkerton outbreak, the pathogen had to survive "a circuitous ecological pathway as [it] traveled from the intestines of cattle, through the surface water pathways, through the soils into the ground water pathways and through the constructed drinking water system to be ultimately consumed by the unfortunate human victim[s]" (Ali 2004:2604). The result was a sharp local spike in infectious disease morbidity and mortality. This case is far from unique; it merely is one among many of growing concern in a world in which profit-driven pressure toward intensified food production is increasing and planetary temperatures are rising. Of course, the two are also related—industrial production is also a primary driver of global warming.

AIR POLLUTION AND LUNG INFECTION

Air pollution is an atmospheric condition in which there is a substance present at concentrations high enough above their normal ambient levels to produce a measurable adverse effect on people, animals, and vegetation. Not only is our air polluted with various substances that are toxic to humans, there is also mounting evidence that pollution is a factor in lung infections. Acute respiratory infections are a leading contributor to the global burden of disease, accounting for more than 6 percent of disease worldwide and an equal level of mortality in developing countries (Singer and Erickson 2013).

Air pollution is usually divided between indoor (e.g., gases given off by heating and cooking devices that use biomass fuels like wood) and outdoor sources (e.g., vehicles, factories). The evidence for a relationship between indoor pollution and respiratory infections, primarily in developing countries, is well established. Family members who spend many hours in the home, particularly mothers, small children, and grandparents, are at greatest risk. Research in Gambia on infant girls who were carried on their mothers' backs during cooking, for example, found the infants have more lower respiratory infections than girls who were not (Armstrong and Campbell 1991). Similarly, among the rural hill region of Nepal, children under two who spent more time next to stoves suffer a higher life-threatening incidence of acute respiratory infection compared to those who spent less time near stoves (Pandey et al. 1989). Parallel findings have been reported for children and adults in various other developing countries as well as in developed countries for children raised in homes with wood stoves in use.

The main pollutant of biomass fuel burning is nitrogen dioxide (NO_2). Our lungs have a number of defense mechanisms against gaseous pollutants like nitrogen dioxide as well as inhaled particulate matter, including various self-clearing mechanisms like aerodynamic filtration, mucociliary clearance, and particle transport. Additionally, *alveolar macrophages* (or "dust cells" as they are also known) in the lungs help to remove pollutants but are also active in providing bodily defense against bacteria and viruses. Existing evidence suggests that exposure to indoor pollution adversely affects lung defense mechanisms, reducing the capacity to control viral infections of the respiratory tract. Research suggests that research suggests that the "ability of different pollutants and particle fractions to cause variable defects in bronchial immunity may ... determine the risk of symptoms following pollutant exposure and infection" (Chauhan and Johnston 2003).

Outdoor air pollutants also play a role in infection. For example, nitrogen dioxide and ozone, outdoor air pollutants from vehicles and industrial production, impair immune response to respiratory pathogens by limiting the clearance of microbes from the respiratory tract and adversely altering the function of macrophages during infection. George Jakab (1998), for example, found that the body's ability to kill *Staphylococcus aureus* bacteria in the lung is impaired at the exposure level of 5 parts per million (ppm) of NO_2 and that this effect occurs at 2.5 ppm or less when NO_2 exposure occurs in lungs that are predisposed to lowered resistance by an immunosuppression drug (such as corticosteroid) commonly used in the treatment of asthma. This research demonstrated that the macrophage phagocytic system, which includes cells in the lungs that destroy invading pathogens, foreign particles, cancerous or diseased cells, and cellular debris, is the defense component of the lungs that is most susceptible to the adverse effects of air pollutants. Consequently, pumping the air with large quantities of diverse toxic pollutants from cars, factories, farms, mining, and other sources is contributing to rising rates of respiratory tract infections worldwide.

Air pollution, and the infectious diseases it facilitates, is not only a product of human technological and social activities; it is also a mirror of the structure of social relationships. Based on research in Hong Kong, Rachel Stern argues that the exposure to and consequences of air pollution reflect relations among unequal social classes: "Everyone does not breathe the same air. Hong Kong's poor both suffer increased exposure to air pollution and bear a heavy share of the economic costs of poor air quality" (Stern 2003:786). As a result, interest has risen in the need for analyses of what J. Timmons Roberts and Bradley Parks (2006, 118) call "the polluting elites"—"those who direct leading sectors of their economies and exercise disproportionate control over national and foreign environmental policies" and practices that affect health.

Water can also be a significant source of infection. This is especially true when the world faces a global water shortage. This widening crisis has sparked a search for alternative water sources, such as the effective and systematic harvesting of rainfall, a practice that is thousands of years old. The identification of microbiological contamination in collected samples, however, complicates the use of rainwater for drinking. A study in Singapore by Rajni Kaushik, Rajasekhar Balasubramanian, and Armah de la Cruz (2012), for example, found four different pathogens in rainwater: *E. coli, P. aeruginosa, K. pneumonia,* and *A. hydrophilia.* Other studies confirm these findings. G. Simmons and colleagues (2001) found that rooftop rainwater systems in four rural areas of New Zealand yield a range of pathogens, including salmonella, aeromonas, and cryptosporidium. The study also found a significant association between the presence of aeromonas and increased gastroenteric symptoms among household dwellers. Dennis Lye (2002) found an association between drinking untreated rainwater from rooftop collection with a range of infectious conditions, including bacterial diarrhea, bacterial pneumonia, and helminth infestations. Between 1978 and 2006 there have been six documented disease outbreaks associated with rainwater consumption. Although it may be appealing to think of rainwater as pure, the ability of micros, including pathogens, to inhabit atmospheric moisture further affirms these organisms' incredible adaptive capacity.

BEYOND RAIN: WATER CONTAMINATION AND HUMAN INFECTIOUS DISEASES

Access to clean water for drinking and sanitary purposes is a precondition for human health and well-being. Yet more than a billion people worldwide do not have ready access to safe water (see Figure 4.5). Water-borne infectious diseases are estimated to cause over 2 million deaths per year around the world as well as 4 billion cases of diarrhea. Although for some of us diarrhea is a mere annoyance, in fact it is among the world's deadliest killers, particularly of small children. It is the second leading cause of death in children under the age of five; in 2011 seven hundred thousand episodes of diarrhea worldwide led to death (Walker et al., 2013). Most of these deaths, caused by a variety of enteric bacteria, viruses, and parasitic organisms that infect the intestinal tract, occur in developing countries.

Almost all human activities can and do adversely affect water. Water quality is influenced by:

- direct point sources (such as specific local discharges from urban wastewater, industry, and fish farms) and

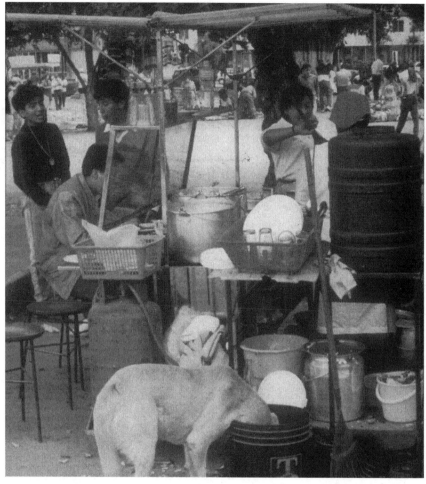

Figure 4.5 Water-borne disease routes, dog drinking from dishwashing bucket at open air market in Quito, Ecuador. (Photo by Linda Whiteford)

- diffuse pollution (pollutants that spread throughout an ecosystem, such as chemical leakage into the environment and its water systems from industrial farms, including agricultural nutrients, pesticides, and fecal microbes).

Water spreads some significant infectious epidemic diseases, such as *cholera*. Cholera is linked to a bacterium of the Vibrio family; it is an acute diarrheal disease that can kill within hours if untreated. Cholera bacteria produce a toxin that flushes the intestines and keeps the human body from absorbing liquids, causing dehydration. This flushing is an adaptation of the bacteria, which clears room in the human intestines, which fauna already heavily populate, for it to latch on and multiply. Interaction between this pathogen and other microbes in the human body is exemplary of the ongoing contestation among microbes that dwell within us that directly affects our health.

The WHO estimates that there are 3 to 5 million cholera cases and 100,000 to 120,000 deaths globally every year. About 75 percent of people who are infected do not develop symptoms, although they can infect others. Among those who do develop symptoms, 80 percent have mild to moderate cases, but the other 20 percent develop acute diarrhea and severe dehydration, possibly leading to death if untreated. People already affected by other health challenges, such as malnourished children or people living with HIV, are at the gravest risk of death from cholera infection.

A major cholera epidemic in 2010 struck the island nation of Haiti, just under seven hundred miles from the United States. Prior to this, the last cholera epidemic in the Western hemisphere occurred in the early 1990s in Peru and sickened about half a million people. The disease spread as far north as the United States but skipped Haiti. Yet Haiti is especially vulnerable to a disease like cholera. The country is one of the poorest in the world, and cholera is very much a disease of poverty. Magnifying the problem, Haiti suffered a devastating earthquake in January 2010 that left a million people homeless and living in crowed tent cities and destroyed hygiene infrastructure. Moreover, people in Haiti had no recent experience with cholera, so many did not know how to prevent transmission or lacked the facilities to do so (see Figure 4.6).

The epidemic began in September in a poor, rural area sixty-two miles north of Port-au-Prince, the capital. By the end of 2012 the Haitian Ministry of Health reported almost 640,000 cases of cholera and about 8,000 deaths with accumulative case fatality rate of 1.6 percent. The infection and fatality rates increased after Hurricane Sandy hit Haiti in the latter part of 2012. Over 5 percent of the country's total population has been stricken with the disease. Overall Haiti's cholera epidemic accounted for 57 percent of all cholera cases and 53 percent of all cholera-related deaths reported to the World Health Organization in 2010 and 58 percent of all cholera cases and 37 percent of all cholera deaths the following year (Barzilay et al. 2013).

The strain of virus found in Haiti was genetically quite similar to the one circulating in Nepal, a country almost nine thousand miles away. Researchers believe that cholera was unknowingly carried to Haiti by Nepalese soldiers deployed there as part of a UN peacekeeping force. This example of the worst cholera epidemic in recent history shows how the movement of people also moves infectious diseases and changes the external microbial environments people inhabit. It further reveals the biocultural/biosocial nature of contemporary

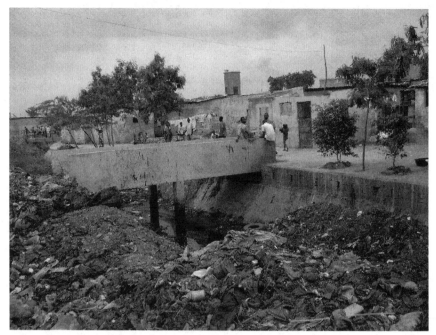

Figure 4.6 Urban breeding ground for infectious diseases, Cite Soleil, Haiti. (Photo by Merrill Singer)

microbial environments. The presence of at least one strain of cholera in Haiti was the product of the structure of social relations among nations that led to the placement of Nepalese soldiers in the distant land of Haiti. Their presence in Haiti unintentionally changed the environment of the island nation by introducing a new pathogen to a socially and biologically vulnerable population. The result has been devastating and is exemplary of the routine failure to consider the infectious disease consequences of human actions in the world (see Figure 4.7).

Although the cholera epidemic in Haiti has been particularly harsh, the disease occurs regularly in the developing world. Yet even the officially reported number of cases is not the full story of cholera, as these statistics likely grossly underestimate the actual global burden of the disease. The best method for combating this grave threat to human life, as Ronald Waldman, Eric Mintz, and Heather Papowitz (2013:593) emphasize,

> The control of the great majority of diarrheal diseases is the strategy that eliminated epidemic cholera from the United States and Northern Europe long before either marketed antibiotics or effective vaccines existed. The development and maintenance of water and sewage

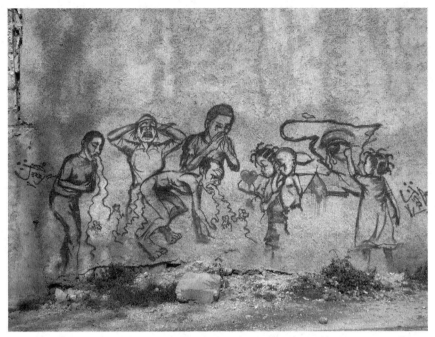

Figure 4.7 Wall mural on cholera epidemic in Haiti. (Photo by Laura R. Wagner)

treatment systems assured safe drinking water and safe disposal of sewage for all, keeping contaminated sewage out of water, foods, and the environment.

This is not just a technical problem but a sociocultural and economic problem that human societies, racked by considerable inequality, must surmount (see Figure 4.8).

PLURALEA INTERACTIONS

Environment degradations of various kinds put human health at risk, but the situation is complicated by *ecocrisis interaction* (Singer 2009a). Rather than being stand-alone threats to human well-being, adverse human impacts on the environment intersect with the potential of causing significant infectious (and other) harms to human health. Called *pluralea interactions,* the intersection and enhanced effects of combined ecological factors are of growing concern in a world with rising temperatures and consequential climatic events. This term is derived from the Latin words *plur,* meaning "many," and *alea,* meaning "hazards," and refers to the growing number of health-related interactions that

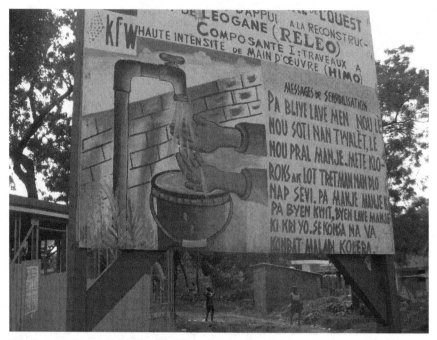

Figure 4.8 Cholera Prevention Billboard in Haiti. (Photo by Laura R. Wagner)

transpire across the full panoply of environmental degradations in our increasingly human-dominated environment.

These interactions are complex and separating "the influence of human-caused temperature increases from natural climate variations or other confounding factors, such as land-use changes or pollution is a real challenge" (Roberts and Parks 2006:118). Yet the tendency has been to avoid this challenge and instead to seek single-cause understandings based on the separation and independent analysis of selected components and processes in the world around us. This approach, however, may lead to faulty conclusions. Even accounts of a major process like climate change involve only the exposed "tip of [a far] broader global sustainability iceberg" that includes numerous other environmental disruptions that are not only coterminous but are also "converging rapidly in a manner not previously experienced" (Spratt and Sutton 2008:xi). Consequently, assessments of environmental impacts on human infectious disease must consider the kinds and nature of interactions among environmental factors that help to shape microbial populations, their locations, behaviors, and human health effects.

The weather event dubbed Superstorm Sandy in 2012 is exemplary of a pluralea interaction and may be representative of major superstorms to come. Sandy began as a tropical wave in the western Caribbean Sea and developed into a hurricane that devastated parts of the Caribbean during a busy hurricane season, the likes of which global warming is likely to cause with increasing frequency. Sandy eventually became the largest, in terms of its diameter, Atlantic hurricane on record, with winds spanning an area of eleven hundred miles. The storm moved ashore the US mainland near Atlantic City, New Jersey, as a post-tropical cyclone with hurricane-force winds. The storm affected twenty-four states, especially New Jersey and New York. In New York City, a thirteen-foot-high flood surge saturated streets, tunnels, and subway lines, cutting power in and around the city. The scale of the damage Sandy caused is estimated to be in the neighborhood of $70 billion, making it the second-costliest Atlantic hurricane in US history after Hurricane Katrina, which struck the United States only eight years earlier. In light of ocean rise caused by global warming of approximately one foot over the last one hundred years along the New Jersey coast, researchers believe that global warming influenced the notable extent of the flooding. That Sandy turned inland along the Atlantic Coast and not out to sea, as such storms historically have, has been attributed to the influence of global warming on the ocean jet stream. Additionally, the hurricane blended with an artic front that some climate scientists attribute to global warming. Adding to the impact of Sandy was the elimination of wetlands and their replacement by concrete in places like Staten Island, which experienced some of the most severe flooding. In short, Sandy was a pluralea event that united several climate and environmental factors influenced by anthropogenic global warming and other human restructuring of the environment.

There are several ways in which a superstorm like Sandy has the potential to increase infectious disease risk. Flooding in places like New York City and its extensive subway system can displace rat populations (which at least equals the human population in the city) and the diseases they carry, including leptospirosis, hantavirus, typhus, salmonella, and plague. Rats that flee flooded areas and settle into new, drier locations are likely to have greater contact with humans. In addition to rat bites and ectoparasites as sources of human infection, rodent feces and urine can spread hantavirus.

Crowding of displaced residents in emergency shelters holds another risk for poststorm infectious disease outbreaks of conditions like influenza, rotavirus, *Kingella kingae*, and *M. pneumonia*. During the poststorm period, which struck during flu season, New York City witnessed a massive increase in visits to health care facilities for influenza-like illnesses, especially among young children. Standing pools of water produced by the storm constitute a third source of infectious disease risk caused by Sandy. Of most concern in urban areas is the bacteria *Escherichia coli*. Found normally in the lower intestine, where it plays a role in digestion, it can be toxic if it enters into the stomach. Floods that carry raw sewage into densely populated areas can be a source of infection with this microbe. Cases of vibrio bacterial infections, which enter the body through open cuts, were reported after Hurricane Katrina, present another infectious disease threat from hurricanes. Finally, as noted earlier, floods cause dampness and create excellent environments for the growth of humidity-loving fungi, some of which can be quite harmful to humans. Although not all of these infectious disease threats were realized with Sandy, climate scientists have predicted an increased frequency of major multifaceted climate events as a result of global warming. Thus, a more storm-stressed population, subjected to the risks of an overtaxed infrastructure, may endure increasing infectious disease outbreaks in our stormier future.

Another example of the infectious disease threat of interactions is the extensive flooding that hit the American Midwest in 2008. In Iowa extensive rainfall led to the flooding of most of the rivers in the eastern part of the state. The "flood stage," which is the point at which a body of water overflows into surrounding areas and causes damage, has been established on the Cedar River near the city of Cedar Rapids as 12 feet above a fixed point near river bottom. The previous record flood occurred in 1929, when the Cedar River rose to 20 feet. In 2008 the Cedar River reached 20 feet and kept rising; weather experts expected the waterway to crest at 22 feet. Ultimately, however, the river crested at 31.3 feet. The intense storm hit cities like Cedar Rapids and Iowa City hard. In Cedar Rapids, for example, the downtown flooded and a railroad bridge collapsed, spilling railroad cars filled with rocks into the river. As a result, some Iowans began using the phrase "Iowa's Katrina" to refer to their experience.

Although heavy rains are not unusual in the Midwest, rainfall and other storms of the magnitude and frequency seen in 2008 are quite unusual. In all, nine rivers in Iowa reached record flood levels during the midyear storms. Flooding of the kind that submerged the Midwest is expected to occur only once every five hundred years, which means that hydrologists, who study the properties, distribution, and circulation of water on Earth, believe that a flood of this enormity has a 0.2 percent chance of occurring in a specific year in a given location. But the 2008 inundation was the second massive flooding of the region to occur since 1993. During the thirty-five years from 1973 through 2008 there were four floods in the Mississippi River basin area that, based on their magnitude, would be characterized as one hundred–year floods. At the same time, relatively large Midwestern storms that used to occur approximately every twenty years now arrive every four to six years (Zabarenko 2008). An analysis of weather data conducted by a group of environmental organizations concluded that there has been a marked increase in the frequency of heavy rainstorms, with the frequency of "extreme rainfall" increasing by 24 percent between 1948 and 2006 (National Wildlife Federation 2008). This emergent pattern of larger, more frequent Midwest flooding has suggested to some climate scientists that in the Midwest we are already seeing the influence of global warming in changing weather patterns. Air warmed by the blanketing effects of the greenhouse gases that now surround Earth are known to be able to carry far more water than cooler air. The effect of this change was again seen in the spring of 2011, when some of the largest floods in the past century occurred on the Mississippi River and created disaster areas in Kentucky, Tennessee, and Mississippi.

Kamyar Enshayan, director of an environmental research center at the University of Northern Iowa, has pointed out that the 2008 disaster was not "natural" for reasons that go beyond climate change: the heavy rains fell on a landscape that humans had radically reengineered. According to Enshayan (quoted in Achenbach 2008:A1), "We've done numerous things to the landscape that took away [its] water-absorbing functions." The changes Enshayan refers to include (1) the replacement of tall-grass prairies, which have now all but disappeared, with plowed fields of corn and soybeans that, unlike prairie grasses, have shallow roots that do not hinder the rapid flow of water run-off as do prairie grasses; (2) the thorough draining of developed fields through the installation of underground pipes; (3) the straightening of streams and creeks, which has reduced the size of their banks while accelerating the speed of water flow; (4) the filling in and development of flood plains; (5) the extension of cultivated land ever closer to the banks of creeks and rivers, thereby eliminating the buffer zones that used to hold back rainfall from moving swiftly from plowed fields to surface water; and (6) because of incentives to produce biofuel, the removal, between 2007 and 2008, of over one hundred thousand acres of land from the Conservation Reserve Program, which pays farmers not to cultivate tracts of potential farmland, the effect of which was a reduction in fallow acreage—when roots grow deep in the soil. As a result of these unrestrained efforts to expand food and biofuel production and human occupation, approximately 90 percent of the wetlands in Iowa have disappeared. This loss is consequential because wetlands play a vital role in reducing the frequency and intensity of floods by acting as natural barriers that slow water flows, absorb great quantities of moisture, and store water in the ground. Wetlands, in other words, are not just scenic sites and wildlife preserves; they limit the health, economic, and social costs of flooding, which is the most common "natural" hazard in the United States.

In the aftermath of the 2008 Midwest floods, public health officials expressed particular concern about several waterborne pathogens, including E. coli, *giardia*, and *cryptosporidiosis*. *Cryptosporidium parvum*, for example, became a major health hazard after the 1993 Mississippi flooding of Milwaukee (Epstein 2005). During a two-week period 25 percent of Milwaukee residents were infected. The individuals suffered from painful stomach cramps, severe diarrhea, high fever, and dehydration, and over one hundred people died, primarily elderly individuals and those suffering from immune conditions. In Iowa in 2008 the Siouxland District Health Department reported that after the storms ended, the Sioux City area was covered in mosquito-friendly pools of stationary water. In Indiana health official reported trapping a number of mosquitoes infected with West Nile virus (Johnson 2008). Heavy rainfall events cause around half of water-borne infectious disease outbreaks in the United States. Research demonstrates a statistically significant association between extreme wet-weather events and infectious disease outbreaks (Atherholt et al. 1998, Curriero et al. 2001).

These examples of pluralea interactions demonstrate how the multiple ways, intentional and unintentional, in which we are reshaping the environment can come together and magnify the likelihood of the occurrence and spread of infectious diseases. As Chapter 6 will explore in detail, infectious diseases outbreaks can interact to form syndemics that further increase threats to human health.

THE IMPACT OF BIODIVERSITY LOSS ON PATHOGENS

There is a growing body of evidence that one way humans enhance pathogen-induced disease is by diminishing *biodiversity,* the variety of life on Earth (Chivian and Bernstein 2010). Anthropogenic activity is known to be a critical source of species extinction and biodiversity loss because humans disrupt environments with activities such as road and damn building, land clearing and deforestation, mining, monocrop agriculture, and urbanization (Singer 2010a). By eliminating some species in an ecosystem, the populations of others may increase. If these expanded species are hosts to human vectors, there will be increases in disease prevalence. Loss of animals like foxes that feed on mice, for example, has contributed to expanded mice populations and the diseases they host, some of which are transmittable to people. In other words, our adverse impacts on other species in the environment sometimes come back to haunt us in the form of increased infectious disease.

This pattern exists with deforestation in the Amazon as well as in East Africa, Thailand, Malaysia, and Indonesia. Although cutting down forests appears to reduce the diversity of mosquito species in deforested areas, those that survive, for reasons that are not yet completely clear, tend to be the best transmitters of diseases such as malaria. In the Amazon region deforestation has resulted in a proliferation of the mosquito species *Anopheles darlingi,* a vector that is highly effective at transmitting malaria. Lost with deforestation were about twenty other mosquito species that were less efficient in malaria transmission. With fewer competitors around, A. dalingi is able to proliferate.

From the standpoint of infectious disease transmission, a highly diverse environment tends to include "more competent" and "less competent" hosts. This language refers to the likelihood that an infected host will transmit a pathogen to a vector. A key question is: What is the likelihood a mosquito will acquire a pathogen when it bites a member of a particular host species? This question is important to infectious disease/environment relationships because greater host species diversity in a particular area is associated in some environmental contexts with a greater proportion of incompetent hosts that are available for vectors to bite. Incompetent hosts, in effect, produce a *dilution effect* that interrupts the infection cycle of a pathogen and reduces the chance that people will become infected in these areas (Pongsiri et al. 2009). Reduction of the dilution effect appears to be a factor in the explosion of Lyme disease in the United States. Studies also have linked low bird species diversity to increased risk or incidence of West Nile encephalitis in the United States (Swaddle and Calos 2008). Consequently, Felicia Keesing and coworkers (2010:651) assert, "biodiversity itself seems to protect organisms, including humans, from transmission of infectious diseases in many cases. . . . Preserving biodiversity . . . may reduce the incidence of established pathogens."

However, this pattern may not hold for all zoonotic diseases or in all situations, and understanding the local composition of reservoir disease hosts and vector species as well as their ecology is critical (Randolph and Dobson 2012). Daniel Salkeld, Kerry Padgett, and James Jones (2013:684), who have completed a meta-analysis of published studies on the dilution effect, argue that "the relationship between biodiversity and zoonotic disease risk is probably idiosyncratic, and that understanding the ecological dynamics of specific disease systems is [most] important in predicting zoonotic disease risk."

NEGLECTED TROPICAL DISEASES

Neglected tropical diseases (NTDs) comprise a group of disabling and often disfiguring infectious conditions that most commonly are found among people living in extreme poverty. The World Health Organization recognizes seventeen NTDS, including dengue, rabies, Chagas disease, leishmaniases, human African trypanosomiasis, Burulli ulcer, yaws, trachoma, and various worm infections. NTDs are responsible for at least half a million deaths per year as well as considerable disability. They affect the lives of as many as 1 billion people worldwide (Hotez et al. 2006). Concentrated in certain geographic and socially marginalized areas and most commonly found in particular kinds of environments, NTDs often are not well known in wealthy and more developed nations—hence their designation as neglected diseases: those that cause considerable loss of health and life but nonetheless attract far less attention in the global health world than do well-publicized infectious diseases like HIV, malaria, and tuberculosis.

The ultimate cause of NTDs lies in the interface between global disparities in power, wealth, and human rights as well as the suboptimal living and working conditions and access to the benefits of public health improvements and health care that result. NTDs, as enduring and debilitating epidemics, are not "natural" in the sense that they are not only biological entities; they are socially produced as major threats to health and are shaped biologically because of this social dimension. Their host populations, locations of concentration, and severe health and social impacts reflect the global, regional, and local structures of unequal social relationships as well as the benefits of inequality for dominant and powerful groups within and across nations. These issues are discussed more thoroughly in Chapter 7.

One factor in the development of NTDs is rural-to-urban migration propelled by hopes among the rural poor and displaced rural populations of finding income in the city or sanctuary in refugee facilities. Human migration as a consequence of environmental change—itself often *sociogenic* in origin—as well because of conflict or extreme poverty has led to increasingly overpopulated urban areas suffering from diseases like leishmaniasis that has been transmitted by canine or sylvatic (e.g., opossum, sloth, anteater) reservoir hosts. A movement of the rural poor to crowded urban areas in Delhi in 2005 is also believed to have caused the reemergence of the *chickungunya* virus. Dengue is an additional NTD found among rural-to-urban migrant populations.

The disease *sporotrichosis,* characterized by pink to purple skin bumps and rashes potentially leading to chronic ulcers, is traditionally associated with agricultural work and floriculture because the pathogenic fungal agent is found naturally in the soil, especially in tropical and subtropical regions. More recently cases of the diseases are being reported in urban areas, such as Rio de Janeiro, Brazil, as a result of zoonotic transmission, especially among adult women. Researchers have learned that in this context the disease begins at the sites of wounds infected by domestic cats and among people caring for sick cats. Cats may become infected while digging in backyard soils. Researchers suspect that environmental changes and an increase in the feline population in Rio have contributed to the urban emergence of this biosocial/biocultural infectious disease (Barros et al. 2008).

Limited government investment in the health and hygiene of poor populations is often a factor in the spread of NTDs. In Pau de Lima, a densely populated slum on the outskirts of Salvador in Northeastern Brazil, for example, people face the risk of being infected with *leptospira,* a life-threatening rat-borne zoonotic disease, found to be inversely associated with the distance of a household from open sewers and uncollected refuse. Poor-quality dwellings with cracks in the walls and roofs allow the disease vectors of other NTDs to enter, such as the kissing bug that transmits Chagas disease (Hotez et al. 2008).

NTDs reflect an adverse feedback loop involving a downward spiral of interlocked poverty and disease, with poverty increasing the risk of exposure and actual infection and the resulting disease contributing to further impoverishment. Thus, in Africa, hookworm and schistosomiasis infections have been found to cause anemia, chronic inflammation, and iron deficiency. Anemia in children in turn leads to growth stunting, malnutrition, fatigue, and impaired cognitive development. Helminth infections like these affect school attendance and educational performance, adversely affecting future earnings and promoting enduring poverty. Similarly, in adults soil-transmitted helminth infection, loss of sight from trachoma, and chronic lymphedema and hydrocele resulting from lymphatic filariasis have been linked to reduced productivity. Over 120 million people are currently infected with lymphatic filariasis, with about 40 million suffering from disfigurement and incapacitation caused by the disease.

In short, NTDs have an enormous detrimental impact on the length and quality of life among the poorest populations of the world. Although they are most common in developing countries with limited health budgets and large debts from development loans, there are parallel "neglected infections of poverty," like the zoonotic diseases toxocariasis and toxoplasmosis, that have been identified among subordinated groups living in disadvantaged enclaves in wealthy countries like the United States.

CONCLUSION: AGENTS AND OBJECTS OF CHANGE

The premise of this chapter is that humans are inescapably part of a larger ecosystem. As a result, changes we make in the environment—whether they are intentional "improvements" like dams and roads, planned extractions like mountain-top removal to mine for valued metals, or unintentional by-products of economic activities such as global warming or pollution linked to social technologies like automobiles—rebound upon us. Our impact on the environment often goes unnoticed, as we tend to assume that the things we see "in nature" are there "naturally"—that they are not a product of human activity.

Urban parks and many suburbs around the United States, for example, are populated by gray squirrels, a species we tend to take for granted as being naturally present in wooded settings. But beginning in the nineteenth century humans started intentionally releasing squirrels in parks and feeding them to ensure they would remain. According to Etienne Benson (2013), a professor of history who has examined how squirrels came to dwell in urban parks, it was culture, not nature, that was most important. Notes Benson, the movement to fill the parks with squirrels "was related to the idea that you want to have things of beauty in the city, but it was also part of a much broader ideology that says that nature in the city is essential to maintaining people's health and sanity, and to providing leisure opportunities for workers who cannot travel outside the city" (quoted in Estes 2013). Yet squirrels spread various infectious diseases to humans, including bubonic plague (see Figure 4.9). Contact with squirrel feces or urine, as happens in house infestations, can lead to both salmonella and *leptospirosis* infections. Although squirrels are not significant vectors of human infectious disease, their presence in many environments characterizes the "built" aspects of what are often thought to be "natural" settings.

Even changes that we intentionally introduce to control infections can backfire. Antibacterial and antifungal soaps, for example, have become popular in recent years, but in the view of the FDA there is no evidence that they prevent the spread of microbes (Perrone 2013). Triclosan is an ingredient in an about 75 percent of antibacterial liquid soaps and body washes sold in the United States; almost all antibacterial soap bars also contain triclosan or related chemicals. However, recent studies suggest that triclosan may interfere with hormone levels in lab animals, promote the growth of drug-resistant bacteria, and disrupt fragile ecosystems. In March 2010 the European Union banned use of the chemical in any products that come into contact with food, such as containers or utensils. Under the pressure of a mounting campaign by consumer groups led

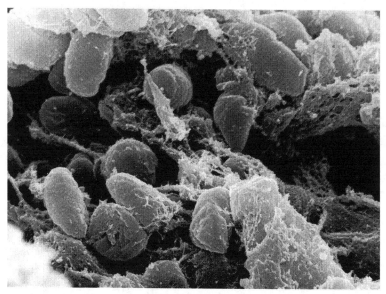

Figure 4.9 Pathogenic agent of bubonic plague. (Photo provided by NIAID)

by Beyond Pesticides and Food and Water Watch, a number of manufacturers have announced they will begin phasing out the chemical from their products.

Overall "the relentless domination of [geographic] space by capital and technology" (Nash 2006:2) has reshaped the planet, producing new risks, ecocrises, and pluralea interactions, some of which trigger or facilitate the spread of infectious diseases. As the extent of our restructuring of all parts of Earth continues at a mounting pace, the consequences of infectious disease are likely to escalate as well.

DISCUSSION QUESTIONS

1. How does deforestation affect infectious diseases?
2. How does loss of biodiversity in some contexts promote human infection?
3. How do both indoor and outdoor air pollution play a role in infectious respiratory diseases?
4. What are some of the Pluralea interactions that promote water-borne infectious diseases?
5. How is mass migration to urban areas affecting the spread of infectious diseases?
6. How might we reduce environmentally mediated infectious diseases?

CHAPTER 5

Emergent, Reemergent, and Drug-Resistant Infectious Agents

"Nothing in the world of living things is permanently fixed."

Hans Zinnser (1935:57)

CHANGING PATHOGENS

Pathogens are in flux. They change along with the environments they inhabit, and human actions now are the primary driver of these transformations. Changing environments and changing human interactions with the environment are contributing to adaptive changes in microorganisms, some of which have very significant repercussions for human health. This chapter examines health-related changes occurring in the microbial world, including:

- the emergence of new human pathogens
- the resurgence of older pathogens
- growing recognition of the role of infectious agents in chronic health conditions
- the development of drug resistance among various pathogenic agents
- the rise of the hospital and other health care settings as critical sites of drug-resistant infection
- continued efforts to eradicate certain pathogens
- the emergent social utility of infection
- the development of engineered pathogens and the field of bioweaponry as sources of growing concern about future infectious disease pandemics

A primary message of this chapter is that our expectations in twentieth century that all infectious diseases could be eliminated from the planet and that our antibiotic arsenal could shield us from harm have fallen victim to new realizations. We have learned a lot about pathogens' ability to breech our pharmaceutical fortress. Research is revealing the role animal reservoirs play in sustaining many infectious agents that cause human disease as well as the self-defeating contributions of our own behaviors in exposing us to new pathogens, renewing older agents of disease, and even intentionally enhancing the virulence of some microbial organisms.

The question we now face is: Have we learned enough to avoid a new era characterized by deadly waves of infectious disease? This question takes us beyond discoveries in microbiology, virology, and infectious disease pathology to anthropological questions about the human capacity for dramatic universally beneficial change.

THE UNEXPECTED TWENTY-FIRST CENTURY

In the 1970s and early 1980s epidemiologists and other health experts at the World Health Organization projected a global convergence of expected human life spans at seventy-five years of age. Events in the world appeared to justify this rosy view of ever-improving estimates for the expected course of human health through time. Countries like the United States, Western Europe nations, and Japan were seeing life expectancy converge at around seventy-five years, whereas developing nations appeared to be gaining control of infectious diseases, an important step in attaining much longer life expectancies for their populations. The landmark eradication during the 1970s of smallpox, one of the most devastating infectious diseases of human childhood, provided powerful support for the prospect of achieving vastly improved global health in the twenty-first century (see Figure 5.1).

Characteristic of this confident worldview is the assertion of the widely respected physician and anthropologist T. Aidan Cockburn in his 1963 book *The Evolution and Eradication of Infectious Diseases*: "We can look forward with confidence to a considerable degree of freedom from infectious diseases at a time not too far in the future. Indeed . . . it seems reasonable to anticipate that within some measurable time . . . all the major infections will have disappeared" (150). A few years later William H. Stewart, the surgeon general of the United States, is alleged to have said during a presentation at the Association of State and Territorial Health Officers in Washington, DC: "It is time to close the book on infectious diseases." In fact, however, Stewart does not appear to have ever made this often-cited statement, but its incorporation into the oral and written history of infectious disease attitudes helps affirm that "the belief that infectious diseases had been successfully overcome was pervasive in biomedical circles" by the late 1960s (Spellberg and Taylor-Blake 2013). By this point funding for infectious disease research had dropped, and attention to infectious diseases in medical school curricula and textbooks was on the wane. In the global north and eventually in the global south as well it was widely presumed in the halls of medicine that infection was on its way to becoming an artifact of history, a minor player in the determination of future human health.

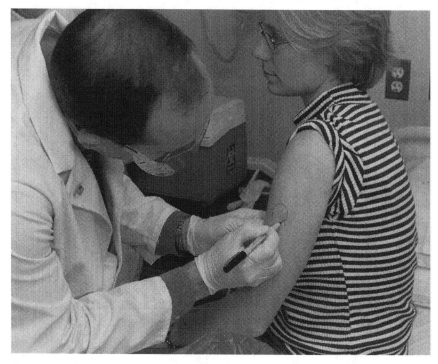

Figure 5.1 Smallpox vaccination. (Photo provided by the University of Rochester School of Medicine)

Of course, this did not occur. With the emergence of HIV disease and many other emergent, reemergent, and resistant infections that followed, we entered into a rather unexpected twenty-first century from an infectious disease perspective. Thinking about infectious disease has shifted dramatically because we recognize that it is likely to play a long and important role in human history (McMichael et al. 2004). Indeed, we now inhabit a world of "viral panic . . . in which a narrative about 'the coming plague'" weighs heavily on people's minds and informs social response to each new wave of influenza or emergence of a novel infectious disease (Herring and Lockerbie 2009:179).

Popular culture reflects and helps amplify this concern. Beginning in 1950, with the movie *Panic in the Streets,* and followed by a host of similar films about menacing infectious disease outbreak, including *Andromeda Strain, Omega Man, The Cassandra Crossing, 12 Monkeys, 28 Days Later, Children of Men, Outbreak, Doomsday,* and *Contagion,* as well as countless zombie movies, the film industry has helped elevate public awareness of and alarm about infectious disease epidemics. Although this heightened focus on infectious disease reflects actual changes going on in human/pathogen relations, perhaps, as Heather Paxson

(2008) has suggested, our uncertainties about how to live with microorganisms echoes our uncertainties and conflicted ideas about how humans ought live with one another or with the other species with which we share the planet.

SINGLE-DISEASE CAMPAIGNS

It is important to realize that although no infectious disease has been totally eradicated in the wild since smallpox in 1978, global public health efforts to eliminate targeted pathogens still go on. The Global Polio Eradication Initiative is an effort spearheaded by the World Health Organization, Rotary International, the US Centers for Disease Control and Prevention, and the UN Children's Fund to achieve a polio-free world. This program, history's largest coordinated public health mobilization, has been implemented in countries around the globe. Since its launch in 1988 it has vaccinated 2.5 billion children against polio infection, many of them multiple times (see Figure 5.2).

By 2003 the initiative appeared to be closing in on its goal, with only 784 new cases reported. The effort soon ran into roadblocks, however. New cases began to rise to about one to two thousand a year; the campaign's objective of eradicating polio suddenly seemed to be in question. In parts of Asia persistent transmission remained highly localized in a few districts, whereas in sub-Saharan

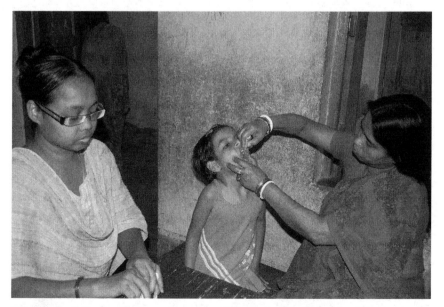

Figure 5.2 Polio eradication campaign, Kolkata, India. (Photo by Gopal Bhattacharee)

Africa polio transmission persisted over a wide area. With continued focused effort by health workers, by 2006 only four countries—Afghanistan, India, Nigeria, and Pakistan—still were unable to stop polio transmission, whereas globally annual new case numbers had decreased by an estimated 99 percent. In 2008 an intensified eradication program was initiated with the goal of finally eliminating the appearance of new cases. Notable accomplishments followed, including a 98 percent immunization rate among children in India. But armed conflict, political instability, the existence of hard-to-reach populations, the adverse impact of rainy seasons on health worker travel, and persistence of poor infrastructure in some countries continued to present challenges. In May 2013 a two-year-old girl from the city of Mogadishu became the first confirmed case of polio in Somalia in more than six years. Within a few months of her diagnosis, however, it was discovered that new polio infections had occurred, paralyzing ninety-five Somali children. Large numbers of children in Somalia still had not been vaccinated because of lack of access to routine preventive care, creating the largest known reservoir of unvaccinated children—approximately 1 million—in a single geographic area in the world (UNICEF 2013).

Cultural factors can also influence eradication efforts. In some countries men cannot work as door-to-door vaccinators because of values about non-relative males interacting with females in a household. Using anthropological research methods, Elisha Renne (2009) examined the community reception and implementation of the polio eradication initiative in Zairia City in northern Nigeria. She found that some residents were fearful that the polio vaccine was harmful and possibly contaminated with HIV virus or antifertility drugs as part of a plot to reduce Moslem populations, a perspective that perceived anti-Moslem motives behind the US wars in Iraq and Afghanistan may have exacerbated. As one woman told Renne, "I heard a rumor that there was something in it. It is said that there is family planning in it. . . . Nothing can change my thinking about this polio vaccine. I don't like it at all" (Renne 2009:522).

For some this fear was caused by previous experience, such as having a child who contracted measles after being vaccinated. Others felt the program was being imposed from outside the community and in a top-down fashion. As a result of such program rejection, in 2003 the governments of three states in northern Nigeria boycotted the polio immunization campaign (see Figure 5.3) and called on parents not to allow their children to be immunized. The boycott lasted for eleven months but was finally resolved through the intervention of the Nigerian federal government and a number of religious leaders (Jegede 2007).

During the eradication campaign, outbreaks in Tajikistan, the Republic of Congo, and China had become more deadly because they hit adults. In some outbreaks half the affected adults died. When the virus infects adults who grew

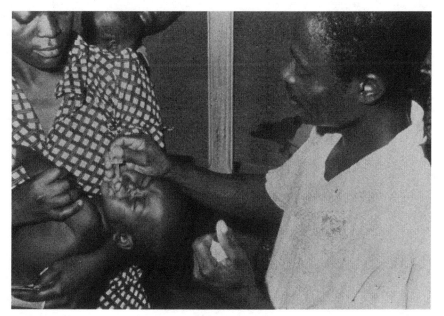

Figure 5.3   Oral poliovirus vaccine administration. (Images from the History of Medicine)

up in areas that previously were polio-free and, as a result, had never been vaccinated, it can be particularly devastating. The mortality rate for polio varies significantly by age of onset: although 2 to 5 percent of children die of infection, among adults the rate is 15 to 30 percent (Atkinson et al. 2012).

Despite enormous challenges and some setbacks, as a result of the coordinated global campaign about 5 million cases of polio in children have been averted (World Health Organization 2012b). Still, anthropologist Svea Closser (2010), who studied and participated in the Global Polio Eradication Initiative, has warned that despite its successes elsewhere, the program is in particular trouble in Pakistan. The reason, she maintains, is not the kinds of cultural factors at play in Nigeria but rather a set of "management issues involving resistance by local level employees of the initiative to mandates handed down by national leaders of the program in the capital city of Abuja." Initiative workers, she found, resist top-down management through "foot-dragging, false compliance, and the use of networks of patron-clientism" (2010:6). Such internal power struggles, conflicted agendas, and corruption—that is to say, social structural factors—and not primarily biological or environmental factors or even cultural beliefs and practices related to fears of the polio vaccination, she argues, have stymied the eradication of polio in Pakistan.

Closser does emphasize one important cultural issue, but it is not one found among the Pakistani recipients of the program. Rather, what she calls a "culture of optimism" pervades entities like the World Health Organization and shapes their implementation efforts. The assumption that everyone should see the inherent value of the eradication program and that "governments will be eager collaborators in eradication programs" characterizes this "culture" (Closser 2010:176). But the Pakistani view of the disease, a perspective held both by members of the general public and health officials, is that there are multiple threats to health in the country; one of every ten children dies before the age of five. In this context Pakistanis do not consider polio, a comparatively rare disease, as urgent as do eradication campaign organizers. Moreover, Closser (2010:170) argues, the "elites who control the governments of many poor countries like Pakistan have little reason to make the health of the poor their first priority, especially given the pressing demands from other quarters." This case demonstrates how the internal politics of inequality and social injustice often trump public health initiatives.

Global political factors also have influenced the eradication program in Pakistan. The intensity of opposition to the campaign increased in 2013 after Pakistan Tehreek-e-Insaf (Pakistan Movement for Justice), a fast-growing nationalist Islamic political party, launched a provaccination drive in Khyber Pakhtunkhwa Province. A number of polio workers in the province were killed in 2013, culminating at the end of the year in the shooting of several health workers at an antipolio vaccination center Pakistan Tehreek-e-Insa operated (Menon 2013). Imran Khan, former cricket star and head of Pakistan Tehreek-e-Insaf, began receiving death threats for supporting the antipolio effort. In response Khan declared that polio workers were mujahid (soldiers of Islam) and announced that he would personally administer the vaccine to children in the province. Adversaries of the vaccination campaign believe that the United States uses the program as a cover for spying. Unsurprisingly, this view was lent greater credibility after it came to light that the CIA had used a Pakistani doctor, Shakil Afridi, to run a (antihepatitis) vaccination campaign as part of military and intelligence efforts to locate Osama Bin Laden in 2011 (Masood 2013).

An even more advanced infectious disease eradication program, led by the Carter Center, founded by former President Jimmy Carter, has targeted Guinea worms, also known as *dracunculiasis*, which comes from the Latin phrase for "afflicted with little dragons." Some interpret the biblical passage in the Book of Numbers 21:6, "And the Lord sent fiery serpents among the people, and they bit the people; and much people of Israel died," as a reference to Guinea worms, although others reject this interpretation (Grove 1994). Guinea worms have been found in the bodies of Egyptian mummies dating to 1000 BCE, suggesting the ancient origin of this human affliction (Tapp 1979). In the mummy labeled

No. 1770 in the museum at Britain's Manchester University, researchers using radiography found evidence of Guinea worm infestation in the female mummy's abdominal wall. The mummy's lower legs had been amputated several weeks before death, possibly because of Guinea worms damage. Symptoms of this "visually spectacular disease" (Moran-Thomas 2013:210) are caused when the adult, impregnated female worm, which averages three feet in length, or about the size of a three-year-old human, begins to migrate downward through the subcutaneous tissues of the sufferer's body, usually to the lower leg or foot. This is achieved by dissolving a pathway through muscle and other tissues, causing intense pain and sometimes leaving the patient crippled for life. At the skin surface the worm provokes the formation of a blister, often compelling suffers to soak their limb in cool, numbing water. On contact with water, such as a pond or stream, the blister breaks, the white-colored worm bores through, and, in an explosive contraction, expels a million or more early stage larvae. These are ingested by water fleas but are not digested (Ruiez-Tiben and Hopkins 2006), so the life cycle repeats itself with subsequent new human infections.

Found today in resource-poor countries, dracunculiasis commonly is transmitted when people drink water contaminated with microscopic water fleas that are infected with larvae of the worm. Acids in the human stomach dissolve the exoskeleton of the water flea, freeing the Guinea worm larvae, which burrows into the intestinal wall, migrates to the connective tissue of the thorax, and begins to grow. Yet anthropological research suggests that people in *endemic* areas may not link Guinea worm and water; rather, as Bernhard Bierlich (1995) found during research in Northern Ghana, Guinea worm may be seen as an innate component of the human body. Instead of an invasive or infectious presence in the body, as understood by epidemiology and biomedicine, among lay people worms are believed to be "in people's blood," a natural feature of human anatomy.

When the anti-Guinea worm campaign began in 1986, there were an estimated 3.5 million cases of the disease distributed across twenty-one countries in Africa and Asia. As with the public health campaign against polio, social conflict has presented a significant challenge to intervention efforts, as has the lack of vaccines or drug therapies for the disease. Reports Michele Barry (2007:2563):

Faced with one of the most imposing barriers to eradication of guinea worm—the civil war in southern Sudan—[former President Jimmy] Carter negotiated a 4-month "guinea worm ceasefire" in 1995, which also allowed public health officials to kick-start Sudan's onchocerciasis [which is second only to trachoma as an infectious cause of blindness] control program. Inadequate security in other countries where guinea worm disease is endemic, inadequate political will on the part of national leaders, and the absence of a "magic bullet" treatment have all presented challenges to the eradication program. Health care initiatives have had to be linked with diplomatic efforts to overcome these challenges.

Cultural issues have triggered some local opposition to the campaign. In Northern Ghana anthropologist Amy Moran-Thomas (2013:207) reports on an incident in which eradication workers sent to treat a local water source with anti-Guinea worm chemicals "were met at the waterway by an angry crowd of local men armed with cutlasses and knives." These individuals believed that the Guinea worm was part of the human body and that it was witchcraft that made the worms come out. Further, they believed that the water treatment chemicals the eradication workers carried enhanced rather then killed the parasite. As anthropologist P. Wenzel Geissler (1998) found in his study of intestinal worms in a Luo community in rural Western Kenya, worms may be culturally meaningful in people's lives, part of the orderly process of birth and decay, emergence and disintegration, as necessary as earth worms breaking down organic matter and forming needed soil for horticulture. In the case of Guinea worms in Ghana, "those who once conserved emerging guinea worms as a sign from their ancestors did not fear the parasite as a symbol of death, but rather often respected it as an angry message from their honored dead, a white finger from another world searing through them in the flesh" (Moran-Thomas 2013:214).

Despite some local opposition, because of the intervention and the participation of thousands of local volunteers (in Ghana alone, 6,500 female Red Cross volunteers assisted the program), by 2012 there were only 542 known cases in four African countries—South Sudan, Chad, Mali, and Ethiopia—representing a 49 percent drop since 2011. By midyear 2013 there remained just 67 known cases of the disease, primarily in isolated locations in South Sudan. According to projections from the Center for Global Development, the campaign has averted more than 80 million cases worldwide since 1986, and Guinea worm infection is poised to be the second human infectious disease to be completely eradicated (Barry 2007; Carter Center 2013). Some see this coming day as a joyous occasion; others, probably not many, oppose the eradication of Guinea worm as an assault on biodiversity.

Although the permanent obliteration of a painful, damaging, or lethal infectious disease is an attractive goal, it remains a significant challenge. Seven major infectious disease eradication programs were launched during the twentieth century—against hookworm, yellow fever, yaws, malaria, smallpox, polio, and guinea worm—but only the effort against smallpox had succeeded by the end of the century. Some other efforts have made significant progress in the early years of the twenty-first century, but the goals of complete eradication remain elusive.

From a cultural perspective one important dynamic created by large global health eradication campaigns is the way in which the appeal of permanently wiping out a major infectious disease has hindered careful analysis of the magnitude of the problems involved in achieving the desired goal. As Closser (2012:397) observes with reference to the Global Polio Eradication Initiative, problems with the campaign "have been minimized or disregarded entirely by international officials." Opposing voices have been ignored, muted, or even more blatantly silenced. With reference to the Bill and Melinda Gates Foundation's embrace of a new campaign to eradicate malaria in 2007, for example, Leslie Roberts and Martin Enserink (2007:1545) noted the importance of the "Gates Effect," the way the considerable sums of money available for health programs from the foundation can "make people reluctant to criticize them or their projects." The Gates' announcement elicited prompt support from the World Health Organization and the Roll Back Malaria Partnership, thereby changing the global health discourse on malaria, "one of the most persistent and pressing global public health problems of our time" (Stratton et al. 2009:854). This surge in enthusiasm emerged from the shadows of the largely failed global malaria eradication efforts implemented in the 1950s through the 1980s (see Figure 5.4).

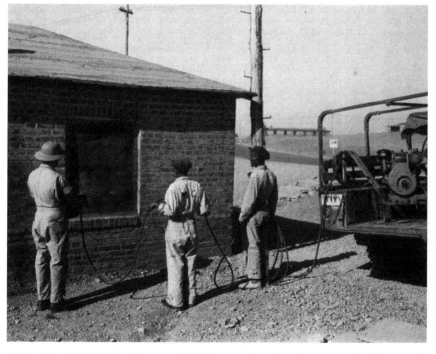

Figure 5.4 1940s Malaria control in Teheran, Iran. (Images from the History of Medicine)

Although great progress has been made in eliminating malaria (with 111 countries now free of the disease and 34 more moving in that direction), the feasibility of completely eradicating this infectious disease in the wild is a hotly debated topic (Liu et al. 2013). Among the many challenges are:

- the emergence of drug and insecticide resistance, what already has occurred in several countries of southeast Asia;
- increasing human mobility, which can lead to the introduction of malaria to previously nonmalarious areas, as has happened in India and parts of Latin America, and to areas where malaria had been eliminated;
- the role of development projects in creating new vector breeding sites;
- the impact of wars and disasters on the disruption of on-the-ground eradication efforts;
- the fact that zoonotic reservoirs endanger all campaigns for eradication of this disease in humans;
- the effects of climate change on the spread of malaria;
- the adverse health care access effects of structural adjustment policies imposed by international lenders on developing countries; and
- the entwinement of malaria and poverty (Stratton et al. 2008).

One hope in the face of these challenges is the development, with financial support from the Melinda and Bill Gates Foundation, of an antimalaria vaccine known as RTS,S. In preliminary human trials the vaccine reduced by 46 percent the number of new malaria cases in children five to seventeen months of age, although only by 27 percent in infants six to twelve weeks (Abdulla et al. 2008; Bejon et al. 2008).

In the successful cases of smallpox, polio, and Guinea worm, in which concerted, large-scale, multicountry public health campaigns have been able to eradicate infection or at least come close, a key factor has been a lack of animal reservoirs for the infectious agent or a lack of direct transmission from animals to people. As discussed in Chapter 3, this does not characterize many infectious diseases that affect humans. For example, influenza, a significant source of human morbidity and mortality, moves among multiple species, including humans, other mammals, and birds and, hence, is not an easy target for this type of eradication campaign.

Assessments of megacampaigns to address infectious disease raise questions about the cost effectiveness of single-disease programs, an issue mentioned in Chapter 1. The Guinea worm initiative incorporated at least some attention to other diseases in the affected populations and in southern Sudan, and as noted, the program facilitated onchocerciasis prevention efforts. In 1996, in fact, the

Carter Center established a program specifically designed to combat oncho-cerciasis in ten countries in Africa and the Americas through health education and distribution of Mectizan, a medicine that can prevent the damaging effects of the disease by killing the worm larvae that causes skin and eye damage. The Guinea worm eradication program has also addressed water quality issues in affected communities, in some cases providing access to safe drinking water where previously none was available. The program also has been linked to in-creased agricultural productivity and food availability in some locations because it reduced labor losses due to Guinea worm infection (Barry 2007).

Critical assessments of infectious disease eradication programs have gener-ated several important lessons, including:

- interventions must be mounted everywhere infection is occurring, no matter how remote or difficult to access a location may be;
- cultural issues must be addressed with sensitivity, including local or even national perceptions that a targeted disease is of comparatively minor importance;
- programs must involve communities and earn local buy-in;
- well-organized monitoring programs must closely track both the disease in question and the implementation and operation of intervention efforts;
- programs must be flexible and act rapidly in response to monitoring find-ings; and
- budgets must account for the recognition that the costs per case will rise sharply as the number of new cases of infection declines. (Hopkins 2013)

Another key lesson is the importance of global political economic relations and inequalities. This factor was highlighted in 2006 when Indonesia staunchly refused to share its samples of the H5N1 avian influenza virus with the World Health Organization's H5N1 influenza surveillance team. Indonesia claimed it possessed *viral sovereignty* over samples collected within the country. Further, the Indonesian government asserted that it would not share its samples until the WHO and wealthier developed countries set up an equitable system for sharing the benefits of knowledge gained from viruses collected in Indonesia, such as the formulation of a vaccine (see Figure 5.5). Central to the Indonesian argument was that samples collected by the WHO surveillance team were distributed to pharmaceutical companies, which, in turn, used them to develop and market patented vaccines that often were too expensive for developing countries to purchase. In response, the countries of the United Nations initiated a series of intergovernment meetings to discuss a new framework for sharing influenza samples (Fidler 2010).

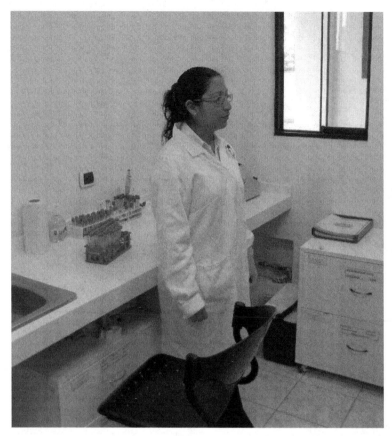

Figure 5.5 Infectious disease researcher, Iquitos, Peru. (Photo by Merrill Singer)

In sum, it is clear that we are not marching along a straight, downhill road that ends at a brighter future world free of infectious disease. Instead, humans, pathogens, and our environments exist together in complex and changing relationships, and the infections and resulting diseases that "plague" humanity will continually emerge, reemerge, and change over time. A more realistic goal focuses on identifying and equitably distributing social, environmental, public health, and medical approaches that limit the adverse impact of pathogens on human health.

DEFINING KEY CONCEPTS: EMERGENT, REEMERGENT, AND RESISTANT

On average three new human infectious diseases are identified every two years, and at least one new pathogen is described in the health literature each week

(GIDEON 2008). Infectious diseases are defined as an *emergent infectious disease* if they are newly identified, have recently appeared in a population, or are rapidly increasing in incidence or geographic range. Emergent infectious diseases can be tracked through daily reports online at ProMED Mail, a website of the International Society for Infectious Diseases (www.promedmail.org). On March 28, 2014, for example, the website reported on a new ebola outbreak in West Africa (see Chapter 7).

In addition to new infectious diseases, various older infectious threats have reemerged as a result of mutation and drug resistance. *Reemergent infectious diseases* are conditions that were contained at one point by available treatment, vaccine, or prevention strategies but have once again begun to increase their incidence and range. Exemplary is tuberculosis (see Figure 5.6). During the period from the late 1980s through the early 1990s there was a dramatic rise in global rates of this ancient disease. In response to the sudden explosion of tuberculosis cases, the World Health Organization declared a Global Tuberculosis Emergency in 1993. This announcement "called into question the assumption that tuberculosis was basically eradicated and unmasked the fact that the illness had never disappeared from impoverished and vulnerable populations" (Koch 2013a:1).

Although various factors contributed to the reemergence of tuberculosis, including the spread of the HIV pandemic, political factors, like the fall of the Soviet Union, were particularly important. In the former Soviet Republic of Georgia, for example, separation from the Soviet Union was ushered in by a collapse of the country's medical infrastructure, a catastrophe that was further exacerbated by civil war and a national energy crisis, "leaving behind facilities lacking basic supplies, health professionals who were 'downsized' or working without salaries, and patients who lost a highly specialized system that they know how to navigate" (Koch 2013b:310). Market-based medical services, mandated by bilateral negotiations with Western countries and multilateral lender institutions, were introduced, based on the assumption that the Soviet system of central planning was inefficient and could be "cleaned up" through an emphasis on the privatization of health care. Privatization as well as other disruptions of social life, however, magnified rather than reduced the spread of tuberculosis in Georgia.

Drug-resistant infectious diseases are infectious agents that, through spontaneous mutation, gene sorting, or epigenetic processes such as dormancy, have successfully adapted to specific pharmaceutical therapies, such antibiotics or other antimicrobial agents, rendering the treatment ineffective. In the contemporary period some infectious agents have gained resistance to multiple drugs, making them especially threatening to host populations. Despite the passage

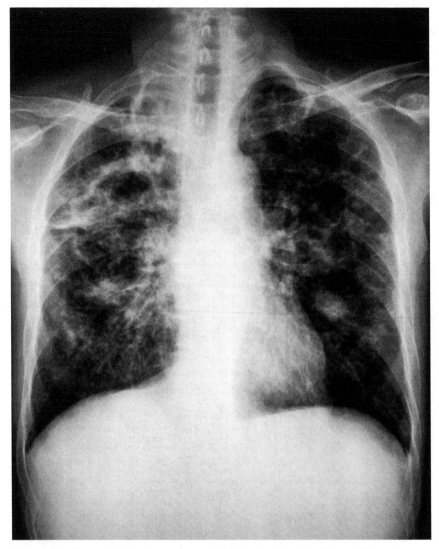

Figure 5.6 X-ray of Mycobacterium tuberculosis infection X-ray. (Photo by Puwadol Vaturawuttichai)

of ten years since researchers learned about the issue of antibiotic resistance, the United States—in contrast with the countries of the European Union—has failed to develop a national plan of response (Bartlett 2013). The Centers for Disease Control and Prevention (2013), however, published an extensive review of the literature on antibiotic resistance in the United States and identified three urgent priority pathogens: carbapenemase-producing Enterobacteriaceae (which can now resist virtually all available antibiotics), *Clostridium difficile* (a source of growing risk in health care facilities among patients made susceptible by antibiotic treatment and the removal of competing gut bacteria), and *Neisseria gonorrhoeae* (the bacterial cause of gonorrhea that, over time, has developed strains that are resistant to first, second, and third generations of antibiotic treatments). The report emphasizes that drug resistance is already a significant problem in the United States. CDC estimates that each year more than 2 million people in the United States suffer from antibiotic-resistant infections, almost twenty-five thousand dying as a result. More broadly it would seem that we live in a time when pathogens have "gone wild" (Singer 2009b). Increasingly they are acting in ways that frustrate human initiative and desire, with adverse consequences for our species. In this they have demonstrated tremendous capacity to adapt to and take advantage of having humans in their world.

These changes in infectious diseases reflect human social alterations, identified in an Institute of Medicine (IOM) assessment of the new face of infectious diseases (Lederber, Shope, and Oaks 1992). Topping the IOM list were five transitions that have occurred in human demographics: (1) population growth, urbanization, and wealth inequality; (2) technology and behavior; (3) economic and land use changes; (4) international travel and the global flow of commerce and commodities; and (5) breakdowns in public health programs.

Shifts in human demographics include unprecedented population growth, increased rates of urbanization globally, and expansion in the number and size of densely crowded, resource-poor slum areas that are now home to impoverished urban residents in many countries. Infectious diseases such as dengue and cholera, characterized by intensified lethality and new more virulent strains, are spreading in vulnerable populations in these social environments. Changes in human behavior, including more lenient sexual practices among youth and young adults and the global spread of injection drug use, contributed to the prevalence of HIV disease as well as other diseases like hepatitis.

The second factor on the IOM list is behavioral changes involving technology and industry, including the emergence of new medical technologies that facilitate the transmission of hospital-acquired infections, overuse and misuse of antibiotics that contribute to the rise of drug-resistant pathogens, and changes in food production that promote outbreaks of food-borne infections. Modifications in the rearing, slaughtering, and processing of cattle for meat and increases in the consumption of ground beef have contributed, for example, to outbreaks of *Escherichia coli* infections. Common practices in the poultry industry are no less a problem. Prior to hatching, chicken eggs are injected with a mixture of vaccines and antibiotics intended to lessen common infectious diseases in the high-volume factory production of 40 billion chickens a year for meat globally. Despite these efforts—or because of the development of drug-resistance in a growing number of pathogens—in 2012 580,000 people in the UK developed *campylobacter* infections, leading to 18,000 hospitalizations and 140 deaths.

Research by Antonio Vieira and colleagues (2011) found significant correlation between resistance to various antibiotics in chickens and E. coli bloodstream infections, which they believe supports the view that bloodstream infections in people are derived from poultry food sources. Based on further analysis, this research team concluded that "the ongoing use of these antimicrobial drugs in mass therapy and prophylaxis should be urgently examined and stopped, particularly in poultry . . . worldwide" (Collignon et al. 2013:1339). Despite such warnings, including frequently expressed public health concerns about both the therapeutic overuse of antibiotics in livestock populations and the nontherapeutic use of penicillin-tetracycline-based and other antibiotics to bolster animal growth and weight gain, the US Food and Drug Administration (FDA) continued to allow dozens of antibiotics to be used in livestock feed. The widespread use of these chemical agents in livestock production, aquaculture, and agriculture has been linked to the emergence of drug-resistant infections in farm settings and the spread of drug-resistant infections in humans (Heuer et al. 2009; Silbergeld, Graham, and Price 2008). In 2014, with public pressure mounting, the FDA announced that most pharmaceutical companies agreed to comply voluntarily with a request to phase out the use of antibiotics as a mechanism designed to promote production in cattle, hog, and poultry production in the United States (Food and Drug Administration 2013). Actual compliance and its effects on rates of microbial drug resistance will be monitored over time.

Sudden outbreaks of infectious diseases also are being tied to practices in other industries. In 1976, for example, there was an outbreak of a severe form of pneumonia at the annual American Legion convention in Philadelphia that was subsequently linked with outbreaks in other human-made environments such as cruise ships. The new disease was christened *Legionnaire's Disease* or Legionellosis and is a potentially fatal form of pneumonia. After the first outbreak it was found to be caused by a bacteria, Legionella, that lives naturally in the environment and thrives in warm water and warm, damp places. In humans the new disease is transmitted by breathing in the bacteria in very fine droplets of water called aerosols. The outbreak of Legionnaire's disease was followed in 1980 by a sudden surge of acute bacterial infections related to superabsorbent tampon use, and occasionally to the use of contraceptive sponges that came to be known as *toxic shock syndrome.* Symptoms of the disease have a sudden onset and proved in some cases to be fatal. A toxin produced by several species of Streptococcus bacteria cause the disease.

Economic development and changes in land use patterns was the third factor on the IOM list of social changes associated with the resurgence of infectious diseases in modern times. Completion of the Aswan Dam in Egypt in 1976, which allowed control of flooding on the Nile River, for example, created a breeding ground for freshwater snails that carry the parasite that causes schistosomiasis. People become infected through repeated contact with snail-dwelling water during irrigation work, fishing, farming, washing of clothes and household utensils, bathing, and recreational activities. Most emergent infectious human diseases are of animal origin and reflect changes in land use and contact with pathogen-bearing animals. As a result of human restructuring of local environments, "formerly isolated microbiological reservoirs of . . . rain forests and mountains have been inadvertently integrated into the food economy of cities—and . . . this 'undercurrent of opportunity' has [led to] a series of viral leaps from animals to humans" (Davis 2005:58). Expanded rice production in Asia, for example, was associated with increased human contact with rodents that served as vectors for the *Hantaan virus* and rising rates of hantaviral disease. This disease, transmitted by human contact with rodents, their urine, or droppings, can cause hantavirus pulmonary syndrome, a potentially fatal condition.

Fourth on the IOM list was the significant rise that has occurred in international travel and the global flow of commerce and commodities. Animals caught or raised in one region of the world and shipped to international markets in the pet trade or for scientific experiments, for example, have contributed to disease outbreaks in various locations. An outbreak of monkeypox in the United States in 2003, for instance, ultimately was traced to a store that had imported Gambian pouched rats for sale to customers desiring exotic pets. Shipment of animals from Africa to China for the food trade was the source of the human SARS epidemic.

A breakdown in public health measures is the final item on the IOM list. In the United States this breakdown reflects the assumption that noncontagious chronic diseases rather than infectious diseases had become the primary concern of health promotion and treatment efforts. Undervaccination for common infectious diseases also occurred as a result of both underfunding of preventive health programs and growing popular concerns about immunization as a cause of autism or other disorders among children. As a result, a level of protection from infectious disease was allowed to slip away, leaving public health and biomedicine poorly prepared for the emergence of new infectious diseases, reemergence of older infectious diseases, and appearance of drug-resistant infectious agents. Together, these far-reaching social changes discussed, which contributed to a dramatic level of environmental transformation, lay the groundwork for a new era of infectious disease, one we all now inhabit. In this era there has been a new "confluence of disease pools" (McNeil 1976) involving the global spread and concentration of infectious agents found historically at separate sites around the world.

The threat to human health from emergent infectious diseases includes emergent infections among wildlife. Research indicates that quite similar factors promote the advent of disease in both human and wildlife populations. There are several implications of emergent infectious disease (EID) among wildlife:

> emerging wildlife diseases cause direct and indirect loss of biodiversity and add to the threat of zoonotic disease emergence. Since human environmental changes are largely responsible for their emergence, the threats wildlife EIDs pose to biodiversity and human health represent yet another consequence of anthropogenic influence [e.g. habitat destruction, fragmentation, encroachment] on ecosystems. (Daszak, Cunningham, and Hyatt 2001:103)

In addition to loss of biodiversity, as seen in infections in Caribbean coral reef populations that have been linked to pollution from Florida (Boyer, Fourqurean, and Jones 1999) and the emergence of zoonotic diseases that began in animal populations but spread to humans, there is also the issue of emergent plant and animal infectious diseases that affect human food sources (see Figure 5.7) and threaten global food security (see Chapter 3; also Anderson et al. 2004). As summarized by Fiona Tomley and Martin Shirley,

> Threats from old and new pathogens [will] continue to emerge, fuelled by changes in the environment (climate, hydrology, disruption of ecosystems, etc.), in agriculture and food production (intensive systems of husbandry, farming monoculture, food processing, etc.) and in the demography and connectivity of the modern "global" village (population growth, urbanization, international trading, world tourism and rapid transportation). (2009:2637)

The appearance in 2012 of a new coronavirus, a member of the family of viruses that includes SARS, affirms this prediction. First reported in Saudi Arabia, the new threat to human health was called Middle East respiratory syndrome (MERS), and it is associated with severe acute infection of the lungs and resultant breathing problems. Of identified cases, 30 percent have died of the disease. Beyond Saudi Arabia, the disease has now been identified in at least seven other mostly contiguous countries in the Arabian Peninsula. The first case of MERS in the United States was confirmed in May 2014 in an individual traveling from Saudi Arabia to Indiana; a second imported case was identified shortly thereafter in another traveler going to Florida from Saudi Arabia. Both of these individuals were health care workers who lived and worked in Saudi Arabia; through treatment both survived. By June 2014 the World Health Organization

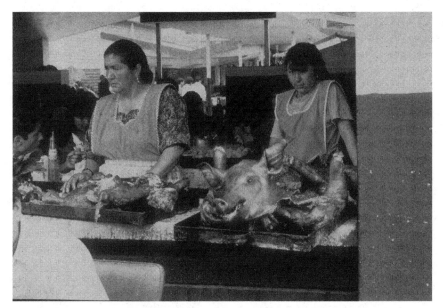

Figure 5.7 Unrefrigerated meat for sale in open air market in Quito, Ecuador. (Photo by Linda Whiteford)

(2014a) reported just over 700 diagnosed cases of MERS and 252 deaths. Based on genetic sequence research, it appears that the virus spread from camels to humans. Additionally, a study of domestic livestock in Saudi Arabia found no antibodies to MERS in sheep, goats, or chickens but found a high prevalence in dromedary camels (Hemida et al. 2013). Consequently the disease may be more common in people who work closely with camels, with subsequent and unsustained human-to-human transmission, including to individuals with no contact with camels.

CHRONIC DISEASES WITH UNEXPECTED INFECTIOUS DISEASE ORIGINS

There was a time, before the 1960s, when infectious and chronic diseases were seen as categorically different kinds of human maladies. Cancer, for example, might be caused by human behavior (e.g., smoking or otherwise consuming tobacco products), industrial air pollution, toxic exposure, genetics or various other factors, but it was not seen as an infectious disease. As our understanding of pathogens has grown, that way of seeing the world of disease is now history. Using available statistics on estimated cancer incidence in the year 2008, Catherine de Martel and coworkers (2012), for example, found that of almost

13 million cancers that occurred in the world that year, 16 percent, or about 2 million new cases, were attributable to infections. Percentages differed by the wealth of the reporting nations. The percentage of cancers linked to infectious agents was highest (23 percent) in developing countries and lowest in developed countries (7 percent). Peak levels were found in sub-Saharan Africa (33 percent). The significance of infectious agents also ranges by cancer site within the body, from 89 percent of cervix cancers attributable to papillomavirus to 1 percent of leukemias attributable to human T-cell lymphotrophic virus (Pisani et al. 1997). A number of different infectious agents have now been linked to cancer, including HCV, HIV, *Helicobacter pylori*, schistosomes, *liver flukes*, and human *T-cell lymphotrophic virus*. With some cancers, such as Epstein-Barr virus and nasopharyngeal cancer, and human herpesvirus-8 and Kaposi's sarcoma, all cases involve the infectious agent. In other cases, such as Epstein-Barr virus and Burkitt/Hodgkin lymphoma, the infectious agent cannot be found in all tumors but the pathogen has been found to play a role in accelerating cancer onset.

Pathogens that remain hidden in human cells in a latent form develop slowly, and only accumulate over the course of decades may be particularly important in the development of chronic diseases like cancer. Generally cancers arise in human cells through a multistep process known as carcinogenesis, involving the accumulation of a series of genetic accidents before cells becomes malignant and multiply to form a tumor. In the case of pathogen-associated tumors one of the damaging events within cells is infection. In human cells infectious agents contribute to carcinogenesis in several ways, including triggering chronic inflammation, inserting a gene—known as an *oncogene*—into the genome of the host cell, inhibiting the body's tumor suppression mechanisms, and stimulating immunosuppression. In the case of schistosomiasis, for example, the development of cancer in infected individuals is tied to a pathogen-induced chronic inflammatory reaction. Bladder cancer associated with *Schistosoma haematobium,* which is most common in Africa and the Eastern Mediterranean, stems from the pathogen's occupation of the small blood vessels that drain the bladder and the ureters, tubes that convey urine from the kidneys to the bladder.

Some pathogens that cause chronic diseases may be transferred between people in ways that previously were unrecognized as routes of infectious disease transmission, including those that are passed from father to child through sperm (a potential cause of miscarriages), persist in a woman's endometrium (the lining of the inside of the uterus), dwell in women's amniotic fluid (causing the birth of preterm infants), and infect nursing children through breast milk (as seen in HIV, which is linked to cancer onset by its suppression of the immune system).

Specific chronic diseases like gastric cancer and peptic ulcer are now routinely linked to infection. Although in the past it was believed that consuming especially spicy food or prolonged life stress were the primary causes of these two conditions, during the 1980s two Australian physicians, Barry Marshall and Robin Warren, discovered that they are proximally caused by a bacteria, *Helicobacter pylori*. This is a spiral-shaped pathogen that lives in the mucus layer of the stomach, duodenum, or, less frequently, the esophagus, and is a very common source of infection around the world, especially in developing countries, where rates of up to 80 percent of adults have been detected (Bardhan 1997). In the United States about 20 percent of people under forty years of age and half of those over sixty years are believed to be infected. Distribution is social class related; in South Korea, for example, researchers have found that 12 percent of children among upper-class families, 25 percent among middle-class families, and 41 percent among lower-class families are infected with H. pylori (Malaty et al. 1996). One feature of socioeconomic status, household crowding and density of community living conditions, has been found to be a primary determinant in the acquisition of H. pylori infection (Khalifa, Sharaf, and Zaiz 2010).

Survival in the severe, acidic-rich environment of the stomach is possible for H. pylori because it secretes an enzyme called urease, which converts the chemical urea into ammonia and carbon dioxide, neutralizing the surrounding acids of the stomach. Also, the pathogen burrows into the less-acidic mucus lining of the stomach, which the body's immune cells cannot penetrate. In this location the pathogen manipulates body cells, allowing it to acquire micronutrients (e.g., iron) from them. Moreover, the pathogen chemically compromises normal immune response, further protecting it from elimination by the body.

When Warren and Marshall began to publish their findings on the pathogenic origin of ulcers and gastritis, they were met with strong skepticism and derision from many of their peers. To prove that H. pylori causes gastritis, Marshall drank a beaker of the microorganisms and, within a few days, began suffering from nausea and vomiting. Examination revealed signs of gastritis and the presence of H. pylori. He was pushed to this rather extreme approach because H. pylori does not infect readily available laboratory animals like mice or rats. In 2005 Warren and Marshall received the Nobel Prize for their research showing the infectious origin of what had previously been conceived of as a set of chronic noninfectious diseases. In assessing why he came to be a part of the discovery of the role of H. pylori in chronic diseases, Marshall (2006) has suggested it was because he came to the work as a generalist within medicine with no background in gastroenterology and, hence, was not trained to limit his thinking to the reigning dogmas of the day.

In recent years we have witnessed a similar transition in thinking about the cause of cervical cancer, anal cancer, and, more recently, some types of oral cancer, for which *human papilloma virus (HPV)* has been identified as the proximal culprit. In this instance the pathogen is sexually transmitted, through vaginal or anal penetration, genital–to-genital contact, and oral sex and, hence, is dependent upon specific intimate human behaviors. In the United States HPV infection is found in at least half of sexually active individuals but not necessarily involving the few strains of the virus most commonly linked with cancer, as there are more than forty different strains of the virus.

Notably, men who have sex with other men are about seventeen times more likely to develop HPV-related anal cancer than are men who only have sex with women (Stine 1999). Gay and bisexual men have been found to have higher rates of both HPV infection and HPV-related disease than their heterosexual counterparts. Studies that include primarily heterosexual men generally have found that 50 percent or less are infected with HPV (Dunne et al. 2006). By contrast, an estimated 61 percent of HIV-negative and 93 percent of HIV-positive gay and bisexual men have anal HPV infections (Palefsky et al. 1998). Men who have sex with men are also at increased risk for anal cancer compared to the general population of men (Palefsky and Rubin 2009). In an Australian study using a community-based sample of 316 men who have sex with men, Claire Vajdic and coresearchers (2009) found near-universal anal infection with HPV, including infection with a wide variety of strains of the virus and co-infections with multiple strains. Anal infection, however, was more prevalent in HIV-positive men than their HIV-negative counterparts.

Overall, approximately 20 million people in the United States are currently infected with HPV. Fortunately there is a vaccine to prevent this disease, although few men get it and ethnic minority women are less likely to get it or to get the full regime than are white women. Public concerns about the side effects of the vaccine have been voiced, an increasingly common issue in a world that characterized by anxieties about infection as well as about the vaccines and medicines developed to contain them. However, in a study in a primarily Latino population in Los Angeles involving parents of seven- to eleven-year-old girls, the most frequent reasons given for not receiving vaccination were desire for more information about the vaccine and inability to attend a clinic when the vaccine was being provided, not outright opposition to vaccination (Yeganeh, Curtis, and Kuo 2010). A second study comparing Latina and non-Latina mothers on this issue found that 97 percent of Latino mothers compared to 68 percent of non-Latino mothers agreed to vaccinate their daughters, whereas 92 percent of Latino mothers and 77 percent of non-Latino mothers agreed to vaccinate their sons (Watts et al. 2009). The existing body of studies suggests that women in the United States are generally willing to have their children vaccinated for HPV, especially if that recommendation comes from a physician who addresses parent concerns and uncertainties (Brewer and Fazekas 2007).

Anthropologist Fouzieyha Towghi (2013:330) studied HPV vaccination of girls in India. The deaths of six girls who had been vaccinated during a free vaccine demonstration project provoked considerable public concern. The pharmaceutical manufacturer of the vaccine asserted that the deaths were not caused by the vaccine but were due to malaria, snakebite, or suicide. The non-government organization responsible for implementing the program also denied that the vaccine was risky, claiming that it had been successfully administered in many locations. Indian health activists, however, questioned the value of the demonstration project and the way the vaccination program was being implemented, seeing the program as a threat to India's public health system and to women's health. Among the popular beliefs that developed was that Indians were being used as guinea pigs to test the HPV vaccine. Health activists were successful in having HPV vaccination promotion advertisements removed from TV and newspapers on the grounds that the drug manufacturers were falsifying the relationship between the vaccine, HPV, and cervical cancer when they claimed that the HPV vaccine was "a vaccine against cervical cancer." In the view of health activists, thinking that the vaccine offers permanent protection from cervical cancer leads women to avoid the preventive screenings that can detect cancer and trigger early intervention. In Towghi's (2013) assessment, "Through their Indian subsidiaries, pharmaceutical corporations are creating a market for the HPV vaccine . . . by initially introducing it into public health programs through free donations." Ultimately, the goal is to establish a pattern of routine vaccination and large-scale vaccine sales to the government and private clinics that will prove highly profitable to the pharmaceutical manufacturer.

Some of the cancers that have now been linked to infectious diseases have high frequencies in particular populations. Bladder cancer, for example, is especially common in Egypt, somewhat more so among men than women, leading to almost eight thousand deaths per year, a strikingly higher rate than in most other parts of the world (Hemmaid et al. 2013). Hepatitis C (HCV), which is common in Egypt, infecting 10 to 20 percent of the population, is now a recognized etiologic agent of bladder carcinomas. Research by Kamel Hemmaid and coworkers (2013) found that HCV-associated bladder tumors occur among younger individuals more than non-HCV-associated tumors. However, the actual route by which HCV facilitates the development of cancer is not yet understood.

The global epicenter of bile duct cancer (cholangiocarcinoma) is a region along the Chi River basin in Northeastern Thailand. In this area infection with *Opisthorchis viverrini,* or parasitic liver fluken is endemic. O. viverrini is a foodborne parasite that is believed to infect more than 40 million people, primarily in Southeast Asia. Raw fish, the immediate host for the parasite, is a staple of the diet in that part of Southeast Asia. In the Chi River area most people have been found to be infected with liver flukes. Although the parasite can be effectively treated with the antihelmintic drug praziquantel, people tend to be re-infected because of their continued consumption of raw fish (Watanapa and Watanapa 2002). Infected individuals pass the eggs of the fluke in their feces, which may be deposited or washed into fresh water sources and continue the complex life stages of the parasite, sequentially involving snail, fish, and human or other fish-eating animal hosts.

Various studies have shown that spouses have a significantly greater chance of developing the same chronic disease as their partners, a pattern that may best be explained by way of an infectious cause, even if the active pathogen has not yet been identified. For example, spouses of people who suffer *sarcoidosis,* an inflammation of the lymph nodes, lungs, liver, eyes, skin, or other tissues, have an incidence rate for this condition that is a thousand times greater than would be expected by chance. Similarly, British researchers have found that men whose spouses suffer from hypertension have a two-fold increased risk of hypertension. They also found that the risk for both male and female study participants persisted after adjustment for other variables, such as diet, suggesting a possible role of pathogens (Hippisley-Cox and Pringle 1998). Further, some research suggests that *cytomegalovirus,* a common infectious virus that is found among 60 to 99 percent of adults worldwide, may be a pathogenic agent cause of high blood pressure (Zhang et al. 2011).

Although the number of specific chronic diseases linked to pathogenic agents remains limited, it is clear that the historic boundaries between infectious and chronic diseases are much more porous than was believed in the past. As Chapter 6 will show in greater detail, one additional group of chronic diseases being heavily investigated in terms of the potential role infectious agents is neurodegenerative conditions, including Alzheimer's disease and multiple sclerosis.

COMMUNICATING WITH EMERGENT INFECTIOUS DISEASES

We have established that infectious diseases are biocultural and biosocial: they exist not just in the bodies of hosts but also in the matrix of how we understand them and communicate about them culturally. These cognitive frameworks are attached to various culturally constituted emotional responses. As anthropologists Ann Herring and Alan Swedlund (2010:1) observe, "As knowledge about pathogens is produced in laboratories and disseminated through various media to enter public consciousness ... anxiety is rekindled about mortality on the scale of historic plagues." The production and dissemination of knowledge about infectious diseases in societies involves the development of cultural narratives about what the disease is, what causes it, where it comes from, what its effects are, and what to do about it. People engage with such narratives when they or those around them fall ill. This process is especially important in the case of emergent infectious diseases, as misinformation can travel as quickly in the world today as accurate information, triggering emotional reactions that are subsequently hard to suppress. Exemplary is the extensive stigma attached in the early years to HIV disease, much of it influenced by popularized inaccuracies about HIV.

Emergent infectious diseases outbreaks are, as a result, social events that can have utility, including being used to advance social agendas and assert social power. As researchers have documented in detail (see also Chapter 7), governments use them as opportunities for imposing mechanisms of population and behavioral control and authority. For example, authorities often are quick to implement laws intended to punish behaviors said to spread new diseases. With regard to HIV/AIDS, the Center for HIV Law and Policy (2010:1) observes,

> From the beginning of the HIV/AIDS epidemic, stigma and fear have fueled mistreatment of people living with HIV. One of the more troubling and persistent issues for people with HIV has been the prospect [and practice] of criminal prosecution for acts of consensual sex and for conduct, such as spitting or biting, that poses no significant risk of HIV transmission.

One pernicious trend from the standpoint of civil liberties is the indefinite detention of an individual with HIV infection under various state sexually violent predator confinement statutes. Such statutes have been upheld by the Supreme Court in *Kansas v. Hendricks* and have been applied to persons with HIV based on sexual activity posing no risk of HIV transmission (Center for HIV Law and Policy 2010).

Infectious diseases also get used socially beyond the realm of governance, as in conservative social responses to the rise of feminism. Individuals and groups who feel that a women's full-time job is in the home raising children and that society fell into decline when women began extending their lives beyond the domestic sphere and entering the workplace in large numbers sometimes express antifeminist sentiments in portrayals of daycare centers as hubs of both older and newer infectious diseases. Thus David Mills (2000:165–166) suggests that "the typical daycare center ... spreads far more infection and communicable disease than the county jail." Similarly, in *The War Against the Family*, William Gairdner (1992:342) itemizes a litany of "daycare-related illnesses" before expressing his assessment of the damage done to society by feminism, whereas Gallagher (1998) maintains that a daycare center is a "breeding ground for infectious disease." By representing daycare centers as "the open sewers of twentieth century" (Robertson 2003:87) and implying that the irresponsible women who put their children in such places are subjecting them to grave threats from monstrous pathogens, opponents of feminism have sought to use infection among children as a means of reestablishing traditional gendered power hierarchies. As this example suggests, the nature of contagion allows it to be adopted as a powerful metaphor for moral campaigns about the threats to the social order. Although there is little doubt that daycare centers—or elementary schools, for that matter—play a role in the spread of childhood infectious diseases, research also shows that children who are walled off from such exposure are more apt to develop autoimmune disorders and allergies.

Emergent infectious diseases, in short, have social utility because, to use an expressive form common in anthropology introduced by Claude Levi-Strauss, they are "good to communicate with." Charles Briggs, in his examination of media coverage of the cholera epidemic in Peru in the early 1990s, observes that press reports on the pending epidemic believed to be spreading from Venezuela "merged images of a frightening, highly infectious disease with images of three populations 'at high risk' for being infected with cholera and for infecting others: the poor; street vendors of food and drink; and indigenous people" (2010:42). These ideas were being expressed in the media even before any cases were reported in Peru. By the time the disease did enter the country, in the public mind cholera was firmly constructed as "a hybrid object—[a] fusion of biomedical pathogens and human 'vectors,'" with the latter comprising subordinate social classes and groups reaffirmed by the epidemic as grave threats to society. The source of media information about the disease was the government, especially the National Office of Epidemiology, which gave reporters regular authoritative updates. Knowledge about the disease, in short, was produced at the top, and reporters and media audiences were consumers of government-shaped messages about hygiene, food procurement, food preparation, and related topics. In effect the epidemic became an arena for the elite of the citizenry to teach proper behavior based on the control and use of disease information (see Figure 5.8).

At the same time, the epidemic allowed the government to imply that poor sectors of society were unsanitary citizens, a designation with significant implications for accessing political and social rights. In their book *Stories in the Time of Cholera: Racial Profiling During a Medical Nightmare*, Charles Briggs and Clara Mantini-Briggs (2004) further analyze the cultural construction in the media that contrasted sanitary and unsanitary citizens in the context of the Venezuelan cholera epidemic. Sanitary citizens were people in society whose appropriate behaviors and mental dispositions seemed to situate them out of the deadly reach of cholera. These people, who were accorded depth and complexity in their

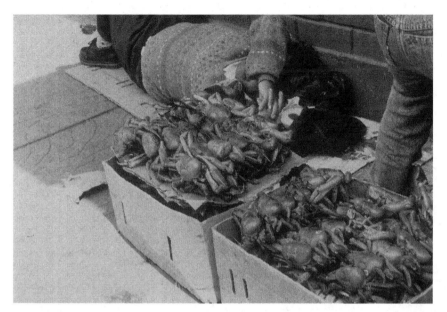

Figure 5.8 In the midst of the cholera epidemic crabs for sale in the open air market in Quito, Ecuador. (Photo by Linda Whiteford)

portrayals, were described in terms of a full package of normative economic, cultural, familial, legal, educational, sexual, and medical characteristics. They were identified by their status as proper Venezuelans rather than being merely depicted in terms of a single characteristic, such as social class. Implied in media coverage was the notion that the state had an obligation to protect them from cholera coming from elsewhere in society. By contrast, unsanitary citizens were narrowly portrayed as lacking the complex of features that would allow them to fit the model of modern citizens; rather, they seem to be "intrinsically linked to a particular package of premodern or 'marginal' characteristics—poverty, criminality, ignorance, illiteracy, promiscuity, filth, and lack of the relations and feelings that define the nuclear family" (Briggs and Mantini-Briggs 2004:33). Their complexity was compressed; they were simply the poor, but implied in this assertion was an ominous quality of danger. Consequently they could be denied access to jobs, legal protections, and even human dignity. Moreover, unsanitary citizens were a specific health threat, and the state had an obligation to protect them "from their own natures and desires—in short, from themselves" (Briggs and Mantini-Briggs 2004:33). Additionally, the state had a responsibility to isolate unsanitary citizens in order to protect sanitary citizens. Written between the lines of these media portrayals were affirmations of the appropriateness of a class-divided and strikingly unequal social structure.

One type of communication that infectious diseases have been especially good for is blaming. Various "blame framing devices" (Blakely 2006) have been invoked in infectious disease epidemics, including those that rely on gender, race/ethnicity, sexual orientation, lifestyle, morality, and type of government. Thus, European Christians burned Jews as the alleged cause of the plague during the Middle Ages; in England and America the Irish were blamed for mid-nineteenth-century cholera outbreaks; the Chinese and Mexicans were deemed responsible for the emergence of plague in California early in the twentieth century; sexually transmitted disease epidemics repeatedly have been attributed to women with loose morals; gay men have been accused of starting the HIV disease; and Mexico was blamed for the 2009 H1N1 influenza epidemic (Alcabes 2009). In the case of the Venezuela cholera epidemic described by Briggs and Mantini-Briggs (2004), the epidemic was racialized, as government and public health officials sought to deflect blame away from themselves and social institutions and onto the victims of the disease. Indigenous culture was blamed because of claims that "it led its bearers to actively reject biomedicine" (Briggs and Mantini-Briggs 2004:42). More broadly, in times of global pandemics there has emerged what anthropologist/physician Paul Farmer (1992) has called an active "geography of blame," involving accusations across national, class, and other borders. These accusations, embedded in the discourse of infectious diseases, have been used to justify national, racial, cultural, and similar maginalizations of people said to be responsible for causing a deadly outbreak.

EMERGENT INFECTIOUS DISEASE AND GLOBAL GOVERNANCE

The effects of expanding trade and travel in increasing the permeability of national borders to the spread of infectious disease has raised concerns about international cooperation, especially in response to emergent pandemics like influenza and SARS. In reaction to the SARS epidemic, in particular, UN member nations, through the World Health Organization, implemented a revised set of International Health Regulations (IHR) in 2005, updating a prior set of protocols that only focused on four diseases. The IHR is a legally binding agreement involving various rights and obligations for nation-states that is intended to enhance coordination during a multinational public health emergency, an increasingly common event in the modern world. In agreeing to the IHR, member nations granted WHO the power to declare the existence of public health emergencies of international concern and to issue recommendations on how countries should best deal with such emergencies. The IHR obligations included mandatory participation in disease surveillance and response; notification and verification to WHO of specified public health events and risks; implementation of health measures for international travelers; requirements for sanitary conditions and services at international ports, airports, and ground crossings; and development of minimum public health facilities for disease surveillance, assessment, response, and reporting for a broad range of risks.

The IHR is considered a governance strategy that is unprecedented in the history of international law and public health because it sends "powerful messages about how human societies should think about and collectively govern their vulnerabilities to serious, acute disease events in the twenty-first century" (Fidler 2005:388). Central to the IHR message is the need in our highly interconnected world to shift from state-centric approaches to unified global responses.

An example of the IHR in operation occurred in the fall of 2008, when Sudan reported an outbreak of Rift Valley fever to the WHO, which, in turn, transmitted information about coordinated prevention and control of this infectious disease to all of the 194 ministries of health of UN member nations. Rift Valley fever is a mosquito-borne viral disease that primarily affects animals but also can strike humans. In accordance with IHR guidelines, the WHO helped to coordinate the response efforts to Rift Valley fever contributed by multiple international organizations, reviewed national action plans, and allocated resources to increase detection of disease spread as well as strengthen disease control. The IHR also was invoked in efforts to eliminate barriers to the polio eradication campaign in Northern Nigeria.

Despite its emphasis on working toward a shared international goal of emergent disease control, implementation of the IHR has been hampered by various constraints, including the sense among less powerful nations that inequality in the world prevails and that they continue to be on the losing end of global economic competition for wealth and resources:

> For resource-constrained countries, which attract few tourists and export minimum commodities, it is perhaps understandable that the IHR are accorded minimal priority. Rather, a large proportion of policy makers in resource-constrained countries perceive that the emphasis of the IHR on the international spread of disease evinces little concern regarding the burden of infectious diseases on the nations in which they occur. This perception is fueled by a long-standing history of selective application and implementation of global health policies in order to support the interests of countries in the developed world (Tomori 2010:205).

In other words, the IHR emphasis is not on the social causes of infectious disease outbreaks but on the spread of diseases across national boundaries and, hence, on the health risks poorer nations present to wealthier ones. Traditionally wealthy states have supported international infectious disease controls as long as they did not interfere with their engagement in global trade, as this is an important source of the flow of wealth into dominant nations. At the same time, less powerful nations traditionally have feared reporting emergent disease outbreaks, as this often has prompted the imposition of unwarranted boycotts and other economically crippling restrictions. Although the IHR introduced a dramatically new paradigm into global infectious disease response efforts, reactions to its implementation have varied based on differing socioeconomic priorities and national perceptions of who most benefits from such international regulation.

An important test of the IHR occurred during the 2009 H1N1 influenza pandemic. An independent review of the WHO response to the pandemic voiced several criticisms, including the decision to keep confidential the names of the people who served on the IHR Emergency Committee that was responsible for providing advice to the director-general of the WHO during the pandemic. This criticism stemmed from a suspicion that there was undue influence from the pharmaceutical industry on the committee. WHO's overstatement of what turned out to be the actual level of health risk the pandemic presented resulted in countries spending billions of dollars to purchase vaccines and antivirals like oseltamivir and zanamivir from already burdened health budgets. Because of the limited impact of the pandemic, many of these drugs wound up unused, sitting in warehouses around the world. As the editor-in-chief of the *British Medical Journal* stated in an editorial, "Given the scale of public cost and private profit, it would seem important to know that WHO's key decisions were free from commercial influence" (Godlee 2010). As it turned out, several scientists who advised the World Health Organization on planning for an influenza pandemic had done paid work for pharmaceutical companies that had developed oseltamivir and zanamivir and stood to reap significant financial gains from the consultation they provided (Cohen and Carter 2010). This case reveals a further challenge to implementing of coordinated global efforts to respond to emergent and reemergent infectious disease outbreaks and the conflicts of interest inherent when the WHO and the global public health system rely on scientific experts who derive income from their work for the pharmaceutical industry. As this suggests, public health, even in confronting emerging infectious diseases, is rarely free of the disruptive effects of conflicted political and economic relationships.

ANTIBIOTICS: THE STILL-TROUBLESOME BIOMEDICAL RESPONSE TO INFECTION

At the beginning of the twentieth century syphilis was one of the most lethal and infectious diseases in Europe. Before 1910 the only treatment available for it was about as painful and damaging as the disease itself—digestion of liquid metal mercury, which could cause death or organ damage. Consequently, when the first clinically tested antisyphilis agent debuted in 1910, it quickly achieved the status of the most-prescribed drug in the world. Even people who had no symptoms but had been sexually active began demanding it from their physicians "just to make sure." The discoverer of the new arsenic-based drug was Paul Ehrlich, of the National Institute for Experimental Therapeutics in Frankfurt, who had shared a Nobel Prize for his work in immunology two years before.

Little did Ehrlich know that he would soon be embroiled in intense controversy. Ehrlich's assistant, Japanese bacteriologist Sahachiro Hata, discovered a way to infect rabbits with the syphilis-causing bacterium *Treponema pallidum,* and, to find possible cures, the duo of Ehrlich and Hata tested several arsenical compounds that Ehrlich and chemist Alfred Bertheim had developed. When Hata injected the sixth chemical in the sixth group of compounds, a substance called arsphenamine, intravenously into live animals, it killed the syphilis bacterium—but not the rabbits.

By September 1910 this drug was on the market under the brand name Salvarsan. This magic bullet, as Ehrlich called it, was expensive and difficult to administer, however, and the side effects—rashes, liver damage, and risks of life and limb, literally—prompted some physicians to denounce Salvarsan. In what historians have dubbed the Salvarsan Wars, Ehrlich and Hata were vilified for profiting from what their detractors saw as a highly dangerous drug (Proto 2010). Some critics claimed that Ehrlich forced prostitutes to undergo Salvarsan treatments to test the drug's efficacy on humans. Ehrlich was condemned both by the police and the Catholic Church, which apparently believed it was morally wrong to cure prostitutes of syphilis. Ultimately Ehrlich was accused of criminal negligence but was eventually exonerated.

In 1912 Ehrlich replaced Salvarsan with a less toxic, easier-to-administer derivative, Neosalvarsan, which became the standard treatment for syphilis until the late 1940s, when penicillin was substituted as a safer alternative. However, neither Neosalvarsan nor, once it was available, penicillin, were provided to participants in the infamous Tuskegee Public Health Service Syphilis Study, a research project that has had lingering effects on people's acceptance of vaccines ever since.

This study was carried out between 1932 and 1972 in Tuskegee, Alabama, by the US Public Health Service (PHS) to assess the natural progression of untreated syphilis in poor, rural black men who did not know they had syphilis and who thought they were receiving free health care from the US government. The study, which came to be seen as the one of the worst ethical violations in post–World War II infectious disease research, was not halted until Peter Buxtun, a PHS venereal-disease investigator, exposed it to the press.

The emergence of drugs like penicillin and other "miracle drugs" in the 1940s and 1950s, although powerful and certainly responsible for saving many lives, have wound up delivering something less than they were originally touted as offering to human health. As noted earlier, recognition of growing drug resistance was one of the factors that activated the modern reappraisal of the threat of infectious diseases. Genes for drug resistance in pathogens, however, are not new; just four years after penicillin was introduced *Staphylococcus aureus* had already developed resistance. Significant clinical resistance is now known for virtually all antibiotics in medical use. Many commentators have noted that antibiotic magic bullets and miracle medicines are losing their effectiveness as a trustworthy protection from infectious diseases at an alarming pace. Resistance to antibiotics is being seen especially in tuberculosis, typhoid, urinary tract infections, and various chest infections.

In 2012, for example, a lethal infection began appearing among patients at the National Institutes of Health Clinical Center, the nation's leading research hospital. Ultimately one patient per week was becoming infected, and six patients died from the disease. But the cause was unclear. The hospital was put on lockdown, scrubbed with bleach, and even plumbing was ripped out and replaced, without benefit. Eventually genome sequencing revealed that the culprit was the drug -resistant pathogen known as *Klebsiella pneumonia,* or KPC (Bartlett 2013). In most instances Klebsiella, a bacteria that lives routinely in human intestines, is not harmful to people with healthy immune systems. But a multidrug-resistant strain had become more common and emerged as a significant threat in intensive care units because it can spread quickly among people suffering from other illnesses that diminish immunocapacity.

In response to mounting data on drug resistance, in her first annual report, Dame Sally Davies (2013:16), the UK government's chief medical officer, noted,

> Antimicrobial resistance is a ticking time-bomb not only for the UK but also for the world. We need to work with everyone to ensure the apocalyptic scenario of widespread antimicrobial resistance does not become a reality. This threat is arguably as important as climate change for the world.

Adds Ian Chubb, a leading Australian scientist, "Once we truly get into the postantibiotic age, people will die from common infections, such as strep throat" (J-A. Davies 2013).

We now realize that, because antibiotics proved on the whole to be relatively safe and effective for bacterial infections, they were widely produced by pharmaceutical companies seeking to have their products approved for multiple diseases and used by physicians and patients seeking cures for diverse diseases, including viral infections. Moreover, antibiotics are heavily used prophylactically in animal husbandry in animal feed supplements as well as in fish farming. Bacteria that survive the initial onslaught of antibiotics exposure, because of their particular genetic makeup or limited contact with the drug (because patients discontinue use once their symptoms subside), however, are increasingly antibiotic resistant. Upon exposure to an antibiotic, the sensitive portion of a bacterial population dies, but then the survivors multiply quickly, they and their offspring are less sensitive to antibiotics in use.

The problem of drug-resistant pathogens is getting worse also in part because big pharmaceutical companies have largely withdrawn from research directed toward new antibiotic discovery. As the Infectious Disease Society of America (2004) has stressed the pharmaceutical pipeline for developing new antibiotics is "drying up." The reason: "Major pharmaceutical companies are losing interest in the antibiotics market because these drugs simply are not as profitable as drugs that treat chronic (long-term) conditions and lifestyle issues" (Infectious Disease Society of America 2004:3). Most of the antibiotics in use today were discovered during the 1940s to 1960s, a period now referred to as the *golden era of antibiotic discovery*. By contrast, the period since the mid-1980s has been referred to as the *antibiotic void* because of the limited additions that have been made to the medical arsenal of antibiotic alternatives (Lewis 2013; Prasad and Smith 2013). This situation has been described anthropologically as reflecting a "values gap" characterized by a growing division between populations that have access to life-saving drugs and the ability to pay for them and populations who lack such access. This gap "is intensified by the choices made by [the pharmaceutical] industry: afflictions whose treatments are relatively easily produced and have ready markets are deemed more worthy of research and development" (Petryna and Kleinman 2006:6). Consequently the question of social good and the power to make life-and-death decisions "filters through every phase of pharmaceutical production, from preclinical research to human testing, marketing, distribution, prescription, and consumption" (Petryna and Kleinman 2006, 7).

The pattern of drug resistance that has been occurring generally is especially far advanced in the case of tuberculosis treatment. As of spring 2011 the WHO reported there were about 440,000 cases of multidrug-resistant tuberculosis (MDR-TB) being identified per year, accounting for 150,000 deaths, including 25,000 cases of XDR (tuberculosis strains resistant to three different antibiotic drugs). At the time the WHO predicted there would be 2 million MDR or XDR cases in the world by 2012. Now there is a strain of tuberculosis in India and elsewhere that is resistant to all twelve of the available drugs, referred to by some as TDR TB—totally drug-resistant tuberculosis (Udwadia et al. 2011).

HOSPITALS AS INFECTION ZONES

In recent years, as alluded to in Chapter 1, new epidemiological patterns have emerged in the contribution of hospitals and other health care institutions like nursing homes and clinics to the transmission of infectious diseases. Referred to as hospital-acquired or *nosocomial infections* among patients being treated for other health problems in hospital settings or hospital staff employed in such settings, these shifts include the spread in hospitals of *multidrug-resistant pathogens*, the appearance in hospitals of pathogens with virulence capacities that facilitate infection in individuals with healthy immune systems, the diffusion of infections from hospitals into surrounding communities, and the circulation of infections from communities into health care settings (McGowan 2000). Hospital-based assessments indicate that there is a growing shift away from more easily treated pathogens toward more resistant strains, allowing for fewer therapeutic options.

Hospital behaviors that promote or prevent the spread of nosocomial infections reflect underlying social structures (e.g., power differentials) and cultural patterns within medical settings. Borg (2014), for example, emphasizes the role of core cultural values held by hospital staff about patient rights, safety, and quality of care. Such values have been found to vary noticeably among hospitals and countries, with some patterns being more conducive to the adoption of effective infection prevention and control measures (Borg 2014). This point has been affirmed through ethnographic research in one pediatric hospital setting in London where S. Macqueen (1995:124–125) found that:

> many of the measures taken to restrict the transmission of infections involved ritualistic theatrical behavior patterns which bore no relevance to inhibiting the transmission of microorganisms. Preventive care was abused by the professionals and seen as unimportant. Explanation as to "why" infection had occurred was inadequate and blamed other people.

In light of such practices, during the 1990s hospitals began to see serious outbreaks caused by pathogens that were resistant to all available antibiotic and antimicrobial resources. Although the first hospital pathogen that was resistant to all antibiotics, a type of bacteria known as enterococci that can cause urinary tract infections among other infectious diseases, was concentrated in patients with compromised immune systems, resistance has developed and is now found in growing numbers of more virulent microbes that can infect patients with healthy immune defenses (Boyce 1997). Eventually antimicrobial-resistant strains of organisms like *Staphylcoccus aureus,* a common cause of skin infections and respiratory infections as well as food poisoning, that first appeared in acute care hospital settings and are now endemic in many hospitals, began to spread into surrounding communities (Gorak, Yamada, and Brown 1999). Some drug-resistant bacterial strains, like penicillin resistant *Streptococcus pneumonia,* are now common in community settings, meaning that incoming patients may carry them into hospitals. Resistant strains of pneumococcus, for example, are now causing infections in hospital and in nursing home settings. These trends in hospital-acquired infection have contributed to increased hospitalization, slower recovery, additional surgery and amputation, increased medical costs, and, in some cases, patient death. They have also raised disturbing social questions about hospital safety and hard-won popular acceptance of hospitals as places where people go to get well rather than places to get even sicker or die unexpectedly.

COMMENSALITY VS. EASE OF TRANSMISSION

For many years biomedical science was dominated by the doctrine of *commensalism*—the notion that the pathogen-host relationship inevitably evolves toward benign coexistence, and the pathogen itself tends over time to evolve toward diminished adverse impact on the host because it is in the microbe's "interest" to keep its host alive (or it will die with it). This view is still commonly found in the literature on infectious diseases. However, Paul Ewald (1994), an evolutionary biologist, has reexamined commensalism in light of Darwinian evolutionary theory. He argues that ease of transmission of the pathogen from one host to another strongly influences the balance between virulence versus mildness in a pathogen.

In this perspective the less-toxic strains of a pathogen will prevail when it is difficult to move from host to host because it is evolutionarily disadvantageous to damage or kill the host before the pathogens have time spread to others, given that reproduction and spread are the driving forces of microbial (and other) life forms. When transmission is instead facilitated by host sickness (e.g., coughing, diarrhea, or even death), natural selection favors virulent strains of the pathogen. The so-called common cold, although admittedly unpleasant, does not tend to be lethal, allowing individuals infected with rhinoviruses to be functional and to readily spread infection to others. In research on the water-borne disease cholera in Latin America, it was found that bacterial strains are virulent in Guatemala, where the water often is not treated, and thus cholera-polluted water can serve as a medium for transmission to new hosts, and mild in Chile, where water quality is good because it is treated and cholera cannot survive in it or be easily transmitted to new hosts when they drink water from public sources. Similarly, strains of the cholera agent isolated from Texas and Louisiana, where drinking waste is purified, produce such small amounts of toxin almost no one who is infected comes down with life-threatening cholera. It is Ewald's belief that if an infectious agent has been present in human populations for many generations but still causes significant levels of sickness and/or loss of life, it is because symptoms and/or death of the host helps produce new infections. In the case of HIV disease, for example, individuals are most infectious at advanced stages of the disease when viral load is highest. Because the virus is beginning to inflict extensive damage to the host's immune system, the virus is able to reproduce rapidly, and the host is highly contagious. In other words, there is selection in HIV for virulence to increase the viral load in preparation for opportunities for transmission (e.g., when the host has sex).

It is for this reason that with HIV disease the slogan "treatment is prevention" makes sense: people on appropriate HIV medications have lowered viral burdens and are less likely to transmit. Conversely, kuru, as we have seen, was a highly lethal non-vector-borne disease. Killing the host makes "evolutionary sense" for kuru because it is in host death—and consumption of part of the host by others—that the prion was transmitted. Otherwise it was very difficult for the prion that causes kuru to be transmitted. From the perspective of evolutionary biology, the most important characteristic is not its virulence but its nature as a self-replicating organism. Conditions of transmission, including routes and the presence of barriers to transmission are among the important determinants of the level of health threat of disease-causing agents. Another pathogen characteristic that affects virulence is the ability to survive outside of a host in a vector for protracted periods. In such cases transmission may be facilitated because hosts become quite sick when infected, making them more available to vector access and less able to prevent vector biting. This fact helps explain why vector-borne diseases like malaria, yellow fever, typhus, and sleeping sickness are so severe.

BIOLOGICAL WARFARE

During the summer of 1942 a small island off the coast of Scotland called Gruinard was evacuated save for thirty sheep that were left behind as part of an experiment. A bomb, filled with highly virulent anthrax spores, was detonated on the island and the outcome observed as part of a test by the British military of bioweaponry. Soon the sheep began to die of anthrax infection—the same disease that set off a major scare in the United States in 2001 (see Chapter 7). The island remained uninhabitable for half a century.

Thus began a new age in the history of infectious diseases, the era of potential systematic, technologically advanced biological warfare. The intentional use of infectious agents as weapons of warfare, if in elementary form, in fact, has a long history. On at least one documented occasion, for example, the British army gave smallpox-contaminated blankets to the Lenape of Delaware, an indigenous Indian population of Canada, during the curiously named French and Indian War of the mid-eighteenth century. In his *Atlas of the North American Indian,* Carl Waldman (1985:108) writes with reference to a siege of Fort Pitt (Pittsburgh) by American Indian forces during the summer of 1763:

> Captain Simeon Ecuyer had bought time by sending smallpox-infected blankets and handkerchiefs to the Indians surrounding the fort—an early example of biological warfare—which started an epidemic among them. [Jeffrey] Amherst [the commanding general of British forces in North America] himself had encouraged this tactic in a letter to Ecuyer.

Other examples of attempts to infect enemies in the course of conflict (e.g., by throwing the bodies of those who died of infection at the enemy) have occurred many times in the course of human history.

The development of the germ theory of disease and twentieth-century advances in bacteriology enabled a significant expansion in the investigation of infectious agents as potential weapons of war. Extensive research began during the Cold War period after World War II and were significantly accelerated after 9/11 (see Table 5.1).

In the United States there was a strong emphasis on developing plant diseases as a way of defeating an enemy by destroying its agricultural base. Biological weapons also were developed to target fisheries and livestock. Offensive biological warfare, including mass production of bioweapons, their stockpiling, and use in conflict, however, was outlawed by an international treaty in 1972 called the Biological Weapons Convention, an agreement signed onto by 165 countries. However, research on biochemical agents continues, nonetheless. Ongoing fears

Table 5.1   Pathogens Studied as Possible Agents for use in Biological Warfare

Type of Pathogen	Biological Agent	Disease
Bacterium	*Bacillus anthracis*Anthrax	
Bacterium	*Yersinia pestis*	Plague
Bacterium	*Francisella tularensis*	Tularaemia
Bacterium	*Brucella* spp.	Brucellosis
Bacterium	*Clostridium botulinum*	Botulism
Bacteria	*Coxiella burnetii*	Q fever
Fungus	*Coccidioides* spp..	San Joaquin Valley Fever
Virus	*Variola major*	Smallpox
Virus	Several ebola viruses	Ebola
Virus	Venezuelan equine encephalitis virus	Encephalomyelitis

about the potential use of biological weapons by nation-states and the use of bioterrorism have become ingrained components of human experience in the modern era, whereas claims of the actual use of bioweapons continue to arise. For example, the United States, at least in part, justified its invasion of Iraq in 2003 on the grounds that Saddam Hussein's government was developing biological weapons. No such weapons were ever found. The issue was raised again several years later during the Syrian Civil War.

CONCLUSION: THE DYNAMICS OF HUMAN INFECTIOUS DISEASES

The agents of infectious disease can be viewed through powerful microscopes that employ an electron beam to illuminate very tiny objects. Advanced microscopes can produce electron micrographs using specialized digital cameras called frame grabbers to produce images of specimens of interest. Consequently, it is possible to take pictures of microscopic pathogens, and these commonly are published in medical journals and popular media and are readily available online. What such pictures—just snapshots of a moment in time—do not show is the incredible dynamic quality of microorganisms, including their ability, through mutation and rapid reproduction under selective pressure as well as gene sharing, to change, interact, and survive in the face of aggressive threats. This capacity allows pathogens to jump across species, gain resistance to antibiotics, adjust to changing opportunities for reproduction and dissemination, respond to shifting physical environments and climatic conditions, and adopt novel routes of transmission to new hosts, including exploiting host behaviors as means of transmission. These qualities empower pathogens as formidable players in the making of human health and disease, which they are likely to be indefinitely. As a result, human communities will continue to be challenged by infectious diseases and must continue to focus on the most productive, equitable, sustainable, and just ways of responding to this substantial challenge (Doyal and Doyal 2013).

Discussion Questions

1. What are some of the challenges infectious disease eradication programs face?
2. From the standpoint of infectious disease, how has the twenty-first century not lived up to twentieth-century expectations?
3. How are infectious disease outbreaks used to "communicate"?

4. Is the historic separation of infectious and chronic disease still meaningful?
5. Is it possible to achieve a pathogen-free world?
6. How do ease and route of transmission affect pathogen virulence?
7. Why, at a time of growing drug resistance among pathogens, are pharmaceutical companies developing so few new antibiotics?

CHAPTER 6

Infectious Disease Syndemics

> Co-infection (where two or more virus, bacteria, protozoa or helminth species concomitantly infect an individual) is the norm in most natural systems.... [Yet a] comparatively understudied risk factor for infection with one organism is co-infection with a second species.
>
> *Lello et al. (2013)*

BEYOND STAND-ALONE INFECTIONS

The *germ theory of disease,* based on the discovery that specific pathogens were linked to specific infectious diseases, was important because it mobilized a major response to human infectious disease. Supplanting earlier medical understanding of disease causation, germ theory proposed that the presence and actions of virulent microorganisms instigated some diseases. The theory radically changed the practice of biomedicine and remains the primary framework that underlies contemporary biomedical treatment of infectious diseases. However, this theory pushed biomedical understanding of the world—and, with it, society's understanding of the world—toward a simplified model of nature: namely, toward the taken-for-granted assumption that there is a single, simple, and identifiable cause of every adverse health outcome. René Dubos (1959) labeled this way of thinking as "the doctrine of specific etiology." In the case of treating an infectious disease, it referred to the existence of a specific pathogenic agent that can be identified and countered through medical action. The doctrine was so appealing that it spread rapidly from biomedical response to noninfectious diseases as well. The resulting biomedical approach to disease has hinged on an effort to isolate diagnostically, study, and treat diseases as if they were distinct entities that existed in nature separate from other organisms and diseases as well as independent of the social contexts in which they arise. There is no doubt that this way of thinking contributed to some important advances, such as the antibiotic treatment of bacterial diseases. Yet, as Dubos observed, although the doctrine of specific etiology "and the theoretical and practical achievements to which it has led constitute the bulk of modern medicine . . . few are the cases in which it has provided a complete account of the causation of disease" (Dubos 1959:102). Further, it hindered recognition of the multiple and consequential ways in which both infectious and noninfectious diseases interact syndemically with each other and with pressing social conditions.

Examining these syndemic interactions and their health implications are the goals of this chapter. Its lesson is that although there is heuristic value in parsing infectious diseases into specific conditions with particular immediate causes, different pathogens cause quite similar diseases, the same pathogens can cause different diseases in different parts of the world or different parts of the body, and, most importantly, diseases do not exist in a vacuum as isolated conditions. Not only do individuals suffer from *co-infections* of two or more diseases, but co-infections also often produce a far greater health burden than the mere additive effect of the involved health conditions. Infectious diseases also produce additive adverse effects through their interaction with noninfectious diseases. In other words, health problems often are made worse through the entwinement of diseases, and social factors facilitate these consequential linkages.

The anthropologically informed concept of syndemics directs attention to the nexus connecting diseases and the social contexts of their sufferers; however, a common misunderstanding is that a syndemic merely labels a situation in which a social condition contributes to ill health or disease. Rather, the term specifically defines damaging biological, biobehavioral, and/or psychobiological interactions between two or more copresent diseases, including infectious diseases, within individuals and within populations that the adverse social, cultural, and environmental contexts in which they occur make possible or worsen. Consequently, syndemics are an essential expression of the biocultural/biosocial conception emphasized in this volume.

This chapter examines the nature and pathways of interaction in infectious disease syndemics, presents a number of cases of this phenomenon, and discusses the importance of environmentally mediated syndemics. It shows that syndemics are not a minor element in infectious diseases but, in fact, are a fundamental component of the human-pathogen story.

DEFINING SYNDEMICS

In the summer of 1833, John Work, an Irish immigrant who lived in Canada, led a Hudson's Bay Company fur animal trapping expedition into central California. In his journal Work recorded his experiences of the expedition, including the health conditions of his party and the Native Americans they encountered en route. He observed that Indian villages that had been filled with people and activities when his party passed through in the beginning of the year were completely deserted when revisited in August. Ultimately whole areas of California lost their indigenous populations to raging disease. By September so many of

Work's own crew also were sick that he described their situation as helpless. At the end of October, Work finally made his way back to Fort Vancouver, but he was "so much exhausted by . . . debilitating disease that I was reduced to a perfect skeleton and could scarcely walk" (Work 1945:71).

What was the debilitating disease event that so affected Work, his crew, and especially the Native American peoples he encountered in central California? Linda Nash (2006:22) notes, "Modern scholars interpret this event as an epidemic outbreak of malaria and typically trace the origins of the disease in central California to Work's own party [as the source] though malaria may have appeared in conjunction with influenza, which could explain the dramatically high death rates." As this interpretation suggests, adverse disease interaction occurring in a moment of considerable sociocultural flux—in this case, interface between a single-celled parasite (the malaria pathogen) and a virus (the influenza pathogen) at a time of intense culture clash—produced a devastating syndemic that dramatically changed the demographic composition of early California and helped to write subsequent state history.

Research suggests that it is difficult to distinguish clinically between patients suffering from malaria alone versus those suffering from malaria/influenza co-infection; indeed, most febrile diseases are notoriously hard to distinguish clinically. In children seen as patients at two hospitals in western Kenya, however, a study carried out by Mark Thompson and co-investigators (2012, 1678) found that coinfection is:

> associated with more severe illness than single infections. At both hospitals, coinfected children aged 24–59 months had longer hospitalizations than children with either infection alone or neither infection. Having a coinfection increased hospital stays by about 1–3 days in settings where the typical stay was 3–5 days. Among patients aged 24–59 months, coinfected children were also more likely to receive blood transfusions than children with malaria only. Chest radiographs were also ordered more often for coinfected vs malaria-only-infected children. . . . It may be that coinfected children presented with a more ill appearance, with signs that we did not capture in our study but that clinicians recognized, prompting more aggressive and prolonged care.

The term syndemic was introduced into medical anthropology and, through it, into public health, allied health, and medical discourses in the early 1990s (Singer 2009c). As this discussion suggests, thinking about health in terms of the existence, nature, and progression of syndemics directs attention to biocultural/biosocial interaction. In infectious disease syndemics four levels of interface are critical:

1. Interactions between humans and their physical environments, including other species that harbor, transmit, or promote disease
2. Interactions between diseases and human bodies, including our immune systems
3. Interactions among diseases within human or animal bodies
4. Interactions between human social systems—and their structures of inequality—and diseases, often as mediated by the environment.

We have come to realize that many of the most damaging human infectious disease epidemics across time and location—from the lethal influenza epidemic of 1918–1919 to the contemporary global AIDS pandemic, and from Black Plague to the European diseases that devastated New World Native American populations—are the consequence not of single disease outbreaks but of several diseases acting in tandem in social and cultural context. Syndemics differ from epidemics in that the latter term generally is applied to the spread of a single disease, whereas a syndemic involves an outbreak of interacting and adversely entwined diseases. Closer examination of many disease events that are labeled epidemics or even pandemics, because they spread globally, however, reveals that they are in fact syndemics involving two or more interacting diseases. Focus on one of the diseases draws attention away from the second disease and the importance of interaction for disease virulence and spread. Measles, for example, which is among the most contagious of infectious diseases, continues to cause severe illness in impoverished settings; case fatality rates reach nearly 10 percent in some sub-Saharan African children. The high death toll associated with measles stems from the fact that it lowers children's resistance to other diseases, allowing for syndemic interaction with herpes simplex virus, adenoviruses, and several bacterial infections as well as malnutrition, including vitamin A deficiency (Perry and Halsey 2004).

In our contemporary world of rapidly emerging, reemerging, and drug-resistant infectious diseases, it appears likely that syndemics will play an important role in shaping the evolving global health profile of the twenty-first century. Suggestive of this outcome is the case of SARS (severe acute respiratory syndrome), which the World Health Organization (2013d) labeled the first serious and readily transmissible new disease to emerge in the twenty-first century. The immediate cause of SARS was found to be a coronavirus that emerged in China in 2002 and ultimately led to the death of about a tenth of the eight thousand people it infected worldwide. Symptoms of the disease included severe respiratory illness, fever, coughing, and breathing difficulties. Its gravest health impacts occurred among people with other health conditions, such as cardiovascular problems or diabetes, indicating that what is of importance from a health perspective is not SARS alone but rather SARS in conjunction with other diseases. Almost 40 percent of those who ultimately became critically ill with SARS during the 2002–2003 epidemic suffered from diabetes (Singer 2009c).

The H1N1 (swine-origin influenza A) influenza pandemic of 2009 also illustrates the importance of biocultural/biosocial factors in syndemics. As both a direct descendent of the virus involved in the most devastating influenza pandemic of the twentieth century and as a genetically unique pathogen that was transmitted originally from pigs to humans and then ultimately transmitted from humans to humans, H1N1 raised considerable concern among public health professionals as well as the public. A product of the assertive mixing of two unrelated swine viruses, the H1N1 virus has, from the standpoint of severe morbidity and population mortality, proven thus far to be a comparatively mild version of its deadly ancestor of ninety years ago. Although the virus affected people in 214 countries, it was only a factor in about 18,500 deaths, a mortality rate far lower than the average annual rate of influenza mortality (Cheng et al. 2012). This pattern, of course, can always change; there remains concern that the virus may re-assort with other existing human influenza viruses, leading to the emergence of more virulent H1N1 viral strains. As David Morens, Jeffery Taubenberger, and Anthony Fauci (2009:225) remind us, since 1918 the H1N1 virus "has drawn on a bag of evolutionary tricks to survive in one form or another, in both humans and pigs, and to spawn a host of novel progeny viruses with novel gene constellations, through the periodic importation or exportation of viral genes."

From a syndemics standpoint, however, data from the United States, Brazil, Canada, Australia, and New Zealand indicate that although ethnic minorities and indigenous populations were not more likely than other groups to be infected with H1N1, they were at a notably higher risk of developing severe disease and dying from H1N1 infection. The CDC (2009), for example, reports that in thirteen US metropolitan areas of ten states monitored for H1N1 cases between April 15 and August 31, 2009, 35 percent of people hospitalized with the disease were black. This is notable because only 16 percent of the combined populations of the areas studied were black. In addition, a study of disabled Medicaid patients found that blacks were three times less likely to receive treatment for influenza with disease-modifying antiviral drugs (Leon et al. 2009). Emblematic of the H1N1 disparity pattern reported by CDC is the city of Boston, where Blacks comprise only 25 percent of the city's residents but accounted for 37 percent of hospitalized H1N1 cases. Latinos, who make up 14 percent of Boston's population, represented one-third of hospitalized H1N1 cases in the city (Parks 2009). In other words, 70 percent of people with more severe infections in Boston were members of ethnic minority populations.

Similarly, Canadian research in Manitoba (Zarychanski et al. 2010), the province with the highest burden of severe H1N1-related cases in 2009, found that indigenous First Nations ethnicity was associated with severe H1N1 disease that required intensive care unit (ICU) admission. In this study the higher the severity level of H1N1 infection, the greater the proportion of individuals of First Nations heritage. First Nations people comprised 28 percent of confirmed H1N1 cases in Manitoba, 54 percent of hospital admissions, and 60 percent of admissions to the ICU. Similar patterns have been observed in aboriginal communities in Australia and New Zealand. Thus, Steven Webb and colleagues (2009) found that in Australia, whereas aboriginal and Torres Strait Islanders account for 2.5 percent of the total population, they comprised 9.7 percent of patients with H1N1 influenza admitted to intensive care units since the beginning of the pandemic. In New Zealand, although the indigenous Māori people represent 13.6 percent of the population, they accounted for 25 percent of patients with H1N1 influenza admitted to ICUs.

In short, compared to majority populations in a number of countries, H1N1's adverse impacts among ethnic minority populations were significantly more severe and appear to reflect broader health and social disparity patterns. Although the majority of cases in all populations proved to be self-limiting, significantly higher rates of hospitalization, intensive care, and death were recorded among low-income ethnic minorities. One important factor in this pattern was the syndemic interaction of H1N1 with other infectious and chronic diseases like tuberculosis and diabetes that, because of disparities in living conditions and access to resources, including health prevention and care, have become comparatively common among disadvantaged groups worldwide. H1N1 influenza, in short, became a global syndemic with heightened adverse outcomes among marginalized minority populations in multiple countries (see Figure 6.1).

An emerging arena of syndemics research concerns neurodegeneration. A growing collection of epidemiologic and experimental studies strongly suggests (but has not yet decisively proven) that chronic bacterial and viral infections, in synergistic interaction with other health conditions, play a role in various neurodegenerative diseases, such as Alzheimer's disease, Parkinson's disease, Huntington's disease, and amyotrophic lateral sclerosis (De Chiara et al. 2012). These diseases, which are characterized by a progressive loss of neurons, are associated with declines in brain function, including cognitive and locomotor control. These diseases differ in a number of ways, including which region of the brain is most affected and which pathogens may be involved in specific neurodegenerative conditions. Current research suggests the potential involvement of enteroviruses and human herpesviruses in the etiology of amyotrophic lateral sclerosis (popularly known as Lou Gehrig's disease), a contribution of Japanese

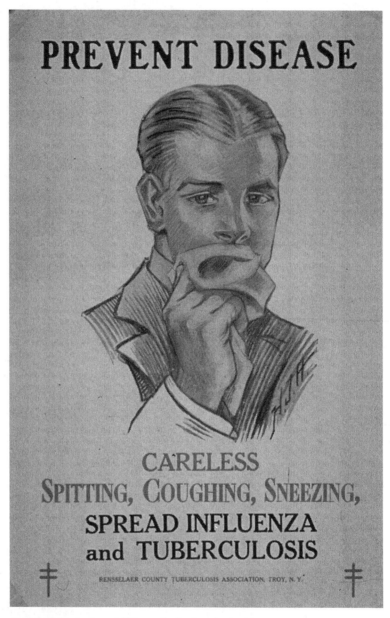

Figure 6.1 Influenza and Tuberculosis Prevention Poster, Rensselaer Country Tuberculosis Association. (Images from the History of Medicine)

encephalitic virus and influenza viruses to the onset of Parkinson's disease, and the involvement of herpes simplex virus type-1 and *Chlamydia pneumoniae* in the pathogenesis of Alzheimer's disease. Additionally, various herpes simplex viruses have been linked to multiple sclerosis. These infectious agents may be increasingly able to penetrate the blood-brain barrier as an individual ages. In addition to age-related alterations of the barrier, increased oxidative stress and impaired energy production may be contributing factors. Aged neurons are more vulnerable to the toxicity of viral or prion proteins. In the case of Alzheimer's disease, neuropathological changes occur in the brain, most notably the development of plaques and neurofibril tangles within nerves that damage nerve cell communication. *C. pneumonia* has been found at high incidence in Alzheimer's disease sufferers' brain cells, especially in close proximity to neurofribrillary tangles. Moreover, in animal studies this pathogen has been found to produce plaque formation in mice brains (Gérad et al. 2006; Little et al. 2004).

In addition to the adverse effects of aging, pathogen interaction with metabolic disorders that interfere with the body's ability to generate needed energy may occur. Factors influenced by social class—high education, active social engagement, physical exercise, and mentally stimulating activity—have been identified as sources of preventive protection from neurodegenerative diseases like Alzheimer's disease, infectious agents notwithstanding (Qiu, Kivipelto, and von Strauss 2009). In other words, neurodegeneration also appears to be a biosocial and biocultural phenomenon.

This section has considered two levels of interaction: between humans and their physical environments and between diseases and human bodies. The remainder of this chapter focuses on two more levels of interaction: among infectious diseases and among infectious and noninfectious diseases. It also explores the social structuring of disease clustering.

PATHWAYS AND CONSEQUENCES OF INFECTIOUS SYNDEMIC INTERACTION

How do infectious diseases interact? There are multiple pathways and mechanisms of disease interaction, including:

- *Alterations or damage done to parts of the body caused by one disease promoting another disease,* as occurs when alterations of the lungs caused by influenza viruses increase the subsequent adherence of pneumococcus bacteria within the lung, facilitating pulmonary infection. As a result, people are more likely to suffer pneumonia, a disease that is estimated to kill over 1 million children under the age of five years every year—more than AIDS, malaria and tuberculosis combined (18 percent of annual child deaths) (World Health Organization 2013c). Similarly changes in the host immune response, such as suppression of acute pro-inflammatory capacity, which facilitates the elimination of pathogens, by one microbe can increase the impact of a second infection. In short, pathogens leave lasting impacts on our anatomy, and these changes, in turn, facilitate the adverse impact of other diseases.

- *One disease enhances the virulence of another disease,* illustrated by the role certain herpes proteins such as ICP-0 and ICP-4 play in improving HIV's ability to replicate, which magnifies infectiousness. Genital herpes, which is linked to the herpes simplex virus 2 (HSV-2), is a sexually transmitted disease found around the world. The immediate symptoms of this infection are reoccurring, painful sores in the genital area. Individuals who are comorbid for HSV-2 and HIV, which ranges in various studies from 50 to 90 percent of HIV patients, experience herpes lesions more frequently than do individuals who are not co-infected. At the same time, co-infected individuals have higher HIV burdens. HSV-2 and HIV-1 have been found infecting the same cells, and several HSV-2 proteins have been shown to up-regulate HIV replication through their interactions with sectors of the HIV genome. Additionally, an HSV-2 protein, known as protein number 16, interacts with the Tat (trans-activator of transcript) protein of HIV in ways that trigger increased HIV transcription, part of the viral reproduction process. Consequently HSV-2 may not only enhance HIV transmission, but it may also have a significant syndemic impact on HIV disease progression in individuals who are dually infected (Chun et al. 2013). In such cases dual infection produces not only the additive effects of two conditions but also the multiplier effects of their biochemical interactions.

- *One disease facilitates the contagiousness of another disease,* as occurs when ulcerations of the genital track caused by sexually transmitted diseases open doorways in the protective epithelial barrier for HIV to enter. As Joanne Lello and colleagues (2013) comment, "Any infection will change the within-host environment in some way, for example by inducing changes in host physiology" such as "creating an ulcerous wound that bacterial opportunists can exploit." Multiple studies, for example, have shown that having a syphilis infection increases one's risk of both acquiring and transmitting HIV. A review of studies on interactions between various sexually transmitted diseases found that infections such as syphilis that cause genital lesions (e.g., herpes, chancroid) increase susceptibility to HIV in both men and women, with a 1.6 times greater effect in men. Sexually transmitted diseases that do not cause genital lesions also increase susceptibility to HIV but at approximately 60 percent the level seen for lesion-causing diseases (Røttingen, Cameron, and Garnett 2001).

- *Two diseases interact to cause a third disease,* which appears to be the case with Burkitt's lymphoma. This is an aggressive cancer of the lymphatic system found in young children. It is common in areas with high rates of *P. falciparum* malaria, but despite a suspected connection between the two diseases, until recently firm evidence had been lacking. Research has shown, however, that Epstein-Barr virus (EBV) infection can be detected in nearly all Burkitt's lymphoma cases located in the equatorial belt of Africa and other areas where malaria is hyperendemic, and it is confirmed as a causative factor in this cancer. EBV is a ubiquitous herpesvirus in human populations that commonly infects B cells, which are lymphocytes that are integral to the adaptive immune system's response to specific identified infectious agents. Research with children in Kenya now reveals that repeated malaria infections in very young children significantly increases the persistence of EBV as well as the risk for the development of Burkitt's lymphoma (Moorman et al. 2005). One likely mechanism involved in malaria's connection with this cancer is that in dually infected individuals it decreases EBV-specific T cell immunological surveillance, a search-and-destroy process carried out by the immune system that detects and eliminates tumorous growths (Moorman et al. 2007). Research by Charles Torgbor and colleagues (2014) reveals that infection with malaria has multiple EBV-enhancing effects on the immune system that together dramatically increase the frequency of Burkitt's lymphoma. In other words, two infectious diseases, Epstein-Barr virus and *P. falciparum,* interact syndemically to promote third disease, Burkitt's lymphoma.
- *Pathogens exchange genes* (i.e., gene assortment), as seen in the movement of genetic material from one strain or subtype of a microorganism to another strain, a factor in the emergence of multidrug-resistant pathogens and the rise of questions about whether we are entering a postantimicrobial era of human history. Nara Figueroa-Bossi and coworkers (2001:260–261) note, "Horizontal gene transfer is widely regarded as the main mechanism driving the evolution of Salmonella." Horizontal transfer involves the movement of genes between two different lineages of this pathogen. Gene flow of this sort among bacteria strains is a primary driver of growing antibiotic resistance. Additionally, genes involved in antibiotic resistance found in one species of bacteria can be transferred

to another species of bacteria or between bacteria and viruses. One way this can occur is a process called "transformation," in which a microorganism releases genetic material into the environment that another microorganism then acquires. Genes also can move across whole groups, such as between bacteria and viruses or between bacteria and yeast cells. In fact, human genes can be found in microorganisms. Although this appears to be rare with regard to bacteria, it has been discovered in the case of sexual disease-causing *Neisseria gonorrhoeae* strains that possess a gene sequence that is 98 to 100 percent identical to the human amino acid encoding nuclear element called L1 (Anderson and Seifert 2011). As yet it is unclear what these genes do—if anything—within the gonococci genome. This finding, however, does further affirm the continued coevolution of humans and microbes.

- *Diseases may interact through behavior,* and as a result people suffering from mental illness may be at heightened risk for sexually transmitted infection because of impaired judgment and resulting participation in risky behaviors. Research has shown that individuals who suffer from loneliness, depression, low self-esteem, sexual compulsivity, sexual abuse, and drug abuse are least likely to benefit from HIV prevention education and most likely to engage in HIV-related risk behaviors. Exemplary is research with men who have sex with other men who have low levels of self-esteem associated with the internalization of societal homophobia and the resulting experience of self-condemnation because of being gay (Stokes and Peterson 1998). These men are more likely to engage in HIV risk taking and to be more likely to be HIV positive than men who have not internalized homophobia. Similarly, a study using data from the 1992 National Survey of Veterans found that the combination of posttraumatic stress disorder symptoms and substance abuse was associated with greater risk for HIV infection (Hoff, Beam-Goulet, and Rosenheck 1997).

- *Medical treatment provided for one disease can affect another comorbid disease,* as seen in the case of measles vaccination leading to primary and secondary vaccine failure among HIV-infected children. Additionally, vaccination against one infectious disease may cause another infectious disease when contaminated drugs are used or when inadequately sterilized syringes are used, as occurred during pre-1986 antischistosomal injections in Egypt that spread hepatitis infection. In 2012 contaminated health care–administered steroid injections were linked to a cluster of fungal infections in the United States, resulting in over 750 infection cases and 64 deaths. In the case of iatrogenic Creutzfeldt-Jakob disease, in 1974 a cornea patient became infected after receiving a transplant from what proved to be an infected cadaver. In subsequent years various new iatrogenic sources of infectious were identified, including blood products and transplant pituitary glands from cadavers. Overall, it is believed that about 450 patients were infected in hospital procedures with this prion-triggered degenerative and invariably fatal brain disorder (Brown et al. 2012).

Infectious diseases are commonly involved in disease interactions in both humans and other animals. Among voles, for example, Sandra Telfer and colleagues (2010) found that patterns of infection risk are significantly affected by the presence of other infections and that these effects were of greater magnitude and explained more variation in infection risk than did characteristics of hosts or environmental factors, which are more commonly considered in disease studies. Similarly, among humans there is growing recognition of the adverse interactive effects of co-infection. For example, there is mounting evidence of interaction between type 2 diabetes mellitus and various infectious diseases, such as hepatitis C. Several factors are known to contribute to the onset of type 2 diabetes, including diet, obesity, and aging. The role of infection, however, is only beginning to be understood. It is well known that risk of infection significantly increases with poor diabetes control, but appreciation of more complex relationships between infection and type 2 diabetes is now emerging as well. Various studies (e.g., Mason et al. 1999), for example, have found that the frequency of type 2 diabetes increases among people who have been infected with the hepatitis C virus (HCV). The Third National Health and Nutrition Examination Survey showed that among people who were forty years of age or older, those with HCV disease were more than three times more likely than those without HCV disease to have type 2 diabetes (Mehta et al. 2001). The specific mechanisms by which HCV leads to type 2 diabetes are not understood, but there is evidence that an HCV-related increase of insulin resistance associated with the overproduction of pro-inflammatory cytokines could play a crucial role.

Based on growing recognition that "interspecific parasite interactions can be a powerful influence on parasite dynamics," Lello and colleagues (2013) investigated three common soil-transmitted helminths—giant roundworm (*Ascaris lumbricoides*), whipworm (*Trichuris trichiura*), and hookworm (*Necator americanus*)—and self-reported fever in school-aged children in Zanzibar, Tanzania. They found that children who were infected with roundworm were at significantly higher risk for whipworm. Similarly children, especially boys, with whipworm were at significant risk for hookworm. Suffering from fever, which suggests bacterial or viral infection, however, was found to be associated with lowered risk for roundworm, or what is termed a *countersyndemic* relationship.

In comparison with the role of co-infection, other factors like host age, sex, and behavior were found to be comparatively low risk for infection. This study affirms that "co-infection can alter disease outcome, parasite transmission potential, and susceptibility of hosts to other infections" (Lello et al. 2013:5).

HIV disease has heightened awareness of the adverse consequences of co-infection. Rapid mutation and enormous variability have conferred a considerable capacity for immune evasion by HIV, a characteristic that has been critical to its grim success as a human pathogen. HIV reproduces at a breakneck pace with a single viron that is one-seventieth the diameter of the white blood cells it commonly infects, replicating billions of copies of itself during a single day. Also of importance in its significant adverse effect is the ability of HIV disease to interact with so many other diseases. In that it targets the immune system, HIV disease has become the premier *syndemogenic* (syndemic-causing) disease of the contemporary world. In Africa, for example, the emergence of HIV has significantly complicated older (pre-HIV) syndemics (e.g., synergistic interaction between helminthic or worm infection and malaria). As discussed below, individuals suffering from worm infestation have been found to be more susceptible to malaria and more likely to develop undesirable clinical outcomes when they are infected by malaria, probably because some infectious worm species diminish the body's ability to develop immunity to the pathogen that causes malaria. Adding HIV disease to this syndemic brew ominously magnifies the threat to the sufferer's health. Worms interact with HIV infection, both increasing susceptibility and exacerbating HIV progression. Similarly, it is known that "HIV fuels malaria and malaria fuels HIV" (Abu-Raddad 2007).

The significance of HIV syndemic interaction in the United States is seen in the Multicenter AIDS Cohort Study (Thio et al. 2002), which divided matched individuals into four groups: those with HIV only, those with hepatitis B only, those co-infected with HIV and hepatitis B, and those who were free of either disease. This study found that liver disease–related deaths were highest in the dually infected subgroup and were especially high in those with low CD4 cell counts, a sign of advanced HIV infection. Men infected with hepatitis B and HIV were seventeen times more likely to die of liver disease than were those infected with just hepatitis B. Similarly, research by anthropologist Bryan Page and coworkers (1990) found that individuals infected with human T-lymphotropic virus (HTLV), a retrovirus associated with the development of leukemia, who were also infected with HIV were three times more likely to die of AIDS than those with HIV disease but not infected with HTLV, suggesting that HTLV adversely affects the course of infection with HIV through synergistic interaction within the human body.

Globally one of the most significant syndemics involves HIV and *Mycobacterium tuberculosis* (MTb) (Kwan and Ernst 2011). Interaction between these two pathogens enhances HIV's *immunopathology* and accelerates the damaging progression of both HIV infection and tuberculosis (TB). HIV and MTb co-infection has become common in US inner-city areas as well as in parts of Africa, South America, and Asia. Research in Côte d'Ivoire in Western Africa, for example, showed that co-infection with HIV and MTb significantly reduced patients' survival time compared to those with just MTb or HIV infection, suggesting a synergistic interaction with deadly consequence for dually infected individuals (Ackah et al. 1995). Research in Haiti found that individuals who were clinically treated for pulmonary tuberculosis were more likely to suffer recurrent infection if they were HIV positive than if they were HIV negative (Fitzgerald et al. 2000). Studies have shown that because HIV damages human immune systems, individuals with HIV disease who are exposed to TB are more likely to develop active and rapidly progressing tuberculosis compared to those who are HIV negative, whose immune systems can keep the disease-causing tuberculosis bacteria in check and in a dormant state. People infected with HIV who are exposed to MTb are eight hundred times more likely than people not infected with HIV to develop active TB (Lockman et al. 2003).

The essential finding in HIV/TB research is that infection is enhanced and more damaging as a result of disease interaction. As emphasized by the World Health Organization, MTb/HIV is a deadly combination that is best conceptualized as a *disease complex* rather than as two copresent conditions. Notably, in Southern Africa, 50 to 80 percent of tuberculosis patients are HIV positive (South African Department of Health 2006), and HIV has played a central role in soaring rates of tuberculosis in the region. The national health consequences of MTb/HIV interaction can be seen in the country of Swaziland, a small, mountainous country landlocked by South Africa and Mozambique that has one of the highest HIV rates in the world. According to Aymeric Péguillan (Medecins San Frontieres 2010), head of the Doctors Without Borders mission in the country:

> Disturbingly, more than 80 percent of TB patients are also co-infected with HIV. Life expectancy has halved within two decades, plummeting from 60 to just 31 years. People are dying in large numbers and tuberculosis is currently the main cause of mortality among adults. As a result, many children are being made orphans and the adult workforce is declining.

Similarly, as suggested earlier, in patients suffering from co-infection with herpes and HIV there is a hurried acceleration of AIDS pathogenesis because of the role the herpesvirus appears to play in speeding up HIV replication (Schacker 2001). *Genital ulceration disease* (GUD) caused by sexually transmitted infection has been found to increase the risk of male-to-female transmission of HIV by a factor of ten to fifty and of female-to-male transmission by a factor of fifty to three hundred. There is strong evidence that "GUD may be responsible for a large proportion of heterosexually acquired HIV infections in sub-Saharan Africa" (Hayes, Schulz, and Plummer 1995:1). One of the important interactions that was not recognized in the early years of the pandemic is between HIV and human papillomavirus (HPV) cervical infection in women. As a result, until the definition of "AIDS" was broadened to include diseases that only or disproportionately strike women, many women died of HIV disease who were never diagnosed as having the disease. It is now known that women who are dually infected with both diseases have 1.8 to 8.2 times higher rates of *viral shedding* (i.e., latent HPV reactivation and recurrence) compared with women not infected with HIV.

More broadly, it is now also clear that sexually transmitted infections (STIs) are among the most significant risk factors for HIV infection internationally because (1) they create openings in the protective mucosal barriers of the body that allow passage of HIV; (2) susceptible immune cells, such as CD4 T-help cells, are attracted to and gather at the body sites of STI infection (Ward and Rönn 2010); (3) they can cause genital bleeding, which enhances sexual risk of exposure to HIV; and (4) immune activation provoked by STIs facilitates HIV access to target cells, leading to enhanced HIV replication, immune system deterioration, and disease progression. In a systematic review of the research on the prevalence of HIV/STI co-infection, Seth Kalichman, Jennifer Pellowski, and Christina Turner (2011) found that the highest prevalence of HIV/STI co-infection was among individuals who were newly diagnosed with HIV during the acute infection phase. This finding reflects the fact that most new STIs are contracted soon after a person has been infected with HIV, although STI co-infections do occur throughout the years of HIV infection. Further, as Zvi Bentwich and colleagues (2000:2078) indicate, "The most important conclusion that can be drawn . . . is that eradication or suppression of concurrent infections may have a major impact on the spread and progression of HIV infection and AIDS," a statement that affirms the critical importance of syndemic interaction in HIV pathogenesis.

As noted above, even without the addition of HIV disease, the adverse interaction of malaria and intestinal helminths is a widespread syndemic in the areas where these two parasitic infections have overlapping geographic distributions. This is certainly the case in sub-Saharan Africa, where this syndemic, which was first described over seventy-five years ago, has been found to be a significant barrier to improving maternal and child health in poor families among whom comorbidity is most common (Singer 2013a). Several hypotheses have been proposed to explain adverse interactions between helminths and malaria. A review of the literature by Tabitha Mwangi and colleagues (2007) highlights the possibility that helminth infection creates a cytokine response that makes individuals more susceptible to clinical malaria. Cytokines are molecules like interleukin that are involved in cell-to-cell communication during body immune responses. They stimulate the movement of immune cells toward sites of inflammation, infection, and trauma. Consequently they are referred to as *immunomodulating agents,* and interfering with their normal operation can create an internal body environment that is favorable to infectious disease. Alternately, Maria Yazdanbakhsh, Anita van der Biggelaar, and Rick Maizels (2001) suggest that the presence of T-regulatory cells increase during helminth infection, which, if present in sufficient numbers, induce a nonspecific immune suppression that facilitates malaria development upon exposure. As yet, given the limited availability of studies, the relative explanatory power of these hypotheses remains uncertain. What is clear, however, is that whatever the specific biological pathway(s), interaction between malaria and helminths is a severe threat to pregnant women and children. The specific helminth species comorbid with malaria, however, may be critical, as some findings suggest a protective or countersyndemic effect with particular types of intestinal worms and a worsening syndemic effect with others. Hookworm, for example, falls into the latter group, which is unfortunate both because its prevalence among pregnant woman in sub-Saharan Africa is high and because on its own it may contribute significantly to anemia, a serious threat during pregnancy. The risk of a woman dying as a result of pregnancy or childbirth is about one in six in the poorest nations of the world, compared with about one in thirty thousand in the wealthy nations of Northern Europe. The United Nations Secretariat (2012) estimated that almost three hundred thousand maternal deaths occurred in 2010, 56 percent of them in sub-Saharan Africa, underlying the fatal consequence of syndemics that diminish health during pregnancy in the region.

HIV also interacts with noninfectious diseases, such as alcoholism. Both of these conditions are known to have damaging effects on brain function, including cognitive and motor impairments expressed as diminished executive functions, memory, visuospatial comprehension, and speed of cognitive processing. Moreover, a growing body of clinical research indicates that in dually diagnosed individuals there occurs an adverse synergism of these two diseases, with resulting drops in brain functioning. Neuropsychological studies of cognitive functioning show that comorbid individuals, those with both diseases, perform worse on standard evaluation batteries than do individuals with a single diagnosis (Samet et al. 2003). Although the precise pathways of disease interaction in this syndemic are yet to be fully defined, it is evident that they involve both behavioral factors, such as drinking to self-medicate the emotional costs of HIV infection and the contributions of chronic drinking to HIV risk behavior, and biological factors, including accelerated hippocampal damage in the brain and alcohol-accelerated HIV disease progression through reduced immunocapacity.

Another example of infectious disease interaction with a noninfectious health condition involves obesity. Research with both animal and human subjects suggests that obesity is associated with impaired immune function. Degradations of the immune system seen in obese individuals include decreased cytokine production, decreased response to both antigen and mitogen stimulation, reduced functioning of macrophage and dendritic cells of the immune system, and impairment of natural killer cell activity. These losses, in turn, have been found to be linked to increased susceptibility to infection involving various pathogenic agents, including community-acquired tuberculosis, influenza, *Mycobacterium tuberculosis,* coxsackievirus, *Helicobacter pylori,* and encephalomyocarditis virus (Karlsson and Beck 2010). The precise pathways linking obesity to heighten infectious disease risk remain to be identified although the contributions of obesity to excessive inflammation, altered adipokine signaling patterns, metabolic changes, as well as impacts on the epigenetic regulation of cells have been suggested as components of such linkage. Conversely, animal research with rodents, chickens, and nonhuman primates reveals that infection with human *adenovirus* leads to the onset of obesity. Test animals have been found to gain fat without changes in their diet. Approximately 30 percent of obese adults suffer adenovirus infection, and rates are even higher in obese children. Findings of this research suggest the role of infection in obesity (Atkinson et al. 2005).

Obesity also has been identified as a risk factor for severe influenza, including increased mortality (Huttunen and Sryjanen 2010). Here too the impact of obesity on adipokine signaling appears to be a pathway of interaction between obesity and infection. *Adipokines* are cytokines, such as adiponectin, leptin, and resistin, that are secreted by adipose or connective fat tissue. They are important in many physiological and metabolic processes, including insulin signaling. Interference in bodily access to and processing of insulin, a hormone involved in glucose metabolism, can affect an individual's ability to fight infection. Research has shown that bodily insulin demands go up with infection (Maloney et al. 2008). Consequently monitoring of patient insulin and clinically increasing insulin levels as needed is recognized as an important strategy for preventing pneumonia in both postoperative and burn patients (Martin et al. 2007).

Like infectious diseases, obesity is shaped by biocultural/biosocial influences, including culturally constituted food beliefs and practices, local food

availability, and social structural factors in food access. Obesity is disproportionate among those living in poverty, for example, because "the poor do not eat
what they want, or what they know they should eat, but what they can afford"
(Aguirre 2000:11). At the same time, various infections may be more common
among the poor because of overcrowding, substandard housing in noxious
environmental settings, and immune-compromising exposures. Thus, obesity-
infectious disease interaction reflects the key role social inequality commonly
plays in syndemic production.

THE SOCIAL STRUCTURING OF DISEASE CLUSTERING

We know that infectious diseases do not exist in a social vacuum nor solely within
the bodies of those they inflict; thus, their transmission and impact is never
merely a biological process. The same is true of their interactions. Ultimately,
as suggested above, social factors such as poverty, racism, sexism, ostracism,
and other forms of *structural violence* may be of far greater importance than the
nature of pathogens or the bodily systems they infect in determining their impact
on human health. Perry Halkitis (2012:1629) notes, "Ecosocial models, including the theory of syndemics . . . delineate that psychosocial burdens created by
inequalities and discrimination are antecedents to disease across our lifetimes."

The concept of *disease cluster,* as it is used in infectious disease syndemics
research, has two interrelated meanings. First, it refers to the concentration of
infectious disease in one segment of a population compared to other segments.
Second, it refers to the copresence of multiple concurrent significant infectious
diseases in a population segment, creating the likelihood that individuals will
suffer not from one but from two or several infectious diseases simultaneously.
It is under these conditions that disease interaction occurs, often—but not always—with adverse health consequences. As Jonathan McCullers (2006:571)
comments with regard to the interaction of two prominent infectious diseases:

> Influenza virus and Streptococcus pneumonia rank as two of the most im-
> portant pathogens affecting humans today. However, it may be that their
> ability to work together that represents the greatest threat to world health.
> The catastrophic influenza A virus pandemic of 1918, which by conserva-
> tive estimates killed 40 to 50 million persons worldwide . . . is an extreme
> example of the impact that this cooperative interaction can have.

At the root of this syndemic interaction is the fact that influenza virus alters
the lungs in a way that predisposes the sufferer to *S. pneumoniade* adherence
and disease development. Additionally, influenza virus chemically changes the

immune response of infected individuals in a way that diminishes the body's ability to clear pneumococcus from the lungs.

The Global Burden of Disease studies, conducted in 1990 and 2000, found that sub-Saharan Africa has the highest total burden of diseases in the world (Murray and Lopez 1996). Within this context an examination of life expectancy across South African ethnic groups shows that the country's quadruple burden of disease is not equally distributed but instead is clustered in the poorer, black population. This type of clustering of multiple diseases and other health conditions in a population is illustrated by the SAVA syndemic.

SAVA

Based on many years of research with drug users, the author (Singer 1996, 1999) introduced the term SAVA, an acronym formed from the terms substance abuse, violence, and AIDS, as these three threats to health "are not merely concurrent, in that they are not wholly separable phenomena" (see Figure 6.2).

Although the link between substance abuse and HIV infection is widely recognized, other interconnections are not as well understood, such as the role of an AIDS diagnosis in enhancing levels of drug use, the impact of violence victimization on subsequent drug use and HIV infection risk, and the conditions under which drug use and drug craving lead to enhanced levels of violence. Although considerable work has been done on patterns of drug use and on the relationship of HIV transmission to specific risk behaviors, violence victimization, which represents a third route for the direct translation of unhealthy social conditions into ill health and suffering, is comparatively understudied. Nonetheless it is clear that in the lives of the urban poor of the developed world and, to an increasing degree, of metropolitan areas of developing countries, mind-altering drugs, violence and its bio-psychological effects, and HIV infection as well as other sexually transmitted diseases, hepatitis, and tuberculosis have significant

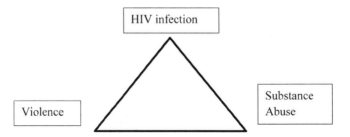

Figure 6.2 The SAVA syndemic.

behavioral and biological connections that amplify the dire health consequences of this deadly triad beyond their individual contributions to social suffering.

Other researchers have stressed the importance of mental health factors in SAVA. Various research teams, for example, have investigated the role of depression in interactions among polydrug use; violence, including child sexual abuse, intimate partner violence, antigay bigotry; and HIV risk behaviors in gay and bisexual men (Halkitis et al. 2013; Stall, Freidman, and Catania 2007). Research in various sites in sub-Saharan Africa affirms that SAVA has added to the disease burden of countries already carrying disproportionate levels of disease clustering. In three cities—Cape Town, Pretoria, and Durban, in South Africa—Charles Parry and colleagues (2009) found that risky injecting behaviors were common among injection drug users, with 20 percent of study participants testing positive for HIV disease. Additionally, testing among patients at emergency rooms in Cape Town, Port Elizabeth, and Durban found that violence-related injuries were more common among drug-involved patients than among patients with other types of injuries in both Cape Town and Durban (Parry et al. 2005). In South Africa drug use has increased as a consequence of globalization and the worldwide flow of drugs. This increase is enmeshed in domestic and gang violence, both of which occur in the context of an explosive HIV epidemic. All of these diseases, in turn, have taken root in a population with high rates of poverty, malnutrition, and considerable social stress.

Another way drug use is involved in the clustering and interaction of diseases under prevailing social conditions is a consequence of the use of syringes in illicit drug consumption and the ability of syringes to both protect and transmit pathogens, as seen with syringe-mediated syndemics.

SYRINGE-MEDIATED INFECTIOUS DISEASE SYNDEMICS

Although the role of illicit drug injection in the spread of HIV disease is generally known, less attention has been paid to the role of syringes in transmitting infectious disease syndemics. In addition to HIV disease, multiperson syringe use has been linked to the spread of a number of other infectious diseases, including hepatitis B (HBV), hepatitis C (HCV), human T-lymphotropic virus types I and II (HTLV), leishmaniasis, chikungunya fever, malaria, and other infections. Individuals who use a syringe recently used by a co-infected individual can acquire two interacting infections at the same time. For example, illicit drug injectors in Southern Europe have been found to be co-infected with HIV and the protozoa that is the proximate cause of leishmaniasis, a disease that can cause skin ulcers or, in its most severe form, visceral leishmaniasis (VL). Clinical expressions of VL include fever, weight loss, enlargement of the spleen, and anemia. If this disease is untreated, severe cases are often fatal. Latent infection may only become clinically manifest years or even decades after initial exposure, especially when infected individuals are immunocompromised for other reasons (e.g. HIV infection). The emergence of the HIV-leishmania syndemic resulted in higher mortality rates and lower mean survival time among dually infected individuals. This occurs because leishmania enhances HIV replication and stimulates the release of inflammatory molecules that play a role in HIV disease progression. At the same time, HIV infection stimulates intracellular growth of leishmania. The introduction of highly active antiretroviral therapy (HAART) has helped curtail the HIV-VL syndemic.

Although HIV-VL was seen among European illicit drug injections (see Figure 6.3), in the United States the HIV-HCV syndemic has been widely spread among injection drug users. In the United States between 15 to 30 percent of HIV patients are co-infected with HCV (Singer 2009c). HCV-triggered liver disease may be especially severe in HIV-infected individuals. Cirrhosis, for example, may be seven times higher in HIV/HCV co-infected patients than in HCV-infected patients not infected with HIV (Soto et al. 1997). Studies of injection drug users have found that "HIV infection modifies the natural history of chronic parenterally-acquired [i.e. injection-related] hepatitis C with an unusually rapid progression to cirrhosis" (Soto et al. 1997:1).

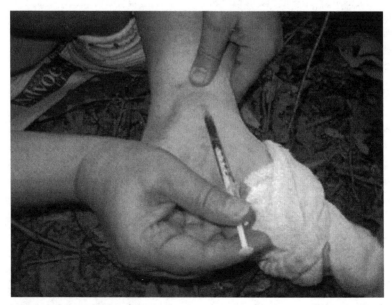

Figure 6.3 Injection drug use emerged as an important route of HIV infection. (Photo by Claudia Santilices)

The social structuring of disease clustering has had particular impact in the interaction of HIV and other diseases or conditions of poverty, such as malnutrition.

MALNUTRITION AND HIV DISEASE IN SOUTHERN AFRICA

In the poorest areas of the world and in very poor populations the world over a fateful interaction occurs between HIV and malnutrition. As a result, Southern Africa is facing a devastating set of co-occurring health and social challenges that includes food insecurity, HIV disease, and poverty. More exactly, the countries of the region are battling a constellation of interacting and mutually exacerbating epidemics and epidemic-enhancing social conditions. At the biological level interaction is centered in the body's host immune system; indeed, malnutrition and HIV infection are the two most common causes of acquired immune dysfunction, and these two conditions are closely linked, especially in regions like Southern Africa. Research suggests that the patterning of immune system suppression caused by malnutrition is similar in many ways to the immune effects of HIV infection (Singer 2008).

We now know that (1) macronutrient (energy-protein) needs to maintain body weight and physical activity levels increase during infection (e.g., by 10 percent for asymptomatic patients with HIV infection and 20 to 30 percent for symptomatic patients); (2) because of its need to replace immune cells expended on responding to pathogens, the immune system is a major consumer of micronutrients; and (3) inadequate nutrition plays an important role in immune dysfunction and the progression of HIV disease. Inadequate diet affects an array of immune system functions, including causing a reduction in the development of antibodies, a loss of delayed cutaneous hypersensitivity, a reduced concentration of immunoglobulin, a decreased presence of lymphocytes, a reduced production of interferon, and lowered levels of natural killer T cells and T cells subsets (e.g., helper cells) and interleukin 2 receptors, which are part of the immune system's signaling system that is instrumental in triggering immune response to infection. All immune cells and their immune active products (e.g., interleukins, interferons, and complements) "depend on metabolic pathways that use various nutrients as critical cofactors for their actions and activities" (Anabwani and Navario 2005:98). Interleukins are important in mounting initial immune responses to HIV, the success of which helps determine the length of the initial, symptom-free stage of HIV disease; interferon inhibits viral replication, especially by RNA-based pathogens, within other cells; and complements are biochemical reactions that clear pathogens from the body.

There are three primary connections between the development of a compromised immune system and inadequacies in the quantity and quality of food intake. First, inadequate protein-energy—and possibly fat—intake affects the immune system's capacity to fight infection, with protein-energy insufficiency being one of the primary causes of immunodeficiency in the developing world. This connection is understandable given immune cells' high energy and amino acid demands for the successful production of normal cells, as occurs during cell division. There are multiple potential immunostatus consequences of macronutrient insufficiency. Protein-energy malnutrition is linked with "a significant impairment of cell-mediated immunity, phagocyte function, the complement system, secretory immunoglobulin A antibody concentrations, and cytokine production" (Chandra 1997, 460). One specific impact of protein-energy insufficiency that has grave importance for the well-being of the immune system is the atrophying of the lymphoid organs, including substantial reductions in the size of both the thymus and the spleen. Lymphocytes produced by the thymus are helper cells that enable lymphocytes derived from bone marrow to differentiate into antibody-forming cells needed to respond to disease.

Second, specific nutrients—like vitamins C and E, selenium, and N-acetlycysteine, as well as dietary compounds like bioflavonoids and proanthocyanidans—help block the development of oxidative stress, a condition that damages the body's cells, including immune cells, and accelerates their destruction. There is a growing body of research suggesting that oxidative stress may contribute to pathogenesis (cell death) by pushing cells into a highly activated state, enhancing viral replication, weakening cell repair activity, decreasing immune cell proliferation, and contributing to loss of immune function. The potential for oxidative stress is rooted in normal oxygen metabolism, which is necessary for survival but puts cells at risk because of the consequent formation of a type of toxic oxygen cell, known as an oxidant, that has less than a full complement of electrons, such as some free radicals and peroxides. Under normal conditions the body's natural antioxidant networks maintain a delicate oxygen balance, limiting oxidant formation and resulting cell damage through enzyme-driven cell repair and oxidant-removal molecules like glutathione, an intracellular antioxidant that promotes T cell proliferation and activation. HIV-infected individuals, however, are under chronic oxidative stress and, as a result, their nutrient needs are elevated. Dietary insufficiency along with environmental exposures to tobacco smoke and other pollutants, excess alcohol consumption, and infectious agents can tip the balance leading to the overproduction of oxidants, oxidative stress, cell damage, and cell demise. In HIV disease patients oxidative stress appears to contribute in several ways to HIV disease pathogenesis, including viral replication, unbalanced inflammatory response, decreased immune cell proliferation, loss of immune function, cell apoptosis, chronic weight loss, and increased sensitivity to the potent toxicities of HIV medications (Singer 2011).

Third, various immune system components and processes depend on the consumption of specific micronutrients, and it is likely that almost all dietary nutrients have quite precise roles to play in maintaining an optimal immune response. Inadequate intake of micronutrients, a condition sometimes referred to as the *hidden hunger*, including vitamins, minerals, trace elements, essential amino acids, and linoleic acid, is known to damage immune system response.

During key developmental stages the multiple and significant connections between malnutrition and damage to the immune system can be particularly harmful. Of particular concern for children is the vicious cycle linking malnutrition and intestinal infection; diarrheal disease, which predisposes children to malnutrition and malnourishment, contributes to a greater incidence, longer duration, and increased severity of diarrhea disease. Consequently Richard Guerrant and colleagues (2008:48) argue that it is not unreasonable to view "malnutrition [itself] as an infectious disease with long-term effects on child development" as well as child and subsequent adult health (e.g., growth stunting). These researchers further argue that to "the 'double burden' of diarrhoea and malnutrition, data now suggest that children with stunted growth and repeated gut infections are also at increased risk of developing obesity and its associated comorbidities, resulting in a 'triple burden' of the impoverished gut" (Guerrant et al. 2013, 220). The impoverished gut is a term used to refer to damaged probiotic microbial life within a person's intestinal tract.

In South Africa in particular malnutrition also has ominously shaped the face of the HIV disease epidemic, with the two conditions in interaction comprising a particularly deadly syndemic. In various parts of sub-Saharan Africa, including South Africa, HIV infection occurs in "an environment of poverty, worsening nutrition, chronic parasite infection, and limited access to medical care. In such circumstances, people are more susceptible to all infectious diseases, however they are transmitted" (Stillwagon 2002:17–18). Consequently there is a consistent patterning of HIV disease as well as other disease clustering among the poor and other subjugated populations with limited resources and restricted life options. James Hargreaves and colleagues (2008:403) conducted a meta-analysis of existing studies and found that "HIV infections appear to be shifting toward higher prevalence among the least educated in sub-Saharan Africa, reversing previous patterns." More generally it is evident that impoverished populations suffering from numerous structural disadvantages and resulting interconnected breakdowns of social infrastructures, interpersonal relationships, and immune defenses are vulnerable to multiple diseases and disease syndemics, and this is the precise set of conditions found today among both rural and urban poor in Southern Africa.

Another social factor that contributes significantly to the cluster and interaction of various diseases is war and armed conflict.

SYNDEMICS OF WAR AND INFECTIOUS DISEASES

By causing physical and emotional trauma in populations, destroying health care and social infrastructures, despoiling the environment, intentionally or unintentionally producing or exacerbating food insecurity and malnutrition, and creating refugee populations, war is another force that promotes infectious disease syndemics. From the recording of infections during the Trojan War, to the fact that infectious diseases linked to poor sanitation killed more people than died in battle during American Civil War, to the global influenza pandemic during World War I mentioned above, to the fact that infection was still the leading cause of death after wounding during the Vietnam War, the importance of war in the frequency of infection is firmly established (Eardley et al. 2010; see also World Health Organization 2014b). It also is well documented that there was a significant jump in dengue in Southeast Asia during and immediately after World War II because of war-related spread of both mosquitoes and, with them, several different strains of the disease into new areas within the region. Similarly the Vietnam War promoted the spread of plague among civilians as a consequence of military-driven deforestation and the collapse of public health and social infrastructure (World Health Organization 2014b).

War and related conflict promotes infection in several identifiable ways, including:

1. The increase of frequency of direct and indirect contact between military and civilian populations, allowing for new disease transmission, including sexually transmitted diseases;
2. The deployment of troops to environmental settings with novel infectious agents for which soldiers have no acquired immunity based on previous exposure;
3. The physical and emotional stress of combat, placing soldiers at heightened risk of infection upon rapid exposure to multiple pathogens;
4. The manner in which infectious epidemics have been known to sweep through army field camps, prisoner of war camps, and other makeshift military settlements; and
5. The unsanitary conditions and militarily enforced population concentration and overcrowding and breakdown of disease control infrastructure (Smallman-Raynor and Cliff 2004).

War also promotes infection by causing malnutrition. The relationships between malnutrition and infectious disease are expressed at both the micro- and macrolevels.

At the microlevel, involving individual biology, the immune system requires an array of macro- and micronutrients to function optimally, and malnutrition compromises immune response. Further, the relationship between malnutrition and infectious disease is bidirectional: malnutrition can promote infection, whereas infection can interfere with the metabolism of nutrients. At the macro- or social level malnutrition can affect an entire population, as occurs in occupied territories and war-embargoed areas, or it can disproportionately degrade the health of vulnerable groups like children, pregnant women, those with preexisting health conditions, and the elderly caught up in a war zone. Under such conditions multiple individual and interacting infectious diseases can spread rapidly across numerous individuals. A study by Augustin Zeba and colleagues (2008) in the post–civil war West African country of Burkina Faso, for example, found a major reduction of malaria morbidity occurred following the administration of vitamin A and zinc to young children, suggesting the role these micronutrients play in containing malarial infection.

Although a malnutrition-infectious disease syndemic is not the only syndemic associated with war, it is of special importance for three reasons. First, war can disrupt access to food in multiple ways, including damaging domestic agriculture and food production, diminishing food transport, restricting access to food through imposed blockades and sanctions, and promoting the displacement of war refugees into areas of food insecurity. Second, because a population's military capacity diminishes with infectious disease progression and pathogenic transmission, disruption of food access has been an enticing weapon of war. The control of food sources or outright destruction of food is a war practice that predates modern times. In 1863, for example, when Lt. Colonel Christopher "Kit" Carson led federal troops against the Navajo for refusing to be confined on a government-imposed reservation, Carson had his soldiers burn Navajo corn fields, cut down their peach orchards, destroy their food caches, and slaughter their livestock. He also dispatched patrols to harass Navajo bands, preventing them from hunting game or gathering wild food plants. Rounded up and force-marched to Fort Sumner, many Navajo died of various causes, including dysentery, pneumonia, and smallpox. It is estimated that en route and while at Fort Sumner over 2,300 Navajo died before they were allowed to return to their homelands (Trafzer 1990).

Finally, interactions between malnutrition and infections in the context of war can affect individuals and populations long after a war has ended, such as adult onset health problems stemming from childhood malnutrition (Ostrach and Singer 2013). Various studies report that children who have been subject to malnutrition as infants suffer immunosuppression that persists over time (Gershwin et al. 2004). Additionally, malnutrition has been demonstrated to be a factor in tuberculosis and HIV co-infection, two diseases that frequently increase in prevalence in conflict zones (Accorsi et al. 2005).

The Somalia civil war in 1992 illustrates the nature of syndemic interaction in the context of war (see also Chapter 2). During the war, blocking civilian access to food led to famine, a collapse of health programs, and mass migration, which further exacerbated the food crisis because of contamination of food supplies. Malnutrition among children ranged between 47 percent and 75 percent. At the same time, diarrheal disease, measles, and *Shigella dysentery*—diseases exacerbated by malnutrition—led to the deaths of hundreds of children under five years of age and produced one of the highest-known mortality rates for civilians in a conflict zone (Moore et al. 1993). As this case indicates, children are at particular risk from syndemics of malnutrition and infectious disease in the context of war because they are passing through critical developmental stages, have specific dietary needs, and possess less developed immune systems.

ECOSYNDEMICS

Syringe-mediated syndemics and war-related syndemics are two of the ways social and behavioral factors can contribute to the spread of interlocked disease complexes. The natural environment, especially degradations of ecosystem health, also can promote what have been called *ecosyndemics* (Singer 2010b). For example, respiratory risks to human health are on the rise around the globe, at least in part because anthropogenic environmental changes are increasing and multiplying the likelihood of respiratory disease comorbidity and disease interaction. Overall, the quality of the air we breathe has diminished in recent decades because of several factors, including discharge from industrial power plants, release of industrial chemicals and gases by manufacturers, exhaust produced by motor vehicles, an increase in forest fires linked to global warming, and an upsurge in pollen from ragweed and other allergy-linked flora, which is also being driven by global warming. Research has shown that exposure to the air pollutant nitrogen dioxide produced by motor vehicles boosts both viral- and bacterial-induced asthma flare-ups. Research based on animal models suggests that exposure to this noxious gas plays a role in impairing immune response to respiratory pathogens by limiting the clearance of microbes from the respiratory tract and altering the function of macrophages during infection (Singer 2013b).

There is now considerable evidence, as C. Murray and colleagues (2006:376) indicate, that "a synergistic interaction [occurs] between allergens and viruses" in the development of asthma attacks. To examine this interaction, Murray and colleagues matched children by age and gender with acute asthma symptoms (the case group) with children with asthma who were not experiencing acute symptoms and children admitted to a hospital with nonrespiratory conditions. Findings showed that participants in the case group were at a significantly higher risk of having been both exposed to and sensitive to allergens and of having a higher respiratory pathogen load than participants in either of the control groups. Multivariate analysis found that a combination of both risk factors—allergy and nasal pathogens—increased the risk of hospital admission by almost twenty-fold. Murray and colleagues (2006, 381–382) concluded that their results "indicate that there appears to be a combined rather than an individual effect of natural virus infection and real life allergen exposure in allergic asthmatic children in inducing asthma exacerbations."

Ecosyndemics of this sort are of particular risk in the time of global warming because of the dramatic and diverse impacts of climate change on local environmental conditions. It is likely that ecosyndemics, as a consequence of diseases' ability to diffuse to new regions, will result in novel infectious disease profiles in diverse populations as the impacts of global warming, air pollution, and other biosphere changes progress and interact over time. For example, although no such ecosyndemic currently is known to be occurring, because Lyme disease and West Nile fever now have overlapping ranges in North America, the potential for adverse interaction exists. However, copresence of multiple diseases does not automatically result in adverse interactions; in fact, as has been noted, in a type of interaction known as a countersyndemic, the presence of one disease may inhibit development of another disease. Examples of this kind of interaction were described earlier with reference to GBC-C and HIV infection (Chapter 2) and roundworm infection and bacterial or viral-induced fever leading to a diminishment of helminth development (this chapter). Recognition of this fact has led to consideration of the use of infectious diseases therapeutically in treating other health problems.

CONCLUSION: SYNDEMICS OF HUMAN AFFLICTION

The occurrence of syndemics offers significant support for the value of conceiving of infectious diseases as products of biosocial and biocultural processes. Social relations promote the concentration, interaction, and spread of infectious diseases. Of particular concern are patterns of social conflict, social inequality and discrimination, and the unhealthy living conditions and lived experiences they foster, including overcrowding, inadequate nutrition, stress and trauma, exposure to industrial toxins, exposure to the elements, environmental disruptions, and breakdowns of health and social infrastructure. Cultural responses to various forms of structural violence, like poverty and discrimination, including the adoption of survival and coping strategies—such as participation in commercial sex activities and illicit drug use and drinking as well as behaviors such as the reliance on household members as caregivers of the sick or burial practices that involve contact with a victim of lethal infectious diseases—can accentuate infectious disease syndemics. Syndemics, in short, are entwined complexes of biological, social, cultural, and often environmental factors. Although understudied until relatively recently, it is becoming increasingly clear that individuals and populations commonly harbor multiple infectious agents and that their impact on health is in no small part a consequence of their diverse interactions. In light of the patterns of infectious disease emergence, reemergence, and growing drug resistance as well as the promotion of disease spread by globalization, infectious disease syndemics have become a health issue of growing importance and a significant force shaping global health. Shifting from traditional one-disease-at-a-time thinking within biomedicine and public health toward a model of syndemic disease interaction allows for the development of new, more comprehensive approaches that enhance our focus on infectious disease in biosocial and biocultural contexts.

Discussion Questions

1. How does a syndemic differ from an epidemic?
2. How does a syndemic differ from a co-infection?
3. How do diseases interact?
4. What are the roles of social and cultural factors in syndemics?
5. Why is HIV called a syndemogenic disease?
6. What kinds of bidirectional interactions occur between malnutrition and infectious diseases?
7. Why does war contribute to the development of syndemics?
8. How significant are syndemics in global health?

CHAPTER 7

Inequality, Political Ecology, and the Future of Infectious Diseases

> Social inequality kills. It deprives individuals and communities of a
> healthy start in life, increases their burden of disability and disease, and
> brings early death. Poverty and discrimination, inadequate medical care,
> and violation of human rights all act as powerful social determinants of
> who lives and who dies, at what age, and with what degree of suffering.
>
> *Nancy Krieger (2005:15)*

THE SOCIAL AND CULTURAL ORIGINS OF INFECTION

This book has emphasized the fact that diseases among humans occur in complex and intertwined biological, environmental, social, and cultural worlds.
Within anthropology this nexus has been referred to as "the social origins of
disease," although, as we have seen, important cultural and environmental elements are always involved. Writing about avian influenza in Central Java, for
example, Siwi Padmawati and Mark Nichter (2008::46) observe that it "is more
appropriate to think of [the disease] as a biosocial and biopolitical challenge for
Indonesia, rather than merely an epidemiological challenge involving a disease
of zoonotic origin." This chapter addresses key factors in the social and cultural
origins, distribution, and differential consequence of infectious diseases. A
focus on the social and cultural nature of health affirms the importance of
understanding and treating infectious disease as much more than a biological
or narrowly medical issue. Although, as has been stressed, infectious agents
like bacteria, viruses, and helminths are the necessary and immediate causes
of infection, who gets infected, under what conditions, and with what health
and social outcomes as well as how sufferer's health problems are culturally
constructed, experienced, and responded to by society involve far more than
the biological aspects of disease. To think of disease solely in term of pathogens, vectors, hosts, and immune systems ignores a great deal about disease,
including how social systems and cultural practices affect pathogens, vectors,
hosts, and immune systems through time, as mediated by the environment,
and in specific local or broader geographic contexts.

This discussion takes on new relevance in a time of growing critique of the historic nature/society dualism within and beyond anthropology coupled with growing efforts to integrate our understanding of the social and biological aspects of the human condition. This surge toward a new synthesis, born of social changes (e.g., various biotechnologies) that have "liberated both the biological sciences and the social sciences and humanities from their old ontological moorings, allowing once divided disciplines to mix in the same melting pot" (Ingold 2013:21), suggests a vital new direction for twenty-first-century anthropology. Already it is clear that a missing link can be found in the literature of this emergent approach within the discipline (Ingold and Palsson 2013, Jablonka and Lamb 2005)—namely, a failure to conduct a political economic unpacking of the social and cultural dimensions that shape mutually constitutive interactions with the biological and environmental domains.

This chapter directs our attention to the ultimate causes of much of the world's infection-related morbidity and mortality: the unequal structures of human social relationships across and within nations, typically in terms of gender, class, ethnicity, sexual orientation, and other often-punishing social divisions. In other words, the chapter focuses on the political economic dimensions of the cultural and social factors in infectious disease health. The concern is with examining what Paul Farmer (2004) broadly has called the "pathologies of power" (i.e., the diseases of inequality) while critiquing efforts that pathologize poverty, characterizing the poor or other marginalized groups as inherently abnormal—indeed, as the cause of their own poor health (Baer, Singer, and Susser 2013). A focus on political economy directs attention to the structural factors within social systems—social class, discrimination, segregation, barriers to political participation, status quo–affirming media messages—that shape infectious disease occurrence, distribution, and outcome (Katz 1990, Royster 2003).

A political economic analysis of contemporary infectious disease must go beyond the broad social determinants of sickness to consider the beneficiaries, "those who benefit from the inequalities that kill" (Navarro 2009: 440). Those who profit from inequality, Vicente Navarro stresses, are the dominant and most powerful social classes, in rich and poor countries alike, that accumulate wealth for their own benefit rather than allow the wealth of the world to benefit the well-being of all of humanity, indeed all of Earth's biologically diverse inhabitants. As Charles Briggs and Clara Mantini-Briggs (2004:8) emphasize, infectious disease epidemics "are 'mirrors held up to society,' revealing differences and power as well as the special terrors that haunt different populations." The International Monetary Fund (IMF), which advises governments on economic growth, has concluded that economic inequality in a society serves as a drag on national economic development: "narrowing of inequality help[s] support faster and more durable growth" (Ostry et al. 2014:25), including expanding access to health resources. Although this perspective has blossomed in recent years in certain economic circles, it is not a new approach at all but rather can be traced to Rudolph Virchow's mid-nineteenth century "Report on the Typhus Epidemic in Upper Silesia" in Germany and his conclusion that the infectious disease outbreak he studied occurred because of "the wretched conditions of life that poverty . . . had created in Upper Silesia" (Virchow 2006:2012). If these conditions of vast social inequality were removed, he asserted, "epidemic typhus would not recur" (Virchow 2006:2012). To understand typhus in Upper Silesia and, by extension, all significant infectious diseases everywhere, Virchow asserted, it is necessary to locate disease distribution and effect in terms of the class structure of society.

This chapter begins by contrasting what historian William McNeil, in a model that various anthropologists have adopted, termed the micro- and macroparasites of human societies, and moves on to examine the politicization of infection and infectious disease research, infections as stigmatizing diseases, the relationship of what Foucault called *biopower* to infection, infectious diseases and human rights, the role of anthropology in addressing the human suffering caused by infectious diseases, and the future of infection in light of contemporary knowledge about how the world is changing.

MICRO- AND MACROPARASITES AND THE CRITICAL MEDICAL ANTHROPOLOGY OF INFECTION

Although biomedical approaches to infectious disease have been concerned especially with biological factors, anthropology seeks to build an understanding that recognizes the relationship of immediate biological factors and the social and political economic factors that turn the possibility of infection into actual disease and disease into an epidemic. A starting point is recognition that "harmful colonization of a host by a microscopic species that uses the host's resources for its own reproduction, is a necessary *but insufficient* cause of contagious disease" (Brown et al. 2012:254, emphasis added). Other factors to consider are the quality of the host's immune system and the living conditions the host faces that affect immune functioning, such as diet, stress, trauma, and treatment access. Consequently understanding the causes of infectious disease outbreaks involves linking the microworld of biological events within bodies to the external social world of events, structural relationships, and environmental conditions and linking these, in turn, to the broader realm of political economic forces that shape the possibilities of human life. In this regard, William McNeil, in his classic book *Plagues and People* (1976), drew an important distinction between what he called:

- *microparasites*—the microbes that serve as the infectious agents of disease, and
- *macroparasites*—*the human social groups and strata that dominate others and live off of their labor and resources*

Here McNeill is using these terms quite differently than commonly is the case in biology, where the key issue is whether a parasite multiplies within their definitive host or not. An important arena of work in the anthropology of infectious diseases is clarifying the nature of the intersection of micro- and macroparasites in McNeil's usage—namely, how they work together to cause disease. This point can be illustrated with several examples.

Since Robert Koch's discovery of the infectious agent in 1882 we have known that *Mycobacterium tuberculosis* causes tuberculosis. The name is derived from the Latin word "tuberculum," a diminutive of tuber or node, and the Greek word "osis," which means abnormal condition. This pathogen commonly enters the body during breathing, although it can be contracted in other ways as well. Frequent exposure to people with the disease—breathing in the air they exhale—substantially increases the risk of infection. There are two stages to the disease. During primary infection the pathogen passes into the body and travels down to the middle and lower lung areas, where it gains access to the bloodstream until it lodges in an organ of the body. Although the body's immune system limits disease development, the body does not rid itself of the pathogen, and thus it can persist in a dormant state, often for decades. During this period the immune system produces macrophages that surround the tubercle bacilli. These cells form a hard shell that keeps the pathogen contained. If the individual is re-infected or if the quality of the body's immune system is diminished because of malnutrition, injury, infection with another microbial agent like HIV, or as a result of childbirth, however, tuberculosis can transition into its secondary, or chronic stage. In this phase it is not the microorganism that causes the primary harm to the body; rather, as the immune system responds to the detected presence of M. tuberculosis by killing the pathogen, there is a steady build-up of dead cells or tubercles, which cause inflammation and destroy body tissues. During the active phase infectious aerosol droplets are expelled through coughing, sneezing, speaking, and spitting, and these transmit the disease to new hosts.

Although this account provides the basic outline of tuberculosis as a disease, it is inadequate. Left out of this description are the social conditions that both promote the transmission of infection from one person to the next and propel the transition from latent (primary) to active (secondary) infection. There was no mention of who gets tuberculosis—and who does not—and under what conditions. Richard Levins and Richard Lewontin (1985) begin to fill in these missing parts of the story by stressing that political economic factors are as much a cause of tuberculosis as *M. tuberculosis*. Addressing the questions of who gets tuberculosis and under what circumstances, Randall Packard, writing of South Africa during apartheid, reports that whites accounted for only 1 percent of new cases each year (1989). In this society, racially segregated by law, most cases occurred among impoverished blacks living in overcrowded and squalid rural slums, subject to harsh discriminatory laws and everyday brutalities, and with restricted access to medical treatment. To survive, many black workers were forced to take jobs in the mining industry, which historically was tightly controlled by South Africa's "Big Six" white-owned mining companies (Anglo American/De Beers, Gencor/Billiton, Goldfields, JCI, Anglovaal, and Rand Mine). Given the nature of South Africa's mineral resources, mining is a labor-intensive job requiring many workers to extract valuable ore, including gold, diamonds, coal, and vanadium. It was in underground mines, under difficult working conditions, that workers often were exposed to tuberculosis; if they fell ill, they were sent "home," taking their infection with them and transmitting it to other family members. In the rural areas "impoverishment undermined the ability of rural Africans to resist ... [tuberculosis] which were transmitted by returning [labor] migrants" (Packard 1989:11).

Social factors also are critical to the spread of tuberculosis elsewhere in the world. As physician/anthropologist Paul Farmer observes, "We cannot understand its marked patterned occurrence—in the United States, for example, afflicting those in homeless shelters and in prison—without understanding how social forces, ranging from political violence to racism, come to be embodied as individual pathology" (1999:13). Living in poverty increases the likelihood of exposure to MTb because of overcrowding in poorly ventilated dwellings. Research in homeless shelters in New York City, for instance, has shown that they are a focal point of tuberculosis transmission among the poor. Once infected, the poor are more likely to develop active tuberculosis both because they are more likely to have multiple exposures to MTb, which may push dormant bacteria into an active state, and because they are more likely to have preexistent immune system damage from other infections and malnutrition. Finally, poverty and discrimination place the poor at a disadvantage in terms of access to diagnosis and treatment for tuberculosis and diminish their ability to adhere to treatment plans due to structurally imposed residential instability and the frequency of disruptive economic and social crises in poor families.

In a parallel case, anthropologist Kris Heggenhougen (2009) describes the situation of Mayan people living in the village of Simajuleu, Guatemala. Denied access by the ruling elite to adequate land to farm and feed their families, men in the village were forced to take out loans. To repay these loans, they were compelled to take farm worker jobs at low wages on wealthy estates in the lowlands, areas that were infested with mosquitoes that transmitted malaria. In this case, although a pathogen and vector were necessary conditions for the transmission of malaria, the prevailing structure of inequality and capitalist mode of production and labor control were equally critical elements in disease transmission.

Writing about his extended ethnographic field work on malaria in Tanzania, Vinay Kamat notes that mothers of children with malaria seen at a local hospital commonly say "maisha magumu—tunahangaika tu!" ("life is hard, we are just struggling") (2013:5). Statements like this, coupled with his fuller experience of watching both malaria and malaria control efforts unfold before his eyes, led Kamat to recognize:

1. the importance of identifying the cultural context of malaria control efforts;
2. the prerequisite to document the lived reality of the malaria illness experience for patients and their families;
3. the need to pay attention to the social and not just the biomedical burden of malaria;
4. the impact of the uncertainty of everyday life, the lack of a social safety net to support people in times of crises, and the social suffering that expresses how people in poor communities experience childhood malaria; and
5. the role micro- and macrolevel social forces like gender discrimination and structural inequalities play in the persistence of malaria among the poor.

Kamat came to realize that "there is more to malaria than mosquitoes, parasites, and medicines"; there are also "existing social, political, and economic realities or structural arrangements that influence people's vulnerability and susceptibility to disease" (2013:5).

More than three decades earlier Milton Terris argued, based on research in India, that to understand the causes of cholera there it is necessary to go beyond the ground level of disease biology and "go back hundreds of years in India's history, to the British invasion and destruction of once-flourishing textile industries; the maintenance of archaic systems of land ownership and tillage; the persistence of the caste system with its unbelievable poverty, hunger, and crowding; the consequent inability to afford the development of safe water supplies and sewage disposal systems; and, almost incidentally, the presence of cholera vibrios" (1979:204).

Indeed, history is rich with additional examples. In 1648 the New World experienced its first epidemic of yellow fever, an acute viral hemorrhagic disease transmitted by mosquito vectors. For the next two hundred years, as Molly Crosby (2006:12) reports, "Yellow fever became the most dreaded disease in North America" and even, because of the toll it took on French troops, played a role when Haiti became the second European colony to win independence. The source was a virus brought to the Americas via the slave trade. By contrast, Asia, which has the vector mosquito *Aedes aegypti* but never had an African slave trade, is not home to the disease. In other words, slavery, a form of human mobility framed around radical differences in wealth and power and intense structural oppression, was critical to the history of yellow fever.

Yellow fever, in fact, is but the tip of the iceberg in the infectious disease legacy of the transatlantic slave trade, a momentous social and environmental reordering that underlines the significant and prolonged disease burden of the intersection of micro- and macroparasites. It has been firmly established that mortality rates of the various components of the slave trade, including within Africa and during passage across the Atlantic, were enormous. Between 1700 and 1850 more than 20 million Africans were traded as slaves, of whom 4 million died in the process (Emmer 2006). Dale Graden (2014) argues that infectious diseases took such an enormous toll on slaves (and slave ship crews) crossing the ocean and, hence, on trader's profits that they played a pivotal role in eventually convincing the wealthy not to invest in the transatlantic slave trade. Nonetheless, two hundred years since the abolition of the trade, infectious diseases, including lymphatic filariasis, schistosomiasis, and onchocerciasis, probably transported from Africa to the Americas during slavery, continue to put people living in poverty at risk in Central and South America and the Caribbean (Lammie et al. 2007).

Lymphatic filariasis remains a health issue in Brazil, the Dominican Republic, Haiti, and Guyana and is a growing problem especially in urban slums. This rise stems from adaptations of one of its vectors, *Culex quinquefasciatus*, popularly known in some areas as the southern house mosquito, that allow it to thrive and proliferate in crowded urban areas with inadequate sanitary, sewage, and drainage systems. In Brazil, for example, lymphatic filariasis is a public health problem in cities within the metropolitan Recife region on the Northeastern coast (Fontes et al. 2012).

Onchocerciasis, or river blindness, is found in Mexico, Guatemala, Columbia, Brazil, Venezuela, and Ecuador. Carried by infected slaves taken from heavily endemic areas of West Africa, it was picked up and spread by local indigenous black fly species such as *S. ochraceum*. "Labor and other migration, and the presence of different vectors in the environment" promoted the regional spread of the disease (Gustavsen, Hopkins, and Sauerbrey 2011). Guatemala ultimately had the largest number of people at risk for onchocerciasis in the Americas. The disease has been most commonly found in what is known as the Central Endemic Zone of Guatemala, an area hospitable to the breeding of vector black flies whose human population "consists primarily of poor, indigenous people of Mayan descent who mostly live and work on small . . . privately owned coffee farms called *fincas*" (Richards 2000:237). A robust campaign for control of the disease throughout the Americas coordinated by the Onchocerciasis Elimination Program for the Americas has made significant gains and holds the potential for eliminating this disease of slavery from the Western Hemisphere.

Schistosomiasis was once quite widespread throughout the Caribbean and South America and was a major source of hepatic fibrosis and death. Millions of people in Brazil, especially those who carry out domestic and social activities in rivers or other bodies of water in the poorer northeast region of the country, are still at risk of infection, although this disease has been contained in other areas. The social process of rural-to-urban migration and the concentration of impoverished migrant populations from endemic areas in urban slums with a lack of sanitation and basic hygienic infrastructure have promoted fecal contamination of aquatic environments and the expansion of schistosomiasis to locations that previously were thought to be disease-free (de Souza Gomes et al. 2012).

These three infectious diseases as well as several others transmitted to the New World by the slave trade continue to take a toll on human life and well-being, especially among those—including, perhaps disproportionately, descendants of slaves—who are forced by existing social hierarchies and inequalities to dwell in deprived and inadequate living conditions long after the last slave-bearing ship hauled its suffering cargo from the shores of Africa.

Issues of inequality are critical not only in disease causation but also in the treatment and prevention of infectious diseases. Unequal access to health services is based on various factors, including social class, ethnicity, gender, sexual orientation, or other axis of overt and built-in social discrimination. For example, research on childhood vaccination in Bangladesh for deadly and disabling infectious diseases like smallpox, poliomyelitis, and measles found that girls were less likely to be immunized than were boys; children whose fathers had a higher-status job with salaried employment were two-and-a-half times more likely to be immunized than children whose fathers held lower-status jobs such as day laborer; and children living in slum areas of cities had the lowest levels of immunization (Chowdhury et al. 2003).

The effects of inequality of risk and access to treatment are found even in the most technologically advanced countries. In the United States Peter Hotez (2008) has described the considerable health burden of a group of chronic and debilitating parasitic, bacterial, and congenital infections among the poor. Termed *neglected infections of poverty,* such diseases are characterized by their chronicity, disabling features, and disproportionate impact on the almost 50 million people who live below the US poverty line. Neglected infections of poverty include a long list of conditions, such as toxocariasis, strongyloidiasis, *ascariasis,* cysticercosis, *trichomoniasis,* leptospirosis, dengue, and cytomegalovirus. Hotez (2008) observes that "tens of thousands, or in some cases, hundreds of thousands of poor Americans harbor these chronic infections, which represent some of the greatest health disparities in the United States." The same pattern occurs worldwide. Poverty creates conditions that promote the spread of infectious diseases and thwart affected populations from obtaining adequate preventive and treatment services. Together poverty and infectious diseases "drive a vicious cycle . . . from which for many there is no escape" (Griffiths and Zhou 2012:12). The Commission on Social Determinants of Health (2008:1) stresses, "This . . . is not in sense a 'natural' phenomenon." Rather, it is created socially through discrimination, exploitation, injustice, and bigotry.

Inequality of access characterizes social hierarchies across nations. Assessment of access to treatment for HIV disease, for example, reflects clear disparities between rich and poor countries. From the perspective of many global health workers, "Addressing the dramatic inequalities between rich and poor countries in access to health care is one of the biggest challenges of this century" (Giuliano and Vella 2007:313). Social inequality can shape treatment of infectious disease in ways that go beyond issues of access to available therapies and preventive measures. Based on ethnographic research in Grahamstown, South Africa, for example, anthropologist Chaunetta Jones (2011) found that people living with HIV disease are forced to choose between a degree of economic security and accessing available *antiretroviral therapy* (ART). As a result, some people refuse ART despite its demonstrated life-saving effectiveness. Under conditions of high levels of poverty, widespread unemployment, and economic suffering—historic products of the South Africa's history of apartheid and its subordinate place in the global economy—people living with HIV disease are forced to rely on disability assistance grants from the government as their main source of income. To receive assistance, an HIV-positive individual must have a significantly damaged immune system as evidenced by a CD_4 count of two hundred or lower. Accessing treatment could result in improved health and increased CD_4 counts, and although this may lead to the patient losing their assistance grant, it will not lead to a job or other source of income. Although not intended to serve as a long-term relief measure, in the absence of other means to alleviate poverty, for many HIV sufferers the disability grant has become a means of immediate economic survival, including having the money for food, shelter, and other necessities of living (Hardy and Richter 2006; Leclerc-Madlala 2006). Consequently, Jones contends, "economic inequalities and structural barriers have created dire situations in which [people living with HIV disease] often are forced to choose between economic and food security and their health security" (2011:68).

All of these cases presented above indicate that *microorganisms and structures of social inequity work in tandem to create infectious diseases and epidemics.* This consistent pattern affirms the need for multidimensional health interventions that address both the biological and social aspects of infectious diseases. These cases, moreover, point to the need for theoretical models in the anthropology of infection that link microlevel social patterns (on-the-ground local conditions accessed through ethnography) and macrolevels social structures (political economic systems of inequality and unequal distribution of power and resources) in light of environmental and biological factors in disease.

Critical medical anthropology (Baer, Singer, and Susser 2013; Singer and Erickson 2013), introduced in the Introduction, provides one such framework for multilevel analysis in the anthropology of infection. Critical medical anthropology focuses on assessing the social origins of disease, such as the ways in which poverty, discrimination, stigmatization, physical violence, and structural violence contribute to poor health and diminish access to treatment. This concern illuminates the existence of a *biology of inequality,* such as the ways social disparity and deprivation get "under the skin" and are inscribed by pathogens on body systems and organs as disease. In other words, "we literally incorporate biologically the world around us," a world we must study to understand fully "who and what is responsible for population patterns of health, disease, and well-being, as manifested in present, past and changing social inequalities in health" (Krieger 2007:668). In such research a critical perspective emphasizes the role of structures of power and inequality in the distributive dimension of health, including health care access, inequalities within health care systems, and the contributions of health ideas and practices, such as the *stigmatization* of various infectious diseases, to reinforcing inequalities in the wider society.

In addition to linking the infectious disease burden of a group or population to patterns of structural inequality, critical medical anthropology examines linkages between the reductions in infectious disease burden in wealthier developed countries and the continued infectious disease burden of poorer countries. The colloquial expression "there's more fruit in a rich man's shampoo than on a poor man's plate" adroitly encapsulates the global pattern of inequalities with reference to nutrition. But beyond this level of association, how exactly are wealthier countries' wealth and health of their middle and upper classes sources of poor health in poorer countries? This relationship is seen, for example, in the drivers and consequences of deforestation. Research conducted by the World Wildlife Fund (2014) indicates the international timber trade is the primary cause of forest loss. This pattern developed rapidly after World War II—All imports increased by almost 1,500 percent in three decades—as wealthier nations began to import tropical hardwood timber from developing nations (Myers 1980).

The pattern continues today. For example, to rebuild following the earthquake and tsunami that hit Japan in the spring of 2011, a disaster that destroyed 100,000 to 150,000 buildings, Japan, a wealthy nation, significantly increased lumber and related wood product imports not only from developed nations like the United States and Canada but also from developing countries like Malaysia and Indonesia. Malaysia has been deforesting at a rate that is three times that of most of the rest of Asia, and deforestation in Indonesia has had an equally devastating impact. The World Wildlife Fund (2014) estimates that half of the forest cover in Sumatra, Indonesia, disappeared from 1985 and 2008, with overall forest cover dropping from 50 to 25 percent. Lost forests and the biodiversity that is diminished when old-growth and tropical forests are cleared contribute to increases in infectious disease in several ways, including increasing contact with disease vectors like rodents and bats, exposing human populations to zoonotic infectious agents, and facilitating flooding and waterborne infection, as discussed Chapters 4 and 5. So too the forced migration to crowded, unsanitary urban centers by forest-dwelling peasants when the forests they have relied on for a livelihood are cut down. This same pattern is repeated across various kinds of resource extraction by affluent countries from poorer ones, a flow of resources that facilitates rising standards of living that diminish infectious disease in developed nations as it promotes poverty and the spread of infectious diseases in developing nations (Parenti 2007). In a world in which the 20 percent of the world's population living in rich countries consumes approximately 80 percent of global resources, the poorest and least healthy pay the health bill for the wealthiest and healthiest people on the planet.

INFECTIOUS DISEASE OF INDIGENOUS POPULATIONS

The case of the Mayan people examined by Heggenhougen (2009) draws attention to the special conditions indigenous populations face in a time of dramatic social inequalities and the global movement of infectious disease. Michael Gracey and Malcolm King (2009) define indigenous peoples as those who are self-identified as aboriginal; who maintain historical continuity and strong links to specific territory; who have distinctive local social, political economic, and cultural systems; and who seek to manage their own affairs separate from centralized states. The approximately 400 million indigenous people worldwide—although they comprise only a small percentage of the total human population today—have been pivotal to the founding of the discipline of anthropology. Consequently there is a considerable anthropological literature on the aboriginal populations of Australia, Native Americans, Inuit, tribal groups of Asia, and indigenous peoples of Africa. This body of research shows that, wherever they are found, indigenous peoples tend to be overrepresented among the poor and disadvantaged and in poor health relative to non-Indigenous counterparts: "Their susceptibility to disease is exacerbated by poor living conditions and water supplies, often with restricted access to fresh and nutritious food, and inadequate health services" (Gracey and King 2009:65).

As a consequence of their marginalized living conditions and subjection to oppressive social relations by dominant groups in societies worldwide, indigenous populations are disproportionately affected by infectious diseases, especially skin infections (e.g., impetigo and tungiasis), eye (e.g., trachoma) and ear (e.g., acute and chronic otitis) infections, dental caries, respiratory and urinary tract infections, diarrheal diseases, and neglected tropical diseases (e.g., intestinal helminth and protozoan infections; zoonotic parasitic infections; neglected bacterial infections like trachoma, leprosy, and yaws; and vector-borne illnesses such as malaria and dengue) (Hotez 2014). This intense clustering of infectious diseases among indigenous populations reflects the critical importance of social inequality, denial of access to needed resources, and racism in the creation of overlapping infectious endemics, epidemics, and syndemic disease profiles.

Indigenous populations have proven to be particularly vulnerable to emergent infectious diseases. Research has shown that emerging diseases that are disproportionately common or virulent among indigenous peoples include several respiratory tract infections, infections associated with antimicrobial-resistant organisms, zoonotic diseases, viral hepatitis, tuberculosis, *Helicobacter pylori*, diseases linked to streptococcus, and meningitis (Butler et al. 2001). Among the Māori, the indigenous people of New Zealand, for example, there has been an epidemic among children stretching for over a decade of invasive meningococcal disease associated with the person-to-person spread of *Neisseria meningitidis* (serogroup B) under conditions of overcrowding. Meningococcal disease is a serious and, without appropriate and urgent care, potentially life-threatening condition. Symptoms include high fever, neck stiffness, mental confusion, nausea and vomiting, lethargy, and skin rash. In 2011 the case fatality rate was approximately 11 percent. The median age of infection among the Māori was two years, compared to eighteen years for New Zealanders of European origin (Lopez, Sexton, and Carter 2012). Additionally, acute rheumatic fever continues to be an important infectious disease health problem among the Māori.

Although the Māori comprise between 5 and 15 percent of the New Zealand population, they suffer almost 60 percent of reported cases. Hardly found any longer among New Zealanders of European origin, the disease is associated with poverty, overcrowding, and hindered access to health care. Individuals who have had acute rheumatic fever are at risk of recurrent infection and of developing chronic rheumatic heart disease if not on preventive medication for at least ten years. Despite the existence of treatments, the incidence of acute rheumatic fever, rheumatic heart disease, and the number of deaths caused by chronic rheumatic heart disease are increasing among the indigenous people of New Zealand as well as among in-migrants to New Zealand from other Pacific Island nations (Best Practices Advocacy Centre 2011).

Although cultural and social conditions vary among indigenous people around the world, disproportionate rates of various infectious diseases tend to be something they have in common, a reflection of the marginalization, displacement, and intolerance they suffer within modern nations.

THE POLITICS OF INFECTION

Once it occurs—or even before that, when it is a threat or imagined threat—disease is always political. It raises questions of causation and responsibility; it entails issues of power and its unequal distribution in society; and it is a source of social strategies and contestations. This is because disease is a point of contact between health and "interest," in the sense of, What is in my own best interest? What are the class, gender, regional, national, or other interests shared by a group in opposition to other groups—say, employers and workers in a labor dispute? For a closer analysis it is appropriate to talk about the politics of infectious disease at two levels: *micropolitics* and *macropolitics of infectious disease.*

Micropolitics of infectious disease can be seen in action, as Gay Becker pointed out, when the body suffers a serious illness: "one's sense of wholeness, on which a sense of order rides, disintegrates. One must constitute that sense of wholeness in order to regain a sense of continuity" (1999:39). Illness, she notes, "necessitates the surrender of the cherished assumption of personal indestructability" (40). Efforts to restore a sense of order and wholeness involve interactions with physicians and other health care providers. Thus, a sufferer of infectious disease must engage in a political and narrative process of explaining to herself: Why did I get sick? How is my sickness related to my life situation, to treatment by others, to decisions I have made? Often, as Howard Waitzkin (2000) stresses, in answer to these questions doctors focus patient attention on proximal issues—lifestyle, exposure to infections—and away from more distal but ultimately more compelling social structural factors in disease. The micropolitics of infectious disease, including face-to-face interaction between healers and sufferers, tends to reproduce the macrolevel of domination in society in the everyday microlevel of interaction of individuals.

Anthropologist Heather Paxson has introduced the term "microbiopolitics" to refer specifically to "the creation of categories of microscopic biological agents; the anthrocentric evaluation of such agents; and the elaboration of appropriate human behaviors vis-à-vis microorganisms engaged in infection, inoculation, and digestion" (2008:17). Such microbiopolitics are expressed in government policies regarding commercial food safety standards for appliances such as refrigerators, mandatory childhood vaccination, hospital mandates concerning the use of rubber gloves and the cleaning of surfaces in health care clinics, and signs in restaurant bathrooms reminding employees concerning policies on hand washing. Another example of microbiopolitics is addressed in Erin Koch's (2006) study of prisoners in post-Soviet Georgia and their participation in bartering for the sputum of tuberculosis patients because a diagnosis of tuberculosis is a ticket to more appealing living conditions in the prison. "Trafficking in sputum," argues Koch (2006:50), "is a form of constrained agency in which disease becomes a survival strategy." This also occurs, of course, among people living with HIV disease in South Africa who refuse treatment as a means of retaining access to food. These cases show that, pressed to the limit, people may choose infectious disease as a means of—at least short-term—survival under harsh social conditions.

Macropolitics, in the case of infectious disease, refers to dominant conclusions about the origin of infection, how those who are infected are portrayed, their social treatment, and their access to care. For example, in discussing tuberculosis among migrants from India and Pakistan in Britain after World War II, John Welshman (2010) notes that the media, public health professionals, and health policy presented the problem as one of migrants from areas with high incidence of tuberculosis coming to Britain already infected. In this rendering migrants are seen as carrying disease with them, which led to encouragement for a policy of administering chest X-rays at ports of entry into the country. As Welshman (2010:133) further notes, "the blame for Asian susceptibility to tuberculosis [was] placed largely on the victim, and actual attempts to tackle the environmental factors in disease remained quite limited." Tuberculosis among Indian and Pakistani migrants was not interpreted as a consequence of contracting the disease in Britain, where migrants were forced to live in poor, overcrowded neighborhoods, endured stressful working conditions, were subjected to social discrimination, and had, as a result of poverty, nutrient-poor diets. Rather than these social conditions, which the dominant society imposed, immigrants were stigmatized as inherently infectious people of color from underdeveloped and unhygienic nations.

The politics of infection extends to the realm of infectious disease research and application. The existence of such a politics is the argument of Bruno Latour's insightful book *The Pasteurization of France* (1993). In this volume Latour asserts that the triumph of the French microbiologist Louis Pasteur, often heralded as the "father of germ theory" for his contributions to infectious disease prevention, can only be understood within the particular historical convergence of competing social forces and conflicting interests in France in the later part of the nineteenth century. In pointing out the fundamental importance of social events and conflicts, Latour hoped to stymie the common fallacy that a "great man [working] . . . alone in his laboratory, alone with his concepts . . . revolutionizes the society around him by the power of his mind alone" (Latour 1993:14). In the case of Pasteur, Latour seeks to dethrone the oft-invoked notion that, through the brilliance of his ideas and force of his character, the renowned microbiologist all but single-handedly brought the nation of France and the surrounding world into sanitized modernity. Instead, Latour demonstrated that the hygienist movement, already afoot before Pasteur, readily adopted him as a prominent scientist who could provide a symbolic rallying point to unify their public health campaign to clean up France's cities, provide clean drinking water to its citizens, and implement a hygienic system for eliminating human waste from urban areas. As Louis remarks, "The microbiological revolution was not a product of Pasteur, but rather, 'Pasteur' was a product of the microbiological revolution" (1989:47).

This same general line of thinking is evidenced in anthropologist Hannah Gilbert's analysis of the "discovery" of HIV-2 as a variant of HIV. Identification of this viral strain began early in the pandemic with the acquisition and testing of blood samples (for HIV-1) from local sex workers in Dakar, Senegal, a process initiated through Professor Souleymane Mboup's Laboratoire de Bactériologie et Virologie at Dantec Hospital. Politically defining the bodies of sex workers as a threat to public health was used to justify bringing their blood under the examination of a state institution. As a result of a set of linkages among major scientific laboratories in France and the United States, Mboup's initially uncertain findings were rapidly transformed into internationally accepted evidence of an important novel viral entity. Gilbert reports,

> the identification of the [HIV-2] virus is not merely the result of a scientific stumbling. It emerged when the movement of certain bodies—local sex workers—was impeded through a process of registration that allowed their bodily products to become untethered from their physical bodies and move about freely from clinic to lab, and eventually across the world. This dynamic exchange, which patterned how HIV-2 as a local biology became visible,

was fed by a strong local moral economy within both the clinic and the laboratory. Contemporary analyses of global research have demonstrated that the incorporation of life into this global biopolitical calculation has led to an intensification of the management of health and vitality, resulting in a different valuation of bodies and life. (2013:354)

In Gilbert's assessment, infectious disease research subjects not just human bodies (e.g., rich vs. poor, white vs. black) but also viruses to differential valuation. For a number of years Mboup's previously obscure laboratory developed close relations with well-funded researchers at Harvard, and large amounts of money from HIV research grants began to flow into the small research center. But all of this initiative more or less collapsed when interest in HIV-2 research among funders evaporated and researchers at Harvard turned to other issues. HIV-2, which never diffused widely outside of Africa, slid off of the global viral research agenda, and without external funding work on it largely halted in Mboup's laboratory. In Gilbert's view this case "demonstrates the degree to which local African science is circumscribed by the inequalities inherent in today's global-scientific economy" (2013:253).

The case of Carlos Chagas further illustrates the heavy hand of "politics" in infectious disease. The Brazilian physician and microbiologist is credited with first describing the epidemiology and clinical manifestations of Chagas disease early in the twentieth century, identifying the insect vector that facilitates spread of disease, and ultimately ascertaining the pathogen (*Trypanosoma cruzi*) that is the proximate cause of the disease, an unparalleled degree of individual accomplishment in infectious disease research. At the front end of this enshrined and complex history of infectious disease discovery is the story of Chagas being sent as a young physician-scientist trained in the epidemiology of malaria to help protect mercantile capitalism's labor force by attending to a mysterious disease outbreak that was slowing progress on the development of a railway. This experience is said to have channeled his interest in the nature of the disease that now bears his name. On the back end is the role of Chagas's work on the economic conquest of the Brazilian environment and the rationalizing of government-directed programs of national development and public health in a time of public leeriness about state power.

Beyond the state-level politics and national economics that created both the conditions for the spread of Chagas disease and efforts to use scientific discoveries about the disease for broader state purposes, there were other politics at play in this case (Bastien 1998). Because of his celebrated accomplishments, Chagas was nominated twice for the Nobel Prize in medicine but was never selected as a recipient, at least in part because of the staunch opposition of Júlio Afrânio

Peixoto, a prominent physician and leader of the nefarious eugenics movement in Brazil at the time. The often-hidden politics of rivalry in science are a key part of the story of Chagas disease, as they are in many other well-known cases of scientific work. Chagas himself played scientific politics. In his historical reexamination of this case François Delaporte (2012) points out that Chagas, with the aid of colleagues and after the fact actively reordered and neatly fitted together his "discoveries" and those of others to create a powerful narrative about the achievements of observation and experimentation in the science of infectious disease. But Chagas's "reconstructions were false" (Delaporte 2012:22). They served as a retrospective justification and affirmation of progressive science. In fact, it appears that Chagas identified a particular developmental stage of *T. cruzi* before he had any suspicion of its linkage to a specific disease. Chagas thus worked from the pathogen to find a disease it caused, and moreover, the pathogen was not found in the vector but in a laboratory animal. Chagas's versions of his own story, however, "for the most part deliberately concealed" the actual chronology of his research (Delaporte 1999:22) and promoted, instead, a politically useful grand narrative that thoroughly reconstructed the actual ordering of his activities.

A somewhat different slant on the politics of infectious disease is provided by Rob Dunn's study of botulism in the former Soviet Republic of Georgia, a country with the highest per capita rate (ninety times that found in the United States) of this potentially fatal food-borne infectious disease linked to the soil-dwelling pathogen *Clostridium botulinum*. Botulism emerged as "peculiarly virulent in . . . postsocialist society, [suggesting] what happens when the carefully ordered elements that make up a regulatory regime are thrown into disarray" (Dunn 2008:244). To understand botulism in contemporary Georgia, Dunn argues, you have to begin by examining how people eat. Traditionally in Georgia, households preserve vegetables in buried wooden or clay casks that, because of the pH level they achieved, were botulism-safe. Canning with glass jars, however, was introduced after World War II as part of an intensive emphasis on industrialization by the Soviet state. Canning was important to the state because it allowed armies to carry food with them (somewhat independent of supply lines), allowed sailors to avoid starvation at sea, limited famines in the general population and the vagaries of supply due to seasonality, and enabled the state to have strong control over the food supply, including by introducing industrial-processed foods only available through the state. National integration and broad social cohesion also was enhanced because glass jars could be produced in standard sizes in Russia, filled and pasteurized according to standards established locally in Georgia, capped with standardized lids manufactured in Armenia, and shipped to Moscow for local consumption and trans-shipment to the rest of the Soviet Union.

In Georgia the introduction of canned goods ultimately altered the way people ate. Canned foods prepared in other locales of the Soviet Union, using local food preparation traditions (e.g., spices, food mixtures, sauces), were introduced into the Georgian diet. How well this geographically and managerially complex system worked in terms of preventing food poisoning due to botulism is suggested by the low rates of this infectious disease prior to 1990. Although traditional Georgian vegetable preservation techniques were not lost, as a result of the national system the routine diet and daily lives of people in Georgia came to reflect patterns found throughout the Soviet Union. Georgians had, in Dunn's words, "developed a taste for the state" (2008:248).

However, the collapse of the Soviet Union in 1991 and the subsequent Georgian civil war radically changed the role and solidarity of the state in Georgian social life and diet. The state government in Georgia was weak and underfunded, leading to the collapse of the infrastructure of Georgian society. The power grid became so degraded that some Georgians did not have electrical power for a decade. Although most state canneries closed, three continued to function but without any government standards or inspection. In this chaos most Georgians were forced to rely on products made at home, not in factories. Now that their diets had changed, however, people did not seek to recreate traditional foods; they began home kitchen canning (now in jars) based on food preferences acquired during the Soviet years. But the techniques of safe canning followed in industrial canneries were virtually unknown in the domestic sphere. One of the things lost in this process was the whole notion of pasteurization—by heating jars to 250°F—to kill *C. botulinum* spores; thus, Dunn observed women using unclean jars in home canning or consuming food from home-canned jars whose lids had swelled (indicating *C. botulinum* production of neurotoxin). The parallels and entwinements of state collapse as a process and botulism as a disease suggest another side to the politics of infectious disease:

The spores of *C. botulinum* are a very different technobiosocial complex than organisms like *Escherichia coli* 0157:H7 or *Listeria monocytogenes,* which flourish in the ecological niches created by consolidated agriculture in the United States. Rather, botulism is a disease of disintegration. The collapsing central nervous system of the patient and the progressive isolation of his or her face, lungs, and limbs mirror the ways that the formerly linked subsystems of the regulatory regime are falling away from each other and losing contact. (Dunn 2008:251)

Rampant botulism in Georgia, Dunn further argues, although certainly a consequence of the poverty and immiseration that befell people as a result of near-state collapse generally, is best understood as a product of the form of poverty that is historically peculiar to the collapse of an industrialized former Soviet republic with its acquired tastes, introduced technologies (jarred foods), managed social patterns, and degraded infrastructure. In other words, the rise and fall of a particular social system at a particular point in time created the epidemic of botulism in Georgia, reflecting again the tight interdigitation of society and infectious disease.

It is evident that both the micro- and macropolitics of infectious disease shape the development of infectious disease outbreaks, how infected individuals are thought about in society, how others treat them, their access to treatment, and their experience of interactions within health care settings. As a result, micro- and macropolitics determine the course and outcomes of infectious disease outbreaks and endemic patterns. In addition, infectious diseases serve as a public arena for justifying and reinforcing particular local expressions of social inequalities and injustices within societies. Warwick Anderson has described a telling example of this process in his analysis of the role of infectious disease medicine during the American colonization of the Philippines in the late nineteenth and early twentieth centuries. Anderson describes how, in response to their devastating encounter in the Philippines with infectious diseases like malaria and yellow fever, American colonizers mobilized the field of tropical medicine both to protect themselves from infectious diseases and to exert colonial control over the Filipino people by "cleansing their newly acquired [territories], attempting to purify not only public spaces, water, and food, but the bodies and conduct of the inhabitants" (2006:1). Fighting infectious disease came to be seen less as primarily a confrontation with pathogens found in the tropics and more broadly as a "civilizing" process that would reform Filipinos' personal hygiene practices and social conduct and make them into acceptable (controlled) biological citizens. Overlooked in such understandings in the Philippines and elsewhere in the world (e.g., Molina 2006), where the presence of infectious disease has been used to rationalize exploitation, expropriation, and reigning structures of inequality, is the fact noted by the World Health Organization in its 1995 Annual Report that poverty, born of such inequality, is the world's deadliest disease and the ultimate cause of a considerable amount of infection (World Health Organization 1995).

In short, the anthropological approach to infectious disease involves both "studying down" to understand the nature and behavior of pathogens in interaction with humans in local contexts and "studying up" to reveal the political economic interests and structures that put people at risk for infection in local and wider contexts. As with the ecosocial approach in epidemiology, this orientation "deliberately fosters analysis of current and changing population [as well as small group] patterns of health, disease and well-being in relation to each level of biological, ecological and social organization" (Krieger 2007:671).

GENDER AND INFECTIOUS DISEASE

A key lesson of feminist anthropology is that people everywhere live gendered lives, and as a result, experiences, behaviors, treatment in society, and health differ along gendered lines. This applies as well to the gendered distribution of infectious diseases, cultural understandings of infectious disease, access to prevention information and resources, and access to health care for infectious disease treatment. Yet for many years in the development of research on the social aspects of infectious disease, a "missing and critically needed perspective in research was the foregrounding of gender" (Manderson et al. 2009:2). It is now well known, for example, that many women died of AIDS before opportunistic diseases only found among women, including invasive cervical cancer, pelvic inflammatory disease, and other gynecological conditions, were included as part of the definition of AIDS in 1993. Similarly the snail-borne disease schistosomiasis discussed in Chapter 4 holds greater risk for women because of culturally defined social responsibilities based on gender, such as washing clothes and cooking utensils and getting drinking water, activities that expose women disproportionately to snail vectors. Such patterns exist across many infectious diseases.

Differences in infectious disease risk among males and females reflect both biological and social factors. Some of the greater biological vulnerabilities women face in the AIDS pandemic, for example, include hormonal and developmental factors. Hormonal changes during menopause increase vaginal susceptibility to lesion development and create a heightened level of fragility of the epithelium, the tissue that lines the cavities and surfaces of structures within the body. Similarly the tissue of the immature genital tract of girls is particularly at risk for tears during sexual activity. Both of these biological vulnerabilities increase the likelihood that HIV will gain access to the body upon exposure, amplifying the likelihood infection will occur (Ostrach and Singer 2012).

Women are put at gravest risk for HIV and other sexually transmitted infectious diseases, however, because of the political economic and power structures that shape their everyday lives, options, and activities. Some examples are:

- economic discrimination at home that drives women to migrate to perform domestic and agricultural labor in environments that are risky for infectious disease;
- the sexual trafficking of women that propels contraction of sexually transmitted diseases;

- rural women who engage in "survival sex" and related infectious disease risk behaviors while their partners are forced to labor in distant urban areas; and
- the increase in so-called free trade and free enterprise zones in developing countries, where factory supervisors may require female workers to perform sexual favors as a condition of employment.

In the Trobriand Islands, for example—a group of inhabited Pacific coral atolls made famous in anthropology by the early ethnographic fieldwork of Bronislaw Malinowski—available data on HIV infection cases indicate increasing gender asymmetry in younger age groups, resulting in cumulative infection rates among adolescent girls and young women that are three and two times greater, respectively, than those among males in the same age groups. The greater HIV/AIDS vulnerability of girls and young women in the Trobriands reflects gender inequalities, gendered violence involving sexual coercion, and involvement of girls and young women in "cross-generational sexual relations with older men who are likely to have increased HIV exposure because of their longer sexual histories" (Lepani 2013:23). For many girls living on these islands vaginal sexual debut precedes first menstruation, increasing the likelihood of tearing of vaginal tissues and HIV transmission if the male partner is infected. Coupled together, biological and social factors put women in the Trobriands and elsewhere at disproportionate risk for infection.

A biosocial/biocultural perspective on HIV/AIDS "highlights the interrelationships between pathogens and social contexts in which it flourishes" (Lepani 2013:25). Indeed, as this book has argued, it is the only approach that explains HIV/AIDS and other infectious disease patterns within and across groups. Moreover, as Cecilia Van Hollen (2013) reveals in her study of poverty, gender issues, and AIDS in Tamil Nadu, India, even biological testing for HIV infection as part of intervention programming can lead to adverse social outcomes, as higher levels of testing among women can lead to accusations that they are the ones responsible for spreading the disease. Social and cultural factors, in short, have significant influence across the continuum that stretches from risk to treatment and health outcome.

THE POLITICS OF STIGMATIZATION

Sometimes those who suffer from infectious diseases are stigmatized, with significant and potentially severe health consequences. Put simply: "Stigma kills. It kills socially because it excludes affected persons from social life by reducing social networks and possibilities to find work, marriage partners, etc.... Stigma also kills literally, as a result of stigma-related social exclusion and treatment delay" (Ribera et al. 2009). The conceptualization of the association between stigma and health is derived from the research of Erving Goffman (1961), beginning with his work in psychiatric hospitals. Goffman defined stigma as the damaged image that a social group creates of a person or group of people based on some physical, behavioral, or social characteristic that is seen as being significantly divergent from established group norms. This socially constructed image of "undesirable difference" provides the rationale for the disqualification of membership in the dominant group, enforced through shunning, ostracism, and other social punishments. Stigma is therefore "a powerful and discrediting social label that radically changes the way individuals view themselves and are viewed as persons" in society (Smart 2005:122). This occurs because individuals who are the target of stigma not only are subject to mistreatment but often come to accept and internalize discredited self-images imposed on them by society. In effect, they come to suffer oppression illness (Baer, Singer, and Susser 2013).

Historically in the United States tuberculosis was a stigmatized infectious disease. Consequently, in a newspaper article entitled "Tuberculosis: A Legacy of Fear," S. Kelleher (1994:3) quotes a California woman who contracted TB in the 1940s, saying, "You have to understand that 50 years ago, TB was like AIDS is today. There was no cure for what you had. People were afraid of it. They were afraid of you." Today US physicians encounter this same attitude among patients from various immigrant and refugee communities. For example, in some East African cultures family and friends traditionally share food and eating utensils. One drinking cup may be used for a group of several people who are eating together, and a family eats with their hands from a single plate of food. When a person becomes symptomatic with tuberculosis, he or she may fear that others will refuse to share food and drink. This fear of social isolation, an intensely frightening experience for people raised to define themselves in terms of their place in the social group and in relationship with others, may lead the person to deny the true nature of the disease to him/herself or to others. As a result, initiation of treatment may be delayed while the disease is being transmitted within the social group.

Furthermore, because antituberculosis medicines were not available until recently—and even today remain expensive and difficult to obtain, especially in rural areas—some people may not realize that the disease is curable. As a result, persons with chronic coughing may refuse to see health care providers for diagnosis and treatment because if they are diagnosed with a stigmatized disease like tuberculosis, they may be forced to use their own cups and utensils, be cut off from various "rituals of social solidarity," and suffer the often intense emotional and health consequences of social marginalization. As social beings, this type of treatment can be very emotionally damaging, creating conditions that exacerbate infection.

Tuberculosis is not just a disease to be treated with antibiotics but also an experience laden with historic cultural meanings. In a set of focus groups reported by Esther Sumartojo (1993), for example, Somalis living in the United States had the following three specific recommendations for how health care providers should address TB in Somali patients: (1) treat the diagnosis of tuberculosis with the same sensitivity and confidentiality you would reserve for sexually transmitted diseases and HIV, (2) educate your patient about the curable nature of tuberculosis and emphasize the good health that will result from treating the disease, and (3) take time to discuss the social ramifications of the disease. Urging the identification of these kinds of emic insights that can enhance the cultural competency of treatment is typical of anthropological contributions to addressing infectious disease.

Stigmatization may be particularly damaging among people who suffer from infections that cause disfiguring wounds. Buruli ulcer disease (BUD), for example, is an infectious disease proximally caused by *Mycobacterium ulcerans* (which is in the same bacteria family as the tuberculosis and leprosy pathogens). In their field notes, based on research in central Cameroon, Joan Ribera and coauthors (2009) describe the case of a man suffering from an advanced stage of Buruli. As these researchers talk to the man, he is

sitting on a wobbly stool repairing an old fishnet. As he limps to add the rags of old clothes he will use later as bandages to a pot of boiling water, the stained bandage covering his oozing wound on his leg and foot becomes apparent. [He asks] "What happened? I was always good in school and worked hard on my fields. I was successful. But it's the jealousy! Someone in the village cursed me with atom (Buruli ulcer) and now I'm here like this! Since then, four years ago, I've had to give up my studies, my wife has left me. It was too much, too long. And now I have to pay for the schooling of my two children as well as for my treatment. I cannot participate in the work groups anymore because of my condition, and so I have no one to help me with my fields which are ruined because of the time I spent at the hospital, waiting for healing. . . . I do have a large family but I have to take care of myself alone now, without their help. But, my life isn't over! I'm still young, I'm strong. My life isn't over!" He is alone. Waiting.

BUD is highly stigmatizing due to its visible lesions but also because of the local attribution of BUD to social transgressions and witchcraft. Indeed, the adverse impact of BUD stigma, a social component, on the sufferer may well outweigh the physical symptoms of the infectious disease, a biological component. Similarly HIV infection patients have told many researchers that mistreatment by other people because of their condition outweighs the actual physical symptoms they suffer from the disease. A study of sixty individuals living with HIV disease in Hartford, Connecticut, for example, concluded,

> visible symptoms that were associated with HIV in particular were those that caused the greatest concern [for study participants]. Some feared that "looking HIV" would lead to discrimination. For others, such signs were evident in others they knew who had not survived; in this case, these clearly signal impending death. As this discussion suggests, AIDS stigma is every bit as and possibly more damaging than HIV disease itself. (Mosack et al. 2005:601)

Stigmas are often labeled "social killers" because the rejection they provoke can lead to isolation from social networks, loss of work, difficulty in finding marriage partners, divorce, damage to personal reputation, discrimination, isolation, ostracism, and even death.

The deleterious effects of HIV disease–related stigma have been under discussion since the mid-1980s and have been a subject of special focus within anthropology. In 1987 Jonathan Mann, as the director of the World Health Organization's former Global Programme on AIDS, noted in a speech to the UN General Assembly that "fear and ignorance about AIDS continue to lead to tragedies: for individuals, families and entire societies. . . . [But] threatening infected persons with exclusion—or worse" will wreak havoc with prevention and intervention efforts (Mann 1987). In December of 2000, as the executive director of UNAIDS, Peter Piot identified a "renewed effort to combat stigma" as first on his list of "the five most pressing items" to be addressed in responding to the global pandemic (cited in Parker and Aggleton 2003:14). A recent study of HIV-disease stigma revealed that suffers living in Burkina Faso, Ukraine, India, and Zambia were associated with different kinds of deviance by others in society. In Burkina Faso infected individuals were seen as being engaged in religious deviance, in the Ukraine with injected drug use, in India with extramarital sexual relations, and in Zambia with prostitution and witchcraft (Chase, Aggleton, and Coram 2001). In their discussion of HIV-related stigma, anthropologist Richard Parker and social psychologist Peter Aggleton (2003, 17) stress, "Stigma always has a history which influences when it appears and the form it takes. Understanding this history and its likely consequences for affected individuals and communities can help us develop better measures for combating it and reducing its effects."

Beyond its particular cultural framing in local contexts, Parker and Aggleton (2003) maintain that it is also critical to investigate how individuals, communities, and the state use stigma to produce and maintain social inequality. They point to the relevance of work by Michel Foucault on the cultural production of difference in the service of power. Conjoined with Goffman's ideas about stigmatization, a theoretical approach emerges for explicating the role of culturally constituted stigmatization as a core strategy in establishing and preserving hierarchal social orders. "Stigma and stigmatization function," they argue, "quite literally, at the point of intersection between culture, power and difference—and it is only by exploring the relationships between these different categories that it becomes possible to understand stigma and stigmatization not merely as an isolated phenomenon, or expressions of individual attitudes or of cultural values, but as central to the constitution of the social order" (Parker and Aggleton 2003:17).

Two additional concepts, *symbolic violence* associated especially with the work of Pierre Bourdieu (1998) and *hegemony* introduced by Antonio Gramsci (1970), are utilized by Parker and Aggleton in their analysis of stigma. Symbolic violence refers to the ways symbolic systems, such as words, meaningful cultural images, and culturally generated behaviors, promote the social-class interests of dominant groups by emphasizing profound distinctions between people in society (e.g., people in different income brackets). Hegemony refers to the role of dominant institutions in society, such as schools, religious organizations, the media, and the government, in promoting the legitimation of social inequality as natural and appropriate, even to those who are the objects of domination and oppression. Stigma operates as a form of symbolic violence that creates and gives valence to distinctions among people, distinctions that, like physical violence, cause real harm. Stigma is given authority and power in society through its reinforcement in the words and actions of major social institutions, resulting in its acceptance and internalization by people in society, including by those who most suffer its consequences. This approach allows "understanding of HIV and AIDS-related stigmatization and discrimination as part of the political economy of social exclusion present in the contemporary world" (Parker and Aggleton 2003:19).

In light of the damage stigmatization of infectious diseases does to sufferers, anthropologists Arachu Castro and Paul Farmer (2005) examined HIV-related stigma in Haiti. Based on studying the effects of improving access to treatment and care, they conclude that "the Haiti experience suggests that improving clinical services can raise the quality of prevention efforts, boost staff morale, and reduce AIDS-related stigma" (57). With new treatments and the implementation of programs to ensure access to them among the poorest and most marginalized members of society, there has been a transformation of HIV disease from an inevitably fatal to a chronically manageable condition. Associated with this change, there has been a dramatic decrease in stigmatization of infected individuals in Haiti, a lesson of global importance.

In another anthropological study that engaged the issue of stigma, Van Hollen examined ethnographically the life experiences of HIV-infected women in Tamil Nadu, India. She reports, "Fears of stigma and discrimination coupled with experiences of sorrow, suffering, and anger framed the contours and filled the content of [her] interviews" with these women (2013:123). A significant arena of stigmatization for them involved interactions with their in-laws, with infected women often being blamed for transmitting infection to their husbands. For women whose husbands had died of AIDS, accusations of promiscuity accelerated, which suggested to Van Hollen (2013:123) a strategic effort by in-laws "to exempt the husband's family from financial responsibility for . . . widows and their children." This emergent cultural pattern is rooted in a gendering of AIDS stigma that reflects a broader and preexisting social ideology of unequal gender social relations. Despite the power of structural and symbolic violence faced by the HIV-positive women she studied, Van Hollen (2013:213) found that although most of the women "still thought that they had to keep their HIV hidden like a shameful secret, some women were beginning to step out into the limelight in their efforts to combat the stigma and discrimination that women living with HIV/AIDS in India face." They began to demonstrate, in short, that entrenched cultural patterns and restrictive social relationships are not strait jackets that nullify the potential resistance and the rise of social movements for change in the midst of an infectious disease epidemic.

BIOPOWER AND INFECTIOUS DISEASE

Another aspect of the politics of infectious disease is seen in Foucault's concept of biopower, first introduced in his three-volume set titled *The History of Sexuality*. Biopower, which constitutes a form of biopolitics, refers to the practice, including both actions and policies, of modern nation-states involving the regulation of their citizens through "an explosion of numerous and diverse techniques for achieving the subjugations of bodies and the control of populations" (1976:140). This includes practices within public health and biomedicine that involve the regulation and management of risk—and people—within society, among other dimensions, such as the social regulation of heredity, sanity, and hygiene (see Figure 7.1). In premodern states brute physical force was the centerpiece of social control, and institutional power involved the implementation and deployment of a relationship of force. In the modern era, where power must be justified both rationally and politically, an emphasis on the

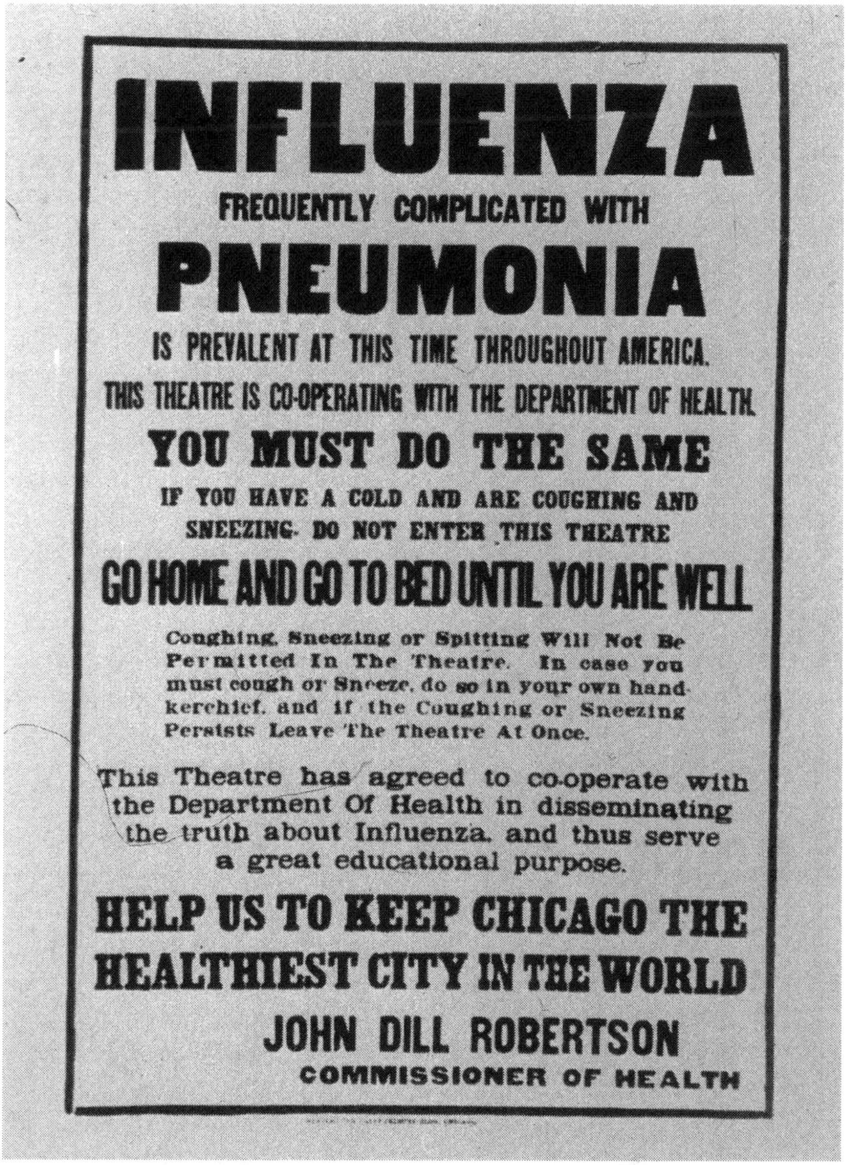

Figure 7.1 Prevention poster used in theaters in Chicago during the 1918 influenza pandemic. (Images of the History of Medicine)

protection of life rather than the threat of death rationalizes biopower. Herein lies the social validation for unjust governance in an infectious epidemic.

The problem lies in the fact that when the state claims the responsibility of protecting the population of citizens, promoting health and stopping disease can be used to justify anything against anyone. Illustrative in microcosm is the case of Mary Mallon, so-called Typhoid Mary, a single Irish woman who migrated to the United States in the 1880s. Mary made her living as a domestic servant for elite families in New York. In the summer of 1906, while she was working for a wealthy banker family, six of eleven family members became ill with typhoid fever, a bacterial infection characterized by diarrhea and a rash that commonly is transmitted through the oral-fecal route (e.g., during food preparation). Wanting to know why they had become infected, the family hired a civil engineer with experience with typhoid to hunt down the culprit who had infected them.

The engineer suspected Mallon was to blame somehow; being of working-class origin, she was inherently untrustworthy in the view of the engineer. By engaging in a form of "shoe leather epidemiology," he traced Mallon's employment record over the previous seven years and found a trail of typhoid among wealthy East Coast families and their servants connected to Mallon's presence. The engineer confronted Mallon, demanding samples of her feces, urine, and blood for testing, but she insisted she had not had the disease and refused him. Under pressure from her employers, however, she was apprehended by the authorities a few weeks later and sent to Riverside Hospital on North Brother Island, in the East River near Riker's Island, home of a US "leper colony," a forced drug rehabilitation center, and a mandated quarantine camp for immigrants diagnosed with infectious diseases. She remained there in custody for the next two years until the Supreme Court heard her habeas corpus lawsuit. The court concluded that because her feces samples—which were taken by force, not volunteered by her—were positive for typhoid, she was indeed a carrier of the disease, someone who can spread an infection without becoming infected. A year later a new health commissioner released Mary, however, and she found a job as a laundress at Sloane Maternity Hospital, which subsequently suffered a typhoid outbreak.

Mary was sent back to North Brother Island for the next twenty-three years until her death in 1938. In an interview with a *Life* magazine reporter (quoted in Gado 2010), she stated, "A few more years of this kind of life and I shall go insane. I have committed no crime, but am innocent. I am doomed to be a prisoner for life!" In effect Mary Mallon represented a triumph for bacteriology as a factor in state governance, as indeed she had broken no laws nor ever been convicted of a crime. Writing of societal sentiment toward and government response to Mary, Judith Leavitt (1996:149), in her book *Typhoid Mary: Captive to the Public's Health*, wrote,

> Mary Mallon, in all of her various levels of culpability, represents pollution, pollution of food, pollution of healthy unsuspecting bodies, pollution of

womanhood and the home. She is a deviant, a threat to the very core of society through the germs that grow in her body and spew out to infect others. She must be shunned. She may stir the pot innocently, but the ultimate result is sickness and death for those who come into contact with her.

The resulting revisualization of the nature of infectious disease and recognition of *healthy carriers* led to new expressions of biopower—efforts to control those within society deemed infectious and programs designed to keep people suspected of being infected with a significant contagious disease from entering the country. In the United States this shift was realized with the AIDS pandemic: the government made efforts to stop individuals who were infected from crossing national borders (e.g., to attend AIDS conferences), despite the fact that the virus was already widely spread in various segments of the US population. The shift is seen as well in government efforts to criminalize HIV transmission. Although more than half of US jurisdictions have specific laws that criminalize the knowing transmission of HIV, there is little evidence available to support the effectiveness of such policies in actually reducing HIV incidence (Lazzarini et al. 2013).

With the rise of new and ever more powerful biotechnologies within ever-larger *biocapital* industries, in the view of Nikolas Rose (2007), the vital biopower issue for the twenty-first century is how to handle "our growing capacities to control, manage, engineer, reshape, and modulate the very vital capacities of human beings as living creatures." One of the products of the emergence of biopower-driven government or institutional approaches to dealing with people and their problems is that people are thought of and are taught to think of themselves narrowly in terms of their biology and to overlook the broader set of political and economic conditions that both diminish the quality of life and the capacity for health.

Another set of issues taken up within the domain of biopower concern the way discourse on infectious diseases in recent years is linked to topics of *bioterrorism, biosecurity,* and *biowarfare* (Collier, Lakoff, and Rabinow 2004). An excess of biopower, Foucault observed, appears "when it becomes technologically and politically possible for man not only to manage life but to make it proliferate, to create living matter, to build the monster, and, ultimately, to build viruses that cannot be controlled and that are universally destructive. This formidable extension of biopower . . . will put it beyond all human sovereignty" (2003:254). We live in an age in which we are on the edge—or even over the edge—in our ability to "build viruses" and other deadly genetically engineered and laboratory-produced bioweaponry, a realization that stirs no small amount of anxiety in the general population (Lowe 2010) (see Figure 7.2). Such fears

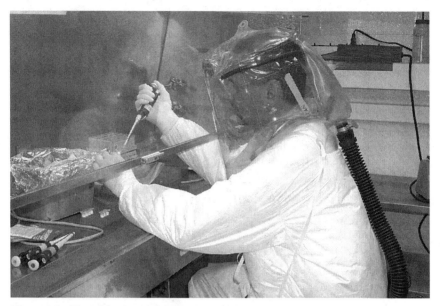

Figure 7.2 Biosafety Level 4 Infectious disease laboratory worker wearing protective gear. (Photo provided by USAMRIID, DoD)

have led anthropologists who work on bioterrorism, like Monica Schoch-Spana (Glass and Schoch-Spana 2002), to argue for a high level of community involvement in bioterrorism response planning to reduce the likelihood of social disruption and discrimination. Utilizing an anthropological lens on health in social and cultural contexts, Schoch-Spana and colleagues maintain that "Community engagement—[involving] structured dialogue, joint problem solving, and collaborative action among formal authorities, citizens at-large, and local opinion leaders around a pressing public matter—can augment officials' abilities to govern in a crisis, improve application of communally held resources in a disaster or epidemic, and mitigate communitywide losses" (2007:8).

Based on his field work in research laboratories studying pandemic influenza, an example of the growing field known as the anthropology of science, anthropologist Carlo Caduff (2012:335) found that concerns about security "loomed large on the horizon of infectious disease researchers in the United States." As a result of fears about bioterrorism, all infectious disease research has become embroiled in increasingly tense controversies about researchers' motivations and the potential nefarious uses of research findings (Lakoff 2008). One consequence of this state of affairs was that in January 2012 an international consortium of scientists representing thirty-nine different laboratories that had been working on the avian influenza virus (H5N1) made a startling announcement. In a letter published in two prominent journals, *Nature* and *Science*, they declared a self-imposed moratorium on their laboratory research, a historically unprecedented act on the part of individuals whose very careers hang on their ability to gain funding, conduct research, and publish their findings. The action was prompted by Netherlands researchers' success in creating an air-borne microbe that combined genetic material from a bird influenza with material from variants of the influenza virus that caused the deadly global pandemic of 1918. The moratorium was temporary, however, and by May of 2013 Chinese scientists published a report on their successful combination of the H5N1 virus with the highly infectious H1N1 human influenza virus (Zhang et al. 2013), once again triggering debate among scientists and concern in the general public about the looming viral monster to which Foucault alluded.

Additionally, the kind of research described above has begun to challenge the very notion of "species," which is a core concept in biology, because it entails the intentional movement of organic material among life forms, using a genetic cut and paste technology, to create new anthropogenic microbial organisms. As Caduff (2012:349) states, "These new creatures call for a relational biology and increasingly disrupt conventional efforts to provide biological bodies with a proper name and a proper place in an evolutionary genealogy of microbial descent." They represent, in effect, a new order of microbial life that, although human-made, carry the potential of slipping free of human control and becoming microscopic sources of mass destruction. In this climate of uncertainty infectious diseases have contributed to a particular "vision of the future, not one of hope but of fear" (Lakoff 2008:401). In this they have regained a position they once held in earlier times, when the causes of infectious disease pandemics were unknown but the consequences were terrifying.

In light of the enormous social focus on bioterrorism in recent years and the considerable expenditure of funds on biosecurity, estimated in the United States in fiscal year 2012 to be $6.43 billion (Franco and Sell 2011; Lam, Franco, and Schuler 2006), Hillel Cohen, Robert Gould, and Victor Sidel (2004) have called into question the entire apparatus of bioterrorism preparedness programs. Rather than actually providing much in the way of security, they see these programs as squandering health resources, increasing the dangers of accidental or purposeful release of dangerous pathogens, and undermining efforts to enforce international treaties to ban biological weapons. They note, for example, that the 2001 release of anthrax spores through the US mail system, which caused twenty-three infections, including five fatalities as well as widespread panic, ultimately were linked to a US military bioweapons research laboratory, "suggesting that the release might not have occurred had the [military's weaponization of] anthrax program never existed" (Cohen, Gould, and Sidel

2004:1667). More broadly, they argue, "bioterrorism preparedness programs are . . . characterized by failure to apply reasonable priorities in the context of public health and failure to fully weigh the risks against the purported benefits of these programs" (1667). Given the inherent difficulties of obtaining and handling anthrax outside of highly controlled laboratory settings, for example, Cohen, Gould, and Sidel deem government plans to spend $1.4 billion for an experimental anthrax vaccine to be a tragic waste of health dollars in light of the pressing array of health issues, such as the neglected infectious diseases of poverty, in the United States. Anthrax is deemed an ineffective bioweapon on a number of grounds: it is not contagious, it very difficult to produce in a form that is useable as a weapon, and anthrax infection is effectively treated with antibiotics (see Figure 7.3).

These researchers also cite the case of smallpox vaccination as part of pre-paredness for the feared use of bioweapons by Iraq, which had no such weapons. Consequently, note Cohen, Gould, and Sidel (2004:1668), "The evidence is highly suggestive that the smallpox vaccination program was launched primarily for public relations rather than public health reasons" as part of an effort to en-hance fear and promote public support for the US invasion of Iraq. Although the planned vaccination effort was never fully implemented because of opposition

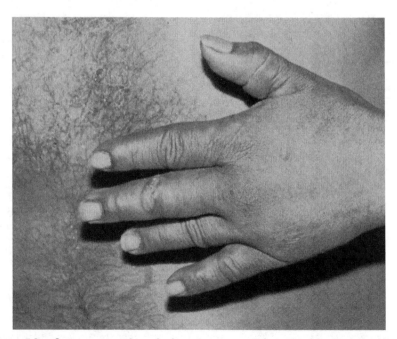

Figure 7.3   Cutaneous anthrax lesions on a man infected with the bacterium Bacillus anthracis. (Photo provided by WHO)

on both safety and political grounds, among those inoculated, the Centers for Disease Control and Prevention (2003) recorded 145 serious adverse events resulting in hospitalizations, permanent disabilities, life-threatening illness, and at least three deaths.

Inherent in Cohen and colleagues' argument is the recognition that bioterrorism preparedness must be added to the list of issues in infectious disease research that can only be fully understood when viewed within a political economic framework that focuses investigation on the operation of power in society.

HEALTH AND HUMAN RIGHTS

In the aftermath of the Second World War and in no small part as a response to the scale of brutalities that occurred during the war, in 1948 the United Nations implemented the Universal Declaration of Human Rights. The foundational principle of this document is the notion that all human beings are equal in dignity and worth and all are naturally endowed with certain unalienable rights that are universal, irrespective of social or cultural setting, and enduring over time. Following passage, the declaration became "the foundation for the creation of an entire framework of international and transnational human rights discourse, within which the most important human rights instruments, nongovernmental organizations, and international publications were established" (Goodale 2006, 487). This discourse provided a language and a framework for specifying various rights, identifying rights violations, and organizing to gain rights by and for subordinated populations. Among the various human rights that have been discussed in this discourse is health. The concept of a right to health has been included in various international agreements beginning with the Universal Declaration of Human Rights (United Nations 1948), which maintains that "Everyone has the right to a standard of living adequate for the health and well-being of himself and of his family, including food, clothing, housing and medical care and necessary social services, and the right to security in the event of unemployment, sickness, disability, widowhood, old age or other lack of livelihood in circumstances beyond his control," and it includes other consensus documents like the International Covenant on Economic, Social and Cultural Rights, the Convention on the Elimination of All Forms of Discrimination Against Women, and the Convention on the Rights of Persons with Disabilities.

This discussion has not been carried out in terms of simplistic assertions of the right of everyone to the same health, because it is recognized that biological factors like genetics make it much easier for some to be healthier than others (while recognizing, as we have seen, that biology, even genes, generally do not act alone in determining health). Rather, discussion of health as a right entails two issues: the right to live and work under social and environmental conditions that are not demonstrably harmful to health and the right to access quality health care. In the words of Alicia Yamin (2009:2), special advisor to Demand Dignity, Amnesty International's global campaign on poverty, "Increasingly, scholars and activists from the human rights community have argued—pointing to obligations regarding economic and social rights, including health rights—that it should not be the case that those on the lowest rungs face not having clean running water, sanitation, nutrition, access to health care or other basic building blocks of human dignity, [and further that in] some cases . . . poverty itself is a violation of human rights." With reference to infectious diseases, this means that people have the right to live and work in conditions that do not foster exposure to the easy spread of communicable diseases and, further, that those who are at risk or suffer from infectious diseases have the right to available quality health prevention and care designed to address infection and the conditions that promote it.

Human rights discourse emphasizes what might be called formal equality, in that this discourse focuses on legal rights that governmental structures enact and enforce. Its primary concern is with state obligations and the extent to which they are being fulfilled. As stressed by the World Health Organization (Solar and Irwin 2007:8), "Rights concepts and standards provide an instrument for turning diffuse social demand into focused legal and political claims, as well as a set of criteria by which to evaluate the performance of political authorities in promoting people's wellbeing." Consequently the emphasis in the human rights agenda is on achieving equality of dignity, legal standing, and legal status rather than an equality that is based on social or economic position. A limitation of this approach, as Nobel prize–winning French poet, novelist, and journalist Anatole France (1894:118) whimsically noted, is that in its majestic equality, "the law . . . forbids rich and poor alike to sleep under bridges, beg in the streets, and steal loaves of bread." Of course, such laws are only ever enforced against the poor because the rich are not forced to sleep under bridges, beg for food, or steal loaves of bread. Thus, beyond rights, there is a critical need to address the social determinants of health in which people are born, grow, live, work, and age in any discussion of health as a human right (Chapman 2010). Often missing from human rights discourse, however, is a conversation about issues like social class and economic status as well as the ways that class structures ensure health inequalities. Also often missing is a deep focus on the issue of power and how it is used to maintain social inequalities because, although they are deeply harmful to large numbers of people, social and economic inequalities ensure great wealth for a small percentage of people. Moreover, as Audrey Chapman (2010:21) observes, "human rights analysis tends to consider the underlying determinants of health individually and sequentially, thus missing the impact their interacting and cumulative effects can have on individuals and communities." This point is highlighted in cases where the law entitles people to certain rights, but when those rights are violated, as they commonly are, individuals often must fight solitary legal battles to have their rights enforced.

In short, although a human rights approach can be a useful tool in seeking to protect communities from infectious disease or calling for access to treatment for existing disease, to achieve infectious disease health equity for all it is necessary to consider the ultimate causes of communicable disease in the entrenched and reigning architecture of society. Additionally it is necessary to recognize that there is commonly a wide discrepancy between legal provisions as written and how those provisions are implemented in practice in light of built-in structural barriers to liberty, social justice, and equality in the institutions of existing societies.

ANTHROPOLOGY AND INNOVATIVE PREVENTION

In light of the discussion of the political economy above, what is the role of anthropology in the world of infection-induced sickness, suffering, and death? What contributions do anthropological approaches make that are not available through other methods (Harper 2006)? Addressing issues of health more broadly, Didier Fassin (2012:114) asks the questions: "Should medical anthropologists be activists in global health? Should their ultimate goal be to reduce global health inequities and contribute to the development of sustainable and salutogenic [i.e., health promoting] systems?" His answer to both questions is no. Whatever we may do to address health issues in our personal lives—for example, volunteering for or donating to programs that directly address infectious disease in a region or population, such as the distribution of antimalarial bed nets—as anthropologists, he asserts (2012:114–115), it is solely as critical thinkers, making "intelligible what often remains obscured, reformulating problems to allow alternative solutions, [and] resisting individualistic and technical models to highlight the social mechanisms and political issues" in health that we "are able to make a difference." Other anthropologists counter, stating that this perspective of the role of anthropologists in the world of health is narrow, excessively academic, and misinformed about the nature and history of applied anthropology (Rylko-Bauer, Singer, and van Willigin 2006). Anthropologists, as anthropologists—and not just in their lives outside of their work or careers—have made useful, practical contributions to the human response to infectious disease, including addressing the issue of social inequality as a factor in disease. Most effectively, anthropologists have carried out this applied work in collaboration with marginalized communities whom structural inequalities have put at risk for enhanced levels of infection. Suggesting that it is not the job of anthropologists to use their knowledge and skills to create more sustainable, health-promoting social systems is the equivalent of saying that biologists who study the loss of biodiversity have no business seeking to protect species from anthropogenic extinction or climate scientists using their understanding of global warming to promote mitigation and adaptation efforts. The question that must be asked in all of these instances is: Whose job is it to seek to improve the world in light of the multiple threats to health from infectious and other diseases, from the loss of biodiversity, and from climate change? Increasingly scientists across disciplines are recognizing and accepting their social responsibilities to apply their knowledge to address problems in a world of mounting risk.

Earlier in the book explicit examples of this kind of work were noted, including Shirley Lindenbaum's contributions to overcoming kuru and the work of numerous anthropologists in developing prevention, intervention, and care programs in the context of global HIV disease. Anthropologists have contributed as well to responses to dengue in various ways, such as identifying local knowledges and practices that might facilitate or hinder infection (Kendall et al. 1991; Whiteford 1997) that can inform effective intervention initiatives. Similarly, in their study of why mothers in Cambodia with children suspected of having dengue delay biomedical treatment, Sokrin Khun and Lenore Manderson (2007) were able to show the reason was a combination of three addressable factors: (1) the cultural assumption that the condition might be mild and responsive to the use of locally available herbs and home remedies, (2) community perceptions of the poor quality of care at both village health centers and public hospitals, and (3) poverty and the limited availability of funds to pay for medical treatment. In all of these instances anthropologists have directly participated in intervention efforts designed to address the infectious health condition that was the focus of their work.

In seeking to address a similar issue, why large numbers of children infected with malaria die because they do not get timely treatment (i.e., within twenty-four hours of onset), Kamat (2009) initiated a sixteen-month ethnographic study in a community (population 5,550) near Dar es Salaam, Tanzania, with high rates of malaria. He found that most children with a fever were not brought to a medical facility until forty-eight hours after the onset of the fever. Rather, when a child develops a fever, most parents (primarily mothers, as fathers tend to stay out of it) take a "wait and see" approach, as there are many causes of fever in the area and most are self-limiting conditions. During interviews parents told Kamat that their first reaction to childhood fever was to assume the symptoms are those of an ordinary illness (*homa ya kawaida*) rather than a life-threatening illness (*homa kali*) or malaria (*homa ya malaria*). Parents commonly spoke about childhood illness as routine, something that is part of everyday life in their world. Even past experience with malaria did not change this pattern, and mothers were surprised when their children were ultimately diagnosed with malaria. Even when their children became quite sick, some mothers did not recognize malaria but thought they had *degedege* (literally: bird-bird), an *ethnomedical condition* characterized by symptoms that mimic malaria and are thought to be caused by a coastal spirit that takes the form of a bird that casts its shadow on vulnerable children and makes them sick. Many parents believed that an injection, such as the one provided for malaria, could cause a child with degedege to go into convulsions, leading to death. Also, parents were concerned about the prohibitive costs of diagnoses that require multiple injections in addition to the costs of having to return to a medical facility multiple times.

Based on these findings Kamat (2009:56) argued, "malaria must be dealt with as an economic and a social issue" with "sociocultural factors [being] central in determining malaria risk, persistence, and popular treatment." Anthropological studies, he reasoned, "can serve as an evidence-based corrective to existing health policies and practices [and] the overly technical and biomedically driven interventions that have come to dominate global malaria control discourse and practice."

In their book *Ebola, Culture and Politics: The Anthropology of an Emerging Disease*, Barry and Bonnie Hewlett (2008) report on their involvement with ebola outbreak response teams affiliated with the World Health Organization (WHO). *Ebola*, thought to be transmitted by the fruit bat, is caused by any of four viruses. First recognized in 1976 in Zaire and Sudan, ebola has one of the highest cases of fatality rates of any known human pathogenic virus; approximately 90 percent of infected individuals die of the disease without treatment. Comparatively small local outbreaks that are of relatively short duration characterize the disease, although the 2014 outbreak in West Africa exhibited a more dispersed pattern over a broad area, with cases showing up in Guinea as well as in neighboring Sierra Leone, Liberia, and Nigeria. This configuration of dissemination has been linked to human mobility patterns in the region and beyond, and to the twenty-one-day incubation period of ebola infection. By October 2014, over 7,000 people had contracted ebola in the largest outbreak on record. Of these, 3,300 people had died. Disease experts projected a worst-case scenario of the epidemic spreading to 1.4 million people by the end of January 2015. By contrast, the previous worst ebola outbreak occurred in 1976 and involved 602 identified cases and 431 deaths. In the first ebola case diagnosed in the U.S, a man who traveled from Liberia to Dallas tested positive for the virus upon visitation to a hospital at the end of September, 2014.

The Hewletts readily acknowledge that the work they eventually did as anthropologists with WHO—an activity they term *outbreak ethnography*—was not part of the original public health mindset about whom to involve in responding to a deadly contagious disease event. Indeed, it was not until twenty-five years after the first outbreak of ebola that anthropologists were first invited to participate on response teams, in no small part because WHO realized it was facing important questions during outbreaks to which it did not know the answers, including:

- Why did people run away from ambulances sent to pick up ebola cases?
- Why did people stop taking sick family members to the hospital?
- How was local culture contributing to infection?

The Hewletts stress that in answering these kinds of questions it is necessary to get to know emic or insider perspectives on ebola and to use ethnography to identify local behaviors that might promote or prevent the spread of the disease. As part of this kind of work, they visited several outbreak sites and conducted interviews, focus groups, and observation, all while wondering how badly they were putting themselves at personal risk for infection. Based on their research, they concluded that understanding culture is critical to responding effectively to the outbreak of a disease like ebola. This is so because local cultural knowledge and practice blends both risky and protective behaviors, behaviors that both promote and limit the spread of infectious disease.

They identified indigenous concepts of contagious disease that, once invoked locally, led people to reduce interpersonal contact, such as cultural rules about avoiding dancing, sex, and handshakes with individuals deemed to be sick, or involving isolation of the sick and burying the dead away from residential areas. These are cultural practices that response teams need to support and encourage, the Hewetts argue. Additionally, they found that people tend to recognize that children are particularly vulnerable and should be kept away from the sick. Moreover, people are willing to help with control efforts if epidemiological team members and public health officials invite them to be involved and treated them respectfully.

At the same time, ethnography identified specific beliefs and practices that enhanced ebola infection. Traditional burial practices, such as washing and dressing the dead, and mortuary rituals, like keeping the corpse in the home for twenty-four hours, that involve physical contact with the bodies of individuals who died of infection could lead to new cases of ebola. Also, individuals were infected when they transported symptomatic family members to the hospital on a cart or bike. Belief that sorcery spreads the disease also may amplify an outbreak by leading to counter-sorcery efforts rather than to seeking treatment. Past colonial relations and continued inequalities led people to be distrustful of "whites" (i.e., outsiders regardless of skin color), including WHO team members, who people sometimes blamed for bringing the disease to them to begin with.

Further, the Hewletts stress that "ebola denial"—tied to the fear of being stigmatized as being a cause of the disease—can be found both at the community level and among government officials. Gender hierarchies may put women at heightened risk by lowering treatment seeking among women and by allowing less access to scientific knowledge about the disease. Consequently the Hewitts maintain that nuanced, fully culturally informed outbreak responses are needed with indigenous culture seen as neither a barrier to disease prevention/intervention nor romanticized as superior to scientific approaches.

Ana Dell'Arciprete and colleagues (2014) also stress the importance of culture in addressing infectious disease, based on their examination of communication between members of two indigenous ethnic communities, the Pilaga and the Wichi, and health care providers in Northern Argentina. These communities are located in endemic zones for Chagas disease, a health threat discussed earlier in this chapter, and efforts to control the disease in these zones have not been effective. Both of these indigenous ethnic groups have higher rates of insect vector infestation and Chagas disease than has been found in the general population in the region. The Wichi, however, have an infection rate that is three times higher than the Pilaga. Whereas the Pilaga have adopted Western hygienic practices and a sedentary lifestyle, the Wichis have emphasized preserving their traditional cultural practices and have resisted change introduced by outsiders. Both of these indigenous communities share health belief systems that differ from the Western notions of medicine. Based on open-ended interviews with members of indigenous communities regarding Chagas disease, including their perceptions of Western biomedical approaches and practices locally, these researchers draw five conclusions that speak to the broader issue of culture and infectious diseases: (1) members of the studied communities tend to see disease as being caused by other people (such as local shamans) or by the disease sufferers' violation of cultural restrictions, rather than in terms of internal biological and infectious disease processes; (2) whereas the Pilaga are more inclined to accept Western medicine, the Wichi tend to favor indigenous ethnomedical practices over biomedicine; (3) members of both of these communities do not link the triatomine (kissing bug) vector with the transmission of the disease and, hence, do not see the need for vector-control activities; (4) members of these communities who undergo diagnostic tests and accept biomedical treatment for Chagas disease often do so without full understanding of the nature and rationale of the treatment; and (5) the patient-biomedical provider clinical encounter in this cultural setting is characterized by misunderstanding and conflict between the expectations of health care providers and those of members of these communities. With regard to perceptions about the insect vector, known locally as *vinchuca*, for example, these researchers comment:

Perceiving vinchuca as a health risk seems to be at odds with cultural heritage. Neither the Pilaga or the Wichi perceive the vinchuca as a health risk, and that has consequences on their attitudes with regards to vector surveillance and control. Due to a lack of information, indigenous people of both ethnicities do not associate it either with the disease, or with sudden death. It is unlikely, therefore, that belief systems that orient indigenous behaviours will encourage the adoption of practices for the prevention of household infestations and consequently Chagas disease. (Dell'Arciprete et al. 2014)

As this statement suggests, the importance of culture in infectious disease understanding and response cannot be overstressed. At the same time, as differences between the Pilaga and Wichi indicate, cultural patterns are always in flux. Moreover, it cannot be assumed that culturally sensitive efforts to improve communication in provider-patients or community-public health interactions will not pay off in terms of disease control; rather, these and a vast array of other ethnographic findings on culture and infectious disease affirm the fundamental importance of knowing indigenous belief practices, respecting the dignity and cultural traditions of communities, recognizing the inequalities of doctor-patient and other cross-sector interactions, and working collaboratively with community members to achieve expressed health improvement goals.

Further, it merits emphasizing that many medical anthropologists have acted as scholar-activists in addressing the many ways, as we have seen, that inequality and injustice promote infectious disease. This has taken various forms, including evaluating infectious disease intervention campaigns, policy work that affects social responses to infectious diseases, actively lobbying for the implementation of public health programs (e.g., syringe exchange programs to prevent the spread of HIV disease), participation in community organizations and campaigns to address the underlying social causes of infection, and contributing to discussions in the public media about infectious disease issues. Guiding such initiatives is a sense of social responsibility and solidarity with marginalized populations and a commitment to use the tools of the trade to develop sustainable, equitable, and health-promoting social systems (Baer, Singer, and Susser 2013).

THE TOMORROW OF INFECTION

Contemporary trends in infectious diseases, including the rise and spread of multidrug-resistant microbial strains that challenge current biomedical responses, the emergence and transfer to humans of zoonotic diseases as a result of our changing place in the world and our interactions with other species, syndemic interactions among infectious diseases and between infectious diseases and chronic noninfectious diseases, the continued and widening gap between the richest and poorest sectors of the world's populations, the global food and water crises, the increasing pace of globalization in its various forms, and global climate change, all suggest a human future shared with significant pathogens. Twentieth-century expectations that the advance of medicine would cast infectious diseases onto the trash heap of world history now seem like misguided fantasies borne of a narrow understanding of biology and culture and their fateful intersection. After a career spent fighting HIV and other infectious diseases, Peter Piot, former executive director of UNAIDS, wondered whether Louis Pasteur had it right when he said, "c'est les microbes qui auront le dernier mot" (it is the microbes who will have the last word) (quoted in Piot 2012:376).

Still, humans have demonstrated an enormous capacity to cope with new challenges, using culture as a creative force for reimagining social and technological possibilities. That humans survived many earlier threats in the course of their evolutionary and more modern history offers a basis for hope; recognition of the multiple challenges to come and the fact that all species eventually face extinction presents an alternative, less sanguine view. However, as Danish physicist Niels Bohr once quipped, "Prediction is very difficult, especially if it's about the future." Explanation of health inequities requires that medical anthropology examine the "central engines in society that generate and distribute power, wealth and risks" (Diderichsen et al. 2001:16). A medical anthropology that fails to engage ultimate social causes of infection, including attribution of responsibility for inequalities in access to needed life resources caused by current patterns of extraction and concentration of wealth, will not make much of a difference in human health. Consequently anthropologists "must move beyond the academy if they are sincere in their desire to address the health-damaging consequences of social pathologies" (Heggenhougen 2009:195).

CONCLUSION

One goal of this book is to consolidate a body of research addressing the question: What is the anthropology of infectious diseases? The conceptual model developed in this book to address this question integrates four interrelated components:

1. The anthropology of infectious disease offers a frame for understanding human-environment relationships that transcends anthropocentric thinking in two ways. First, it recognizes that humans interact extensively and constantly with other species and that these interactions include both mutual interdependence as well as "conflict." Second, we have quite literally become the beings we are through ongoing processes of co-evolution with other species, both within and outside the boundaries of our skin.

2. Human infectious disease, however, is far more than an issue of the biological interaction of species; it also entails cultural configurations and structures of social relationships that shape our interactions with and understandings of each other, the environment, and disease. So entwined are the biological and the cultural that we must move beyond the idea that they are two separate factors interacting and see them instead as inseparable within a biocultural and biosocial paradigm.

3. Consequently the anthropology of infectious disease requires an ecosocial understanding of health as a product of synergistic environmental health factors such as anthropogenic environmental change, pluralea interactions, and ecosyndemics.

4. It also requires a political economy of health that addresses the social role of infectious diseases in the production and reproduction of social and economic inequality.

This type of complex approach can help guide the further development of anthropological infectious disease research and theory because it recognizes the fundamental importance of assessing dynamic relations involving biology, the environment, culture, and social structure and is informed by modern ethnographic approaches for assessing the on-the-ground worlds of human activity and experience as well as the wider fields of globalization and power. This holistic and integrated bicultural/biosocial vision enables anthropologists to raise important but often otherwise unasked questions about infectious disease as an enduring, dynamic, and influential force in human life and provides direction for finding useful answers.

Discussion Questions

1. What does the concept "social origin of disease" mean?
2. How do microparasites and macroparasites work together to create disease?
3. What are social factors in the transition from latent to active tuberculosis?
4. What are the social functions of infectious disease stigma?
5. What are the infectious disease effects of biopower?
6. What kinds of contributions have anthropologists made to infectious disease research and to the development of social responses to the proximate and ultimate causes of infectious disease?

GLOSSARY

Adaptive immune system—a multicomponent defensive system involved in the creation of an immunological memory after initial exposure to a pathogen; white blood cells that are part of this system mount agent-specific immune responses.

Adenoviruses—a large group of double stranded DNA viruses that are involved in a range of diseases, from mild respiratory and eye infections (e.g., tonsillitis, croup, conjunctivitis) to life-threatening conditions like pneumonia, viral meningitis, and encephalitis.

Adipokines—hormone-like substances like adiponectin, leptin, and resistin secreted by adipose (fat) tissue.

Aflatoxin—a highly toxic substance produced by two related fungi species, Aspergillus flavus and A. parasiticus, that grow on various food crops.

Air-borne pathogens— infectious agents that can be transmitted through breathing, coughing, or sneezing.

Alveolar macrophages—also called "dust cells"; are found in the lungs, where they help to remove pollutants but are also active in providing bodily defense against bacteria and viruses.

Anthropocentric—a narrow focus on humans, placing them at the center of analyses, that ignores issues of co-evolution, zoonotic diseases, and other forms of significant interspecies interaction.

Anthropogenesis—refers to the significant role of humans in shaping pathogen behavior and evolution.

Antibiotic void—limited discovery of new antibiotics since the mid-1980s and reduced effort to identify new antibiotics.

Antiretrovial therapy (ART)—medicines designed to treat viral infections, often by disrupting viral reproduction.

Applied anthropology—the use of anthropological methods, concepts, and personnel in solving pressing health and social problems.

Archaea—a kingdom of single-celled microorganisms that have no cell nucleus.

Atherosclerosis—cholesterol-related "hardening of the arteries"; a chronic health condition that appears to have an infectious origin.

Ascariasis—an infectious disease of humans caused by the parasitic roundworm *Ascaris lumbricoides*.

Aspergillosis—the most common infectious mold; it causes allergic reactions, lung infections, and infections in other organs.

Assortative sociality or homophily—selective association with some people, defined as being like self and avoidance of others seen as being different (e.g., associating primarily with people of one's religious group).

Atopic dermatitis—also known as eczema, AD is a relapsing, noncontagious skin inflammation.

Autoimmune disease—diseases, sometimes triggered by pathogens, that involve the immune system attacking the body's own cells.

Avian influenza—an influenza caused by viruses initially adapted to living in birds.

Bacteria—an ancient kingdom of single- or multicelled and micro-organisms that, despite their small size, are so numerous that collectively they form a biomass that is greater than that of all plants and animals.

Bacterial or viral déjà vu—terms used to explain why some people appear to be particularly susceptible to more intense impacts from a particular pathogen because of prior exposure.

Bacteriophage—a virus that infects bacteria.

Behavioral immune system—social behaviors and psychological orientations that provide protection from infectious disease agents and guide the management of infectious diseases when they occur.

Biocapital—the production of commodities for profit based on the laboratory manipulation of components of living organisms, such as gene and tissue.

Biocultural—the interaction of biology, including infectious disease biology, with the configuration of beliefs, meanings, norms, values, and stylistics of local behavior that give distinctive flavor and pattern to human lifeways.

Biodiversity—the rich variety of life forms found on Earth.

Biofilm—multicellular interacting communities of microbes, such as dental plaques, that adhere to biological or nonbiological surfaces.

Biology of inequalty—the impacts of social inequality on human biology through diet, disease, stress, and related factors.

Biome—used often as a synonym of ecosystem, the term refers to organisms living in the same climatically and geographically defined conditions.

Biopower—the practice of modern nation-states that involves the regulation of their citizens through numerous and diverse techniques for achieving the subjugation of people's bodies and the control of populations.

Biosecurity—the state of preparedness for effectively stopping or responding to bioterrorism and state-sanctioned biowarfare, including the development of vaccines and the organization of health care responses.

Biosocial—the interaction of biology, including infectious disease biology, with hierarchical structures of social relationships.

Biosphere—the world of all living things.

Biotechnology—technologies based on the manipulation and modification of components of living organisms, such as genes and tissues.

Bioterrorism—the manipulation and use of infectious diseases as weapons by nongovernment forces targeted at civilian populations.

Biowarfare—the manipulation and use of infectious agents as weapons against people, animals, or agriculture.

Buruli ulcer disease (BU)—an infectious disease proximally caused by *Mycobacterium ulcerans* that can be disfiguring and, hence, is socially stigmatized.

Campylobacter—a corkscrew-shaped bacteria responsible for food-borne disease.

Carcinogenesis—the transformation of normal cells into cancerous cells, sometimes involving pathogenic agents.

Card sorting—a research method in which study participants are asked to sort labeled cards into piles based on degrees of similarity and difference in the item listed on each card (e.g., the names of various diseases).

Cat-scratch disease—a bacterial disease transmitted by scratches, bites, and other close contact with felines, especially kittens.

Chickungunya virus—a pathogen transmitted to humans by mosquitoes that causes illness with similar symptoms as dengue, including fever, headache, and joint pain.

Cholera—an acute diarrheal disease, proximally caused by a bacterium of the Vibrio family, that can kill within hours of infection if untreated.

Clostridium difficile infection—an intestinal disease that causes more deaths in the United States than all other intestinal infections combined.

Coccobacillus—a group of bacteria, including *Chlamydia trachomatis*, that have the shape of a short rod.

Co-infection—suffering from more than one infectious disease at the same time.

Commensalism—the idea that the pathogen-host relationship inevitably evolves toward benign coexistence, and the pathogen itself tends to evolve toward diminished adverse impact on the host.

Communicable disease—a disease that can be transmitted person to person or animal to person through various methods.

Contingency genes—genes with a high mutation rate that appear to be responsive to environmental pressures.

Countersyndemic—interaction between two diseases that results in a reduction of the pathogenesis of one or both, thereby reducing the burden of disease.

Creutzfeldt-Jakob disease—known popularly as "mad cow disease"; a prion-related disease of the brain.

Critical medical anthropology—the theoretical perspective in medical anthropology that emphasizes the importance of political economy in health while focusing attention on interactions between the microlevel of biological process and local social patterns and broader systems of power.

Cryptosporidiosis—a water-borne infectious disease caused by *Cryptosporidium parvum*.

Cultural consensus analysis—a research method used for assessing agreement among study participants about issues of concern and for discerning the patterning of differences in cultural knowledge within and across social groups.

Cultural factors—refers to the configuration of beliefs, meanings, norms, values, and stylistics of local behavior that give a distinctive pattern to each of the various human lifeways.

Cysticercosis—a disease caused by infection of the brain or muscle tissues by the helminth *Taenia solium*, the pork tapeworm.

Cytokines—molecules involved in cell-to-cell communication in immune responses that stimulate the movement of immune cells toward sites of inflammation, infection, and trauma.

Cytomegalovirus—an infectious viral disease which in humans is caused by human herpesvirus-5.

DALY—Disability Adjusted Life Year; epidemiological measure of loss of "healthy life" or disease burden that combines data on disability and loss of life.

Dengue—a painful and debilitating viral infection spread by a mosquito vector.

Despeciation—refers to the breakdown of boundaries between two groups previously seen as comprising distinct species.

Dilution effect—the presence of less competent host species in an environment that lowers the likelihood of infectious disease spread by vectors.

Disease—clinically identified biological conditions involving tissue damage and body system disruption.

Disease cluster—refers both to the concentration of infectious disease in one segment of a population compared to other segments and the copresence of multiple significant infectious diseases in the same population segment.

Disease complex—a set of interlocked diseases, alternately known as a syndemic.

Diseases of poverty—diseases that are particularly prevalent among the poor because of the social conditions of poverty.

DNA methylation—a biochemical process entailing the addition of a methyl group of molecules to two of the four DNA nucleotides, namely cytosine or adenine, that is believed to be a component of an ancient genomic immune system.

Dracunculiasis—also known as Guinea worm, this helminth infection can case intense pain and leaves sufferers permanently crippled.

Drug-resistant infectious disease—disease caused by pathogens that have adapted to antibiotic drugs, rendering them ineffective; also known as treatment-resistant infectious disease.

Dynamism—refers to the fact that pathogens and the diseases they induce are not static but rather continue to change over time and place.

Ebola virus disease—a zoonotic human disease that is caused by four of the five known ebola viruses.

Ecocrisis interaction—the intersection and amplification of multiple anthropogenic environmental crises; also called pluralea interactions.

EcoHealth perspective—an approach to health that focuses on how changes in human ecology, including human-promoted changes in Earth's ecosystems, affect human health.

Ecological imperialism—the global spread and rise to dominance of Europeans, European animals, European plants, and European infectious diseases.

Ecological web of causation—the complex of social, cultural, environmental, and biological factors that, acting together, produce infectious disease.

Ecosocial theory—a theoretical perspective in epidemiology that emphasizes the interaction of political, economic, social, and environmental factors in disease.

Ecosyndemic—a syndemic that is mediated by environmental factors, such as the role of global warming, facilitating the movement of vector-borne pathogens to new areas where they might interact syndemically with local pathogens.

Ectoparasites—parasites that live on the skin and hair of their hosts.

Emergent infectious disease (EID)—newly identified or newly diffused infectious diseases.

Emic—the term used in cultural anthropology to refer to the insider's perspective.

Endemic—diseases that are well entrenched in a population or region.

Endocarditis—an infection of the inner layer of the heart or endocardium.

Endothermy—internal heat generation seen in mammals that frees them from reliance on the absorption of heat from external sources like the sun.

Environmental anthropology—is the applied study of human/environment relationships with the intention of improving human wellbeing and environmental sustainability

Environmentally mediated infectious disease—changes in infectious diseases due to anthropogenic environmental changes.

Epidemic—unexpected increases in the incidence of a particular disease.

Epidemiological transition—large-scale changes in the types of diseases afflicting all or large sections of humanity.

Epigenetic—reproduction that does not involve genes, as seen in prions.

Erythema migrans—the so-called bull's eye skin rash associated with Lyme disease.

Ethnography—the long-term observational and participatory field study of people and issues in social and environmental context.

Ethnomedicine—indigenous, folk, and ethnic healing systems, including, historically, biomedicine, although the latter has become global and cross-cultural in its distribution.

Free listing—a research method designed to investigate targeted cognitive domains, which involves having study participants list all of kinds of a particular category (e.g., "infectious diseases" or "causes of illness") they can think of.

Fungi—a large group of eukaryotic organisms (i.e., cells containing a nucleus and other organelles enclosed within membranes) that includes microorganisms such as yeasts and molds, mushrooms, and infectious agents that spread by producing spores.

Fusarium—a group of molds that include pathogenic species.

Gene assortment—the movement of genes among microorganisms, including pathogens, that may lead to enhanced virulence or drug resistance in the recipient microbe.

Genetic mixing—an aspect of microbial traffic involving the movement of genetic information across pathogen strains and species.

Genital ulceration disease—lesions in the genital area caused by sexually transmitted disease and other factors such as trauma, adverse drug reactions, and nonsexually transmitted infections.

Germ theory of infectious disease—the understanding that disease can be causes by microscopic infectious organisms like bacteria and viruses.

Giardia—a protozoan pathogen that can colonize the intestines and cause giardiasis, a disease characterized by diarrhea, stomach and abdominal cramps, dehydration, and nausea.

Golden era of antibiotic discovery—the period from the 1940s to the 1960s when numerous new antibiotics were discovered.

Global mixing bowl—the mixing together in local sites of pathogens and other species of diverse origin.

Global warming—a heating of Earth caused by the build-up of human-produced greenhouse gases that is contributing to the spread of vector- and water-borne pathogens.

Globalization—the ever more rapid contact, exchange, and communication occurring across societies and regions of Earth, involving the movement of corporations, commodities, technologies, ideas, people, and infectious diseases around the planet.

Gut flora—bacteria that inhabit the gastrointestinal track, with a combined weight of three to five pounds.

Hantaan virus—a pathogen transmitted by contact with mice, mice urine, or mice droppings that can cause Hantavirus Pulmonary Syndrome, which can be fatal.

Health—level of well-being across multiple biological, psychological, and social dimensions.

Healthy carrier—someone infected by a pathogen who suffers no ill effects but can pass infectious agents on to others who do become ill.

Hegemony—the role dominant institutions in society play in promoting the legitimation of social inequality as natural and appropriate, even to those who are the objects of domination and oppression.

Helicobacter pylori—a bacteria that causes gastric cancer and peptic ulcer.

Hemorrhagic fever—a diverse group of animal and human disease caused by various viral species, characterized by bleeding, fever, shock, and, possibly, death.

Hepatitis A—an acute infectious disease of the liver caused by the hepatitis A virus.

Hepatitis B—an infectious inflammatory illness of the liver caused by the hepatitis B virus.

Hepatitis C—an infectious disease primarily affecting the liver that is caused by the hepatitis C virus; chronic infection can lead to scarring of the liver and, ultimately, to cirrhosis.

Herpes simplex virus—two forms of evasive virus (called 1 and 2) that infect humans; while type 1 produces cold sores, type 2 is a sexually transmitted disease.

Hidden hunger—inadequate consumption of micronutrients, such as vitamins, minerals, trace elements, and essential amino acids; known to be a factor in less-than-optimal immune functioning.

HIV—Human immunodeficiency virus; a slowly replicating retrovirus, meaning that its genetic nucleus consists of RNA strands. It replicates in a host cell through the process called reverse transcription.

HIV disease—disease produced by infection with the human immunodeficiency virus, ranging along a continuum from initial infection and mild symptoms to more extensive immune system damage and, if untreated, death in most sufferers.

Hookworms—a parasitic helminth that inhabits the small intestines of its mammalian hosts, including humans.

Host—the organism occupied by a pathogen; pathogens are themselves hosts to their own set of pathogens.

Host-pathogen coevolution—mutual responsive changes between pathogens and immune systems.

Human papilloma virus (HPV)—an infectious agent linked to the onset of cervical cancer and some types of organ cancer.

Hunter Theory—a theory of the zoonotic jump of the virus that evolved into HIV as a result of contact with chimpanzees during the hunting for bushmeat.

Hydatid disease—a potentially lethal parasitic infection caused by the larval stages of several tapeworm species.

Hygiene Hypothesis—the theory that lack of early childhood exposure to pathogens increases susceptibility to allergic diseases.

Hyperendemicity—the simultaneous and overlapping circulation of multiple strains of an infectious disease agent within a population.

Illness—culturally shaped experience and meaning of being sick.

Immune reactivity—the reaction of the adaptive immune system to the detection of a foreign entity in the body.

Immune system—the body's multilayered defense mechanism against pathogens and other foreign organisms and tissues, including cancerous cells.

Immunomodulating agents—molecules that regulate the operation of the immune system.

Immunopathology—ability of a pathogen to downgrade the effectiveness of the body's immune system.

Infection—presence in the body of a pathogen that may be dormant or active in causing local tissue damage or other changes in body systems.

Infectious agents—also known as pathogens; organisms that are the proximate causes of infectious diseases.

Infectious disease—active and adverse presence of pathogens that are causing damage to body tissues and systems and degrading sufferer health.

Influenza—a rapidly mutating viral disease that exists within and across species and causes annual epidemics of varying magnitude.

Innate Immune System—the body's first line of defensive response to pathogens, composed of various features that are present at birth, including skin, mucous membranes, the vernix, a fatty substance covering the fetus that has antifungal properties as well as macrophages.

Interspecies mutualistic symbiosis—an interaction among two species in which both benefit from the relationship.

Kuru—a debilitating and generally lethal disease caused by a prion that was only found among the South Foré people of New Guinea.

Legionnaire's disease—a disease caused by Legionnaire's disease bacteria, which are spread by inhaling infected water mist, and cause the development of a form of pneumonia.

Leptospira—a life-threatening, rat-borne zoonotic bacterial disease.

Leptospirosis—an infectious bacterial disease that is among the world's most common zoonotic diseases; infection can lead to meningitis, liver damage, and renal failure, commonly occurring during contact with water contaminated by animal urine.

Liver flukes—a parasitic helminth that has been identified as a causal agent in bile-duct cancer.

Lyme disease—a tick-borne viral disease that has generated considerable controversy concerning its appropriate treatment.

Lymphatic filariasis—a disfiguring and incapacitating infectious disease involving significantly swollen limbs that begins when filarial parasites are transmitted to humans through mosquito bites.

Lyssaviruses—named for the Greek goddess of rage and frenzy, this is a group of viruses that includes rabies.

Macroparasites—a term introduced by the historian William McNeil to refer to human social groups and strata that dominate others and live off of their labor and resources.

Macrophage—cells that are part of the immune system that consume entities that are identified as foreign to the body, including pathogens.

Macropolitics of infectious disease—in the case of infectious disease, refers to dominant conclusions about the origin of infection, how those who are infected are portrayed, their social treatment, and their access to care.

Malaria—a mosquito-borne infectious disease of humans and other animals caused by parasitic protozoans; infection is debilitating and can cause death, particularly in children.

Mamavirus—the largest known virus.

Medical anthropology—the branch of anthropology that studies health-related issues in human societies and lived experiences.

Medical ecological theory—an explanatory approach that stresses health implications of the ways societies respond to the challenges and opportunities presented by the physical environments and climatic conditions they face.

Meningitis—an infection of the protective membranes covering both the brain and spinal cord.

Microbiome—a term used to refer to humans and the many microbes that dwell within them as a single biological unit.

Microbial traffic— the flow of pathogens to new host populations, including from animals to people, people to other animals, and between human populations.

Microparasites—a term introduced by the historian William McNeil to refer to the microbes that serve as the infectious agents of human disease.

Micropolitics of infectious disease—the political and narrative process of explaining to oneself: Why did I get sick? How is my being sick related to my life situation, to treatment by others, to decisions I have made?

Mimivirus—a very large bacteria-like virus, capable of producing proteins.

Mitochondriam—tiny, rod-like structures found in most of our cells that help us break down glucose into usable energy.

Modern Synthesis—the unification of understandings about genetics, random mutation/diversity, and natural selection into what has been the dominant scientific model of biological evolution (now being challenged by epigenetic research).

Multidrug-resistant pathogens—a pathogen's acquired capacity to resist a number antimicrobial drugs, suggesting the possibility of the rise of a postantimicrobial era in human history.

Mutual causation process—co-evolving interspecies response processes in which changes in one species lead to changes in another, which in turn provoke changes in the first species and so on.

Mycobacteria—pathogens known to cause serious diseases in mammals, including tuberculosis.

Mycotoxins—poisonous substances produced by molds.

Narrative analysis—an approach for analyzing the underlying cultural themes and cultural logic of the stories we tell each other in cultural context.

Necrotizing fasciitis—also known as flesh-eating disease, this is an example of what is known as Group A Streptococcus, a fast-moving and tissue-damaging infection caused by the bacterium *Streptococcus pyogenes*.

Neglected infections of poverty—infectious diseases concentrated in poor populations in developed countries, characterized by chronicity and disabling features.

Neglected tropical diseases (NTDs)—a group of disabling and often disfiguring infectious conditions that most commonly are found among people living in extreme poverty and, hence, historically receiving less attention in international health efforts directed by wealthier nations.

Nipah and Hendra—members of the *Paramyxoviridae* family of viruses that are transmitted by bats to humans.

Non-government organizations (NGOs)—local, regional, national, and international organizations that are freestanding and address health and social issues.

Norovirus—a genetically diverse group of single-stranded RNA viruses that is the most common cause of gastroenteritis.

Nosocomial—an infection acquired as a patient, employee, or visitor to a hospital, nursing home, or other health care facility.

Onchocerciasis—also known as River Blindness; a parasitic disease that is a primary cause of blindness. Disease is caused by roundworms, the nematode of the black fly, that is infected with the parasite *Wolbachia pipentis.*

Opportunistic infections—infections that are only able to colonize a host when its immune system is deficient, including as a result of an immune-damaging pathogenic agent.

Oncogene—a gene, sometimes inserted by a pathogen into the genome of a cell, that has the potential to cause cancer by triggering proliferation and preventing normal cell death.

Orgel's second rule—the recognition that the long-term trial-and-error course of evolution does not require the need for invoking an "intelligent designer" to explain the diversity or configuration of life forms.

Osteomyelitis—an infection of the bone or bone marrow.

Outbreak ethnography—a term that refers to on-the-ground ethnographic research to understand and help to respond to an epidemiological outbreak of an infectious disease

Paleopathology—the archeological and paleontological study of ancient diseases based on impacts left on bones or through the identification of ancient DNA.

Pan troglodytes troglodytes—the Latin scientific name for chimpanzees.

Pandemic—a very widespread infectious disease outbreak, potentially global in its diffusion.

Paramyxovirus—an RNA-based virus involved in a number of human and animal diseases, including mumps and measles as well as bronchiolitis and pneumonia in children.

Parasite—an organism that feeds on and is sheltered on or in a different organism while contributing nothing to the survival of its host.

Parasite-stress theory of sociality—the biosocial theory that asserts that the variable adoption of in-group and out-group sociocultural tactics (e.g., in-group badges of membership like clothing styles) occur in response to the local threat of infectious disease agents and serve to create social space from out-groups who may harbor infectious threats.

Pathogen-host interactions—reciprocal adaptations between pathogens and their hosts, sometimes described as a biological arms race.

Pathogen latency—the adaptive ability of some pathogens to avoid detection by remaining in a dominant state in response to a healthy immune system.

Pathogen-pathogen interactions—syndemic interaction among pathogens of the same or differing life forms.

Pathogenic or infectious burden—the health deficit suffered by a person through their life course due to infectious diseases.

Pathogen pollution—anthropogenic movement of infectious agents outside their natural geographic or host species range.

Pathogens—disease-linked microorganisms and parasites.

Persister cells—dormant cells that do not develop and divide, enabling them to persist after antibiotic assault.

Phenomenological and related meaning-centered theory—explanatory approaches that draw attention to the subjectivities of illness and the ways they are experienced, interpreted, and made meaningful in human societies.

Plague—while the term is sometimes used in a general sense to refer to lethal epidemics, it is more narrowly applied to refer specifically to bubonic plague or Black Death, as it came to be called in medieval Europe.

Plastisphere—the dense and diverse microbial communities living on anthropogenic plastic debris found in the ocean.

Pluralea interaction—adverse interactions between anthropogenic ecocrises.

Political economy of health—the theoretical perspective that sees the interface of social structure and the economy as the primary force shaping society.

Prions—pathogenic variants of proteins that are naturally produced in nerve cells and certain other cells.

Proteobacterium—a diversely shaped group of bacteria named after the Greek god of the sea, Proteus, because in mythology he is depicted as being capable of taking on many different shapes.

Protozoa—a diverse group of unicellular microorganism, some of which are mobile through the use of a tail or foot-like structure, and some of which are pathogenic.

Psyllid—a tiny insect that feeds on citrus trees and serves as vector of the citrus-destroying bacteria *Candidatus liberibacter*.

Quorum sensing—the ability of microorganisms to sense the presence of other microorganisms, allowing the initiation of social behaviors.

Rapid ethnographic assessment—use of ethnographic approaches in highly focused, short-term research designed to address specific issues of concern.

Red tide—conglomerations of algae and infectious bacteria that have become a growing source of human disease because of the effects of global warming and agricultural runoff of fertilizers and other chemicals into the oceans.

Reemergent infectious diseases—diseases that were previously under control through the use of antibiotics but are once again emergent and spreading.

Retrotransposable elements—parasitic strands of DNA that may be a factor in cancer and aging.

Risk environments—social and physical environment that promote involvement in risky behaviors.

Roundworms—widely dispersed and varied helminths of animals and humans tied to a number of diseases such as ascariasis, which is thought to infect about a fourth of humanity.

Sarcoidosis—an inflammation of the lymph nodes, lungs, liver, eyes, skin, or other tissues that may be caused by a pathogenic agent.

SARS—Severe Acute Respiratory Syndrome; an acute viral zoonotic disease with lethal potential, especially among individuals suffering from other significant diseases.

SAVA—a syndemic involving adverse interaction among substance abuse, violence, and AIDS.

Shigella dysentery—an infection of the digestive system, also known as Shigellosis, that is caused by Shigella bacteria. The bacteria are only found in humans.

Shigella flexneri—a bacteria that causes dysentery in humans and primates.

Siderophore pyoverdine—a chemical released by bacteria that can facilitate the acquisition of iron from its environment.

Simian Foamy virus—an infectious disease agent among primates that has jumped to human hosts.

SIVcpz—SAVchimpanzee; a simian immunodeficiency virus found in chimpanzees and believed to be the zoonotic source of HIV-1.

SIVgorilla—a simian immunodeficiency virus found in gorillas.

Sociogenic—health problems caused by social arrangements and structures of social inequality.

Species barrier—internal biochemical and cellular differences between species that hinders the movement of pathogens across host species.

Sporotrichosis—a fungal skin disease characterized by pink to purple skin bumps and rashes, potentially leading to chronic ulcers.

Status incongruity—the stressful tension (that has been linked to transitions from latent to active infectious diseases) between the social status an individual holds using a traditional cultural model versus the social status an individual can achieve as a result of the influx of foreign cultural elements.

Stigmatization—the extreme disapproval and labeling of a person or group as different, inferior, and dangerous.

Strongyloidiasis—a chronic parasitic infection of humans caused by *Strongyloides stercoralis.*

Structural violence—assaults on human dignity and well-being, including poverty, discrimination, stigmatization, and unequal access to resources, that are built into and naturalized as parts of social systems rather than the acts of identifiable culprits.

Successive infection—tissue and immune system changes wrought by one infectious agent that facilitate the impact of subsequent infectious agents, even by different pathogens, such as a viral disease followed by a bacterial disease. Successive infection is one type of syndemic.

Swine influenza—an infectious disease caused by a virus that was initially adapted to pigs but was often zoonotic.

Symbolic violence—the ways symbolic systems, such as words, meaningful cultural images, and culturally generated behaviors, promote the social-class interests of dominant groups by emphasizing profound distinctions between people in society.

Syndemic—two or more adversely interacting diseases in the context of social inequality and other disease-promoting social conditions.

Syndemogenic—diseases like HIV infection that tend to interact adversely with other diseases.

Taeniasis—a disease caused by infection of the intestines by the helminth *Taenia solium.*

T-cell lymphotrophic virus—an infectious agent that has been linked to some cases of leukemia.

Threadworms—also known as pinworms; small, white intestinal helminths, peculiar to humans, that cause itching.

Toxic shock syndrome—a sudden onset and sometimes fatal disease associated with tampon use that is caused by a toxin produced by several species of *Streptococcus bacteria.*

Toxocariasis—a zoonotic infection caused by the larvae of the roundworm, variable in its expression depending upon the host's immune response and the level of the parasitic load, but symptoms can include fatigue, weight loss, fever, headache, and rash.

Toxocariasis—an infectious and zoonotic disease in humans caused by a larvae (immature worms) of either the dog roundworm, the cat roundworm, or the fox roundworm.

Transmission dynamics or transmission factors—the various different ways infections are spread from one person to others or from other species to humans (and vice versa).

Treponema pallidum—the bacterial agent of syphilis.

Triatomins—also known as conenose bugs, kissing bugs, and assassin bugs, these insects tend to feed on the blood of other species and are potential vectors of Chagas disease.

Trichomoniasis—an infectious sexually transmitted disease caused by a single-celled protozoan parasite; it is the common cause of vaginitis.

Trypanosoma—a family of parasitic protozoa that includes the pathogens associated with sleeping sickness and Chagas disease.

Tuberculosis—an ancient, still common, and, in many cases, lethal infectious disease caused by various strains of mycobacteria.

Typhoid fever—a bacterial disease characterized by diarrhea and a rash that is commonly transmitted through the oral/fecal route.

Vector-borne pathogens—pathogens transmitted to a new host by vector species like mosquitoes, blackflies, sandflies, ticks, and fleas.

Viral shedding—the process of successful viral reproduction, expulsion of virons (or single virus particle) from host cells, and further host-cell infection, also used to refer to viral movement from one part of the body to another or from a host body into the environment.

Viral sovereignty—the national right, first claimed by Indonesia, to control viral samples collected within its borders rather than be obliged to turn them over to the World Health Organization surveillance program.

Virgin population—a population being exposed to a spreading infectious disease for the first time and, consequently, having no prior immunity that has developed in response to the disease agent.

Virulence—refers to the aggressiveness of a pathogen in causing disease.

Virus—a microscopic infectious agent that replicates only inside the living cells of other organisms by commandeering host-cell materials needed for reproduction but not possessed by the virus.

Water-borne pathogens—infectious agents that live in water or water-dwelling organisms that facilitate their contact with new hosts.

Wind-blown pathogens—infectious agents that are carried to new hosts by the wind

Yellow fever—an acute viral hemorrhagic disease transmitted by mosquito vectors.

Zoonoses—an infectious disease agent that successfully transferred from an animal population host to a human population host.

REFERENCES

Abdulla, Salim, Rolf Oberholzer, Omar Juma et al. 2008. "Safety and Immunogenicity of RTS,S/AS02D Malaria Vaccine in Infants." *New England Journal of Medicine* 359: 2533–2544.

Abi-Rached, Laurent, Matthew Jobin, Subhash Kularni et al. 2011. "The Shaping of Modern Human Immune Systems by Multiregional Admixture with Archaic Humans." *Science* 334 (6052): 89–94.

Abu-Raddad, Laith. 2007. "HIV and Malaria: A Vicious Cycle." *SCitizen*. http://scitizen.com /aids/hiv-and-malaria-a-vicious-cycle_a-26-313.html.

Accorsi, S., M. Fabiani, B. Nattabi et al. 2005. "The Disease Profile of Poverty: Morbidity and Mortality in Northern Uganda in the Context of War, Population Displacement and HIV/ AIDS." *Transactions of the Royal Society of Tropical Medicine and Hygiene* 99 (3): 226–233.

Achenbach, Joel. 2008. "Iowa Flooding Could Be an Act of Man, Experts Say." *Washington Post*. June 19: A1.

Ackah, A., D. Coulibaly, H. Digbeu et al. 1995. "Response to Treatment, Mortality, and CD4 Lymphocyte Counts in HIV-Infected Persons with Tuberculosis in Abidjan, Côte d'Ivoire." *Lancet* 345: 607–610.

Adamson, Rosemary, Vasudha Reddy, Lucretia Jones et al. 2010. "Epidemiology and Burden of Hepatitis A, Malaria, and Typhoid in New York City Associated with Travel: Implications for Public Health Policy." *American Journal of Public Health* 100 (7): 1249–1252.

Aguirre, Patricia. 2000. "Socioanthropological Aspects of Obesity in Poverty." In *Obesity and Poverty: A New Public Health Challenge*, edited by Manuel Peña and Jorge Bacallao, 11–22. Washington, DC: Pan American Health Organization.

Aichbhaumik, Niladri, Edward Zoratti, Ronald Strickler et al. 2008. "Prenatal Exposure to Household Pets Influences Fetal Immunoglobulin E Production." *Clinical and Experimental Allergy* 38: 1787–1794.

Albenberg, Linsey, and Gary Wu. 2014. "Diet and the Intestinal Microbiome: Associations, Functions, and Implications for Health and Disease." *Gastroenterology* 146 (6): 1564–1572.

Albers, Bruce, Alexander Johnson, Julian Lewis, Martin Raff, Keith Roberts, and Peter Walter. 2002. *Molecular Biology of the Cell*. 4th ed. New York: Garland Science.

Alcabes, Philip. 2009. *Dread: How Fear and Fantasy Have Fueled Epidemics from the Black Death to Avian Flu*. New York: Public Affairs.

Ali, S. Harris. 2004. "A Socio-Ecological Autopsy of the E. coli O157:H7 Outbreak in Walkerton, Ontario, Canada." *Social Science and Medicine* 58: 2601–2612.

Allan, Brian, Felicia Keesing, and Richard Ostfeld. 2003. "Effect of Forest Fragmentation on Lyme Disease Risk." *Conservation Biology* 17 (1): 267–272.

Alvarez, Lizette. 2013. "Citrus Disease with No Cure Is Ravaging Florida Groves." *New York Times*. May 9. www.nytimes.com/2013/05/10/us/disease-threatens-floridas-citrus -industry.html?pagewanted=1&_r=1&adxnnlx=1388530803-4Sb5HcX6GihvCNFs FU6NcA&/.

American Veterinary Medical Association. 2008. "One Health: A New Professional Imperative." One Health Initiative Task Force Final Report. Schaumburg, IL: AVMA.

Anabwani, Gabriel, and Peter Navario. 2005. "Nutrition and HIV/AIDS in Sub-Saharan Africa: An Overview." *Nutrition* 21: 96–99.

Anderson, Mark, and Hank Seifert. 2011. "Opportunity and Means: Horizontal Gene Transfer from the Human Host to a Bacterial Pathogen." *mBio* 2 (1): e00005–11.

Anderson, Pamela, Andrew Cunningham, Nikkita Patel, Francisco Morales, Paul Epstein, and Peter Daszak. 2004. "Emerging Infectious Diseases of Plants: Pathogen Pollution, Climate Change and Agrotechnology Drivers." *Trends in Ecology and Evolution* 19 (10): 534–544.

Anderson, Warwick. 2006. *Colonial Pathologies: American Tropical Medicine, Race, and Hygiene in the Philippines*. Durham, NC: Duke University Press.

Appadurai, Arjun. 1990. "Disjuncture and Difference in the Global Cultural Economy." *Theory Culture Society* 7: 295–310.

Armelagos, George. 1997. "The Viral Superhighway." *The Sciences* (Jan/Feb): 24–29.

Armelagos, George, and Kristin Harper. 2005. "Disease Globalization in the Third Epidemiological Transition." In *Globalizing, Health, and the Environment: An Integrated Perspective,* edited by G. Guest, 27–33. Walnut Creek, CA: AltaMira Press.

Armelagos, George, and Kristin Harper. 2010. "Emerging Infectious Diseases, Urbanization, and Globalization in the Time of Global Warming." In *The New Blackwell Companion to Medical Sociology,* edited by William Cockerham, 291–311. Malden, MA: Wiley-Blackwell.

Armelagos, George, Thomas Leatherman, Mary Ryan, and Lynn Sibley. 1992. "Biocultural Synthesis in Medical Anthropology." *Medical Anthropology* 14 (1): 35–52.

Armstrong, Joana, and Harry Campbell. 1991. "Indoor Air Pollution Exposure and Lower Respiratory Infections in Young Gambian Children." *International Journal of Epidemiology* 20: 424–429.

Armstrong, N. R., and J. D. Wilson. 2006. "Did the 'Brazilian' Kill the Public Louse?" *Sexually Transmitted Diseases* 82 (2): 265–266.

Aronowitz, Robert. 1991. "Lyme Disease: The Social Construction of a New Disease and its Social Consequences." *Milbank Quarterly* 69 (1): 79–112.

Atherholt, T. B., M. W. LeChevallier, W. D. Norton, and J. S. Rosen. 1998. "Effect of Rainfall on Giardia and Cryptosporidium." *Journal of the America Water Works Association* 90 (9): 66–80.

Atkinson, R. L., N. V. Dhurandhar, D. B. Allison et al.. 2005. "Human Adenovirus-36 Is Associated with Increased Body Weight and Paradoxical Reduction of Serum Lipids." *International Journal of Obesity* 29: 281–286.

Atkinson, William, Jennifer Hamborsky, Arch Stanton, and Charles Wolfe, eds. 2012. *Epidemiology and Prevention of Vaccine-Preventable Diseases*. Washington, DC: Public Health Foundation.

Baars, Bernard. 1997. *In the Theater of Consciousness: The Workspace of the Mind*. New York: Oxford University Press.

Bäckhed, Fredrik, Hao Ding, ting Wang, Lora Hooper, Gou Koh, Andras Nagy, Clay Semenkovich and Jeffrey Gordon. 2005. "The gut microbiota as an environmental factor that regulates fat storage." *Proceedings of the National Academy of Sciences of the United States of America* 101(44): 15718–15723.

Baer, Hans, and Merrill Singer. 2009. *Global Warming and the Political Ecology of Health: Emerging Crises and Systemic Solutions*. Walnut Creek, CA: Left Coast Press.

Baer, Hans, and Merrill Singer. 2014. *The Anthropology of Climate Change: An Integrated Critical Perspective*. New York: Routledge, Earthscan.

Baer, Hans, Merrill Singer, and Ida Susser. 2013. *Medical Anthropology and the World System*. 3rd ed. Westport, CT: Greenwood Publishing.

Bardhan, Pradip. 1997. "Epidemiological Features of *Helicobacter pylori* Infection in Developing Countries." *Clinical Infectious Diseases* 25 (5): 973–978.

Barrett, Ron. 2010. "Avian Influenza and the Third Epidemiological Transition." In *Plagues and Epidemics: Infected Spaces Past and Present,* edited by Ann Herring and Alan Swedlund, 81N94. New York: Berg Publishers.

Barros, Mônica, Armando Schubach, Tânia Schubach, Bodo Wanke, and S. Lambert-Passos. 2008. "An Epidemic of Sporotrichosis in Rio de Janeiro, Brazil: Epidemiological Aspects of a Series of Cases." *Epidemiology and Infection* 139 (6): 1192–1196.

Barry, Michele. 2007. "The Tail End of Guinea Worm: Global Eradication Without a Drug or a Vaccine." *New England Journal of Medicine* 356: 2561–2564.

Bartlett, John. 2013. "Advances in the Highly Kinetic Field of Infectious Diseases." Medscape Multiplicity. www.medscape.com/viewarticle/815114_1.

Barzilay, Ezra, Nicolas Schaad, Roc Maglorie et al. 2013. "Cholera Surveillance During the Haiti Epidemic: The First 2 Years." *New England Journal of Medicine* 368: 599–609.

Bastien, Joseph. 1998. *The Kiss of Death: Chagas' Disease in the Americas.* Salt Lake City: University of Utah Press.

Bateson, Mary Catharine, and Richard Goldsby. 1988. *Thinking AIDS.* Reading, MA: Addison-Wesley.

Battershell, Lauren. 2011. "Zoonotic Diseases." The Encyclopedia of Earth. www.eoearth.org /view/article/157228/.

Becker, Gay. 1999. *Disrupted Lives: How People Create Meaning in a Chaotic World.* Berkeley: University of California Press.

Bejon, Philip, John Lusingu, Ally Olotu et al. 2008. "Efficacy of RTS,S/AS01E Vaccine Against Malaria in Children 5 to 17 Months of Age." *New England Journal of Medicine* 359: 2521–2532.

Benson, Etienne. 2013. "The Urbanization of the Eastern Gray Squirrel in the United States." *Journal of American History* 100 (2): 591–710.

Bentwich, Zvi, Gary Maartens, Dina Torten, Altaf Lal, and Renu Lal. 2000. "Concurrent Infections and HIV Pathogenesis." *AIDS* 14: 2071–2081.

Bernard, H. Russell. 1995. *Research Methods in Anthropology.* Newbury Park: Sage.

Best Practices Advocacy Centre. 2011. "Rheumatic Fever in Māori: What Can We Do Better?" *Best Practices Journal* 37. www.bpac.org.nz/BPJ/2011/august/rheumatic.aspx.

Bierlich, Bernhard. 1995. "Notions and Treatment of Guinea Worm in Northern Ghana." *Social Science and Medicine* 41 (4): 501–509.

Bierne, Hélène, Mélanie Hamon, and Pascale Cossart. 2012. *Epigenetics and Bacterial Infections.* New York: Cold Spring Harbor Perspectives in Medicine. Online at: http://perspec tivesinmedicine.cshlp.org/content/2/12/a010272.full.

Bindon, James. 2007. "Biocultural Linkages: Cultural Consensus, Cultural Consonance, and Human Biological Research." *Collegium Anthropologicum* 31 (1): 3–10.

Blakely, Debra. 2006. *Mass Mediated Diseases: A Case Study of Three Flu Pandemics and Public Health Policy.* Lanham, MD: Rowman and Littlefield.

Bloom, Peter. 2008. *French Colonial Documentary: Mythologies of Humanitarianism.* Minneapolis: University of Minnesota Press.

Bloudoff-Indelicato, Mollie. 2012. "Fortified by Global Warming, Deadly Fungus Poisons Corn Crops, Causes Cancer." *Scientific American.* www.scientificamerican.com/article .cfm?id=deadly-fungus-poisons-corn-crops.

Boles, Blaise, Matthew Thoendel, and Pradeep Singh. 2004. "Self-Generated Diversity Produces "Insurance Effects" in Biofilm Communities." *Proceedings of the National Academy of Science* USA 101: 16630–16635.

Bonds, Matthew, Andrew Dobson, and Donald Keenan. 2012. "Disease Ecology, Biodiversity, and the Latitudinal Gradient in Income." *PLoS Biology* 10 (12): e1001456. doi:10.1371 /journal.pbio.1001456.

Borg, M. 2014. "Cultural Determinants of Infection Control Behavior: Understanding Drivers and Implementing Effective Change." *Journal of Hospital Infection* 86 (3): 161–168.

Bourdieu, Pierre. 1998. *Practical Reason: On the Theory of Action*. Stanford, CA: Stanford University Press.

Boyce, John. 1997. "Epidemiology and Prevention of Nosocomial Infections." In *The Staphylococci in Human Disease*, edited by Kent Crossley and Gordon Archer, 309–329. New York: Churchill Livingstone.

Boyer, Joseph, James Fourqurean, and Ronald Jones. 1999. "Seasonal and Long-Term Trends in the Water Quality of the Florida Bay (1989–1997)." *Estuaries* 22: 417–430.

Bray, R. S. 2004. *Armies of Pestilence: The Impact of Disease on History*. Cambridge: James Clarke and Co.

Brewer, Noel, and Karen Fazekas. 2007. Predictors of HPV Vaccine Acceptability: A Theory-Informed, Systematic Review." *Preventive Medicine* 45 (2–3): 107–114.

Briceño-León, Roberto. 2007. "Chagas Disease and Globalization of the Amazon." *Cadernos de Saúde Pública* 23: 33–40.

Briggs, Charles. 2010. "Pressing Plagues: On the Mediated Communicability of Virtual Epidemics." In *Plagues and Epidemics: Infected Spaces Past and Present*, edited by Ann Herring and Alan Swedlund, 39–59. Oxford, UK: Berg.

Briggs, Charles, and Clara Mantini-Briggs. 2004. *Stories in the Time of Cholera: Racial Profiling During a Medical Nightmare*. Berkeley: University of California Press.

Brown, Paul, Jean-Philippe Brandel, Takeshi Sato et al. 2012. "Iatrogenic Creutzfeldt-Jakob Disease, Final Assessment." *Emerging Infectious Diseases* 18 (6): 901–907.

Brown, Peter. 1998. "Cultural Adaptations to Endemic Malaria in Sardinia." In *Understanding and Applying Medical Anthropology*, edited by Peter Brown, 79–92. New York: McGraw-Hill.

Brown, Peter, George Armelagos, and Kenneth Maes. 2012. "Humans in a World of Microbes: The Anthropology of Infectious Disease." In *A Companion to Medical Anthropology*, edited by Merrill Singer and Pamela Erickson, 253–270. Malden, MA: Wiley.

Browner, Carole. 1999. "On the Medicalization of Medical Anthropology." *Medical Anthropology Quarterly* 13 (2): 135–140.

Brundtland, Gro. 2001. United Nations Association's Global Leadership Awards. www.who.int/director-general/speeches/2001/english/20010419_UNAawardsdinnernewyork.en.html.

Brunham, Robert, Francis Plummer, and Richard Stephens. 1993. "Bacterial Antigenic Variation, Host Immune Response, and Pathogen-Host Coevolution." *Infection and Immunity* 61: 2273–2276.

Butler, Jay, Sue Crengle, James Cheek et al. 2001. "Emerging Infectious Diseases Among Indigenous Peoples." *Emerging Infectious Diseases* 7 (1): doi:10.3201/eid0707.017732.

Caduff, Carlo. 2012. "The Semiotics of Security: Infectious Disease Research and the Biopolitics of Information Bodies in the United States." *Cultural Anthropology* 27 (2): 333–357.

Calisher, Charles, James Childs, Hume Field, Kathryn Holmes, and Tony Schountz. 2006. "Bats: Important Reservoir Hosts of Emerging Viruses." *Clinical Microbiology Reviews* 19 (3): 531–545.

Caprara, Andrea. 1998. "Cultural Interpretations of Contagion." *Tropical Medicine and International Health* 30 (12): 996–1001.

Caraco, Thomas, and Ing-Nang Wang. 2008. "Free-Living Pathogens: Life-History Constraints and Strain Competition." *Journal of Theoretical Biology* 250: 569–579.

Carmichael, Mary. 2006. "How It Began: HIV Before the Age of AIDS." *Frontline*. www.pbs.org/wgbh/pages/frontline/aids/virus/origins.html.

Carter Center, The. 2013. Guinea Worm Disease Eradication. www.cartercenter.org/health/guinea_worm/mini_site/current.html.

Castro, Arachu and Paul Farmer. 2005. Understanding and Addressing AIDS-related Stigma: from Anthropological Theory to Clinical Practice in Haiti. *American Journal of Public Health* 95(1): 53-59.

Center for HIV Law and Policy. 2010. *Ending and Defending Against HIV Criminalization: A Manual for Advocates.* New York: Center for HIV Law and Policy.

Centers for Disease Control and Prevention. 2003. "Update: Adverse Events Following Civilian Smallpox Vaccination—United States, 2003." *Morbidity and Mortality Weekly Report* 53: 106–107.

Centers for Disease Control and Prevention. 2009. "2009 H1N1 and Seasonal Flu and African American Communities: Questions and Answers." www.cdc.gov/h1n1flu/african_americans_qa.htm?s_cid=ccu121409_AAQandA_e.

Centers for Disease Control and Prevention. 2012. *Fungal Pneumonia: A Silent Epidemic Coccidioidomycosis (valley fever).* Atlanta, GA: CDC.

Centers for Disease Control and Prevention. 2013. *Antibiotic Resistance Threats in the United States, 2013.* Atlanta: CDC.

Center for Strategic and International Studies. 2012. "Infectious Disease: A Persistent Threat." www.smartglobalhealth.org/issues/entry/infectious-diseases.

Chandra, Ranjit. 1997. "Nutrition and the Immune System: An Introduction." *American Journal of Clinical Nutrition* 66: 460–463.

Chapman, Audrey. 2010. "The Social Determinants of Health, Health Equity, and Human Rights." *Health and Human Rights* 12 (2): 17–30.

Chase, Ellen, Peter Aggleton, and Thomas Coram. 2001. Stigma, HIV/AIDS and Prevention of Mother-to-Child Transmission: A Pilot Study in Zambia, India, Ukraine and Burkina Faso. UNICEF, Panos Institute AIDS Programme.

Chauhan, Anoop, and Sebastian Johnston. 2003. "Air Pollution and Infection in Respiratory Illness." *British Medical Bulletin* 68 (1): 95–112.

Chaves, Luis, Justin Cohen, Mercedes Pascual, and Mark Wilson. 2008. "Social Exclusion Modifies Climate and Deforestation Impacts on a Vector-Borne Disease." *PLoS Neglected Tropical Disease* 2 (2): e176.

Checkley, William, Leonard Epstein, Robert Gilman et al. 2000. "Effects of El Niño and Ambient Temperature on Hospital Admissions for Diarrheal Diseases in Peruvian Children." *Lancet* 355 (9202): 442–450.

Cheng, Vincent, Kelvin To, Herman Tse, Ivan Hung, and Kwok-Yung Yuen. 2012. "Two Years After Pandemic Influenza A/2009/H1N1: What Have We Learned?" *Clinical Microbiology Reviews* 25 (2): 223–263.

Chivian, Eric, and Aaron Bernstein. 2010. *How Our Health Depends on Biodiversity.* Cambridge, MA: Center for Health and the Global Environment, Harvard Medical School.

Chowdhury, A. Mushtaque, Abbas Bhuiya, Simeen Mahmud, Abdus Salam, and Fazlul Karim. 2003. "Who Gets Vaccinated in Bangladesh?: The Immunization Divide" *Journal of Health, Population and Nutrition* 21 (3): 193–204.

Chromel, Burno, and Ben Sun. 2011. "Zoonoses in the Bedroom." *Emerging Infectious Diseases* 17 (2): 167–172.

Chua, Kaw Bing. 2003. "Nipah Virus Outbreak in Malaysia." *Journal of Clinical Virology* 26: 265–275.

Chun, Helen, Robert Carpenter, Grace Macalino, and Nancy Crum-Cianflone. 2013. "The Role of Sexually Transmitted Infections in HIV-1 Progression: A Comprehensive Review of the Literature." *Journal of Sexually Transmitted Diseases* 2013: 1–15.

Closser, Svea. 2010. *Chasing Polio in Pakistan: Why the World's Largest Public Health Initiative May Fail.* Nashville, TN: Vanderbilt University Press.

Closser, Svea. 2012. "'We Can't Give Up Now': Global Health Optimism and Polio Eradication in Pakistan." *Medical Anthropology* 31: 385–403.

Clutton-Brock, Juliet. 1994. "The Unnatural World: Behavioural Aspects of Humans and Animals in the Process of Domestication." In *Animals and Human Society: Changing Perspectives*, edited by A. Manning and J. Serpell, 23–35. London: Routledge.

Cockburn, Aidan. 1963. *The Evolution and Eradication of Infectious Diseases.* Baltimore: Johns Hopkins University Press.

Cohen, Deborah, and Philip Carter. 2010. "WHO and the Pandemic Flu 'Conspiracies.'" *British Medical Journal* 340 (7759): 1274–1279.

Cohen, Hillel, Robert Gould, and Victor Sidel. 2004. "The Pitfalls of Bioterrorism Preparedness: The Anthrax and Smallpox Experiences." *American Journal of Public Health* 94 (10): 1667–1671.

Coimbra, Carlos. 1988. "Human Settlements, Demographic Pattern, and Epidemiology in Lowland Amazonia: The Case of Chagas's Disease." *American Anthropologist* 90 (1): 82–97.

Collier, Stephen, Andrew Lakoff, and Paul Rabinow. 2004. "Biosecurity: Towards an Anthropology of the Contemporary." *Anthropology Today* 20 (5): 3–7.

Collignon, Peter, Frank Aarestrup, Rebecca Irwin, and Scott McEwen. 2013. "Human Deaths and Third-Generation Cephalosporin Use in Poultry, Europe." *Emerging Infectious Diseases* 19 (8): 1339–1340.

Commins, Scott, and Thomas Platts-Mills. 2013. "Tick Bites and Red Meat Allergy." *Current Opinion in Allergy and Clinical Immunology* 13 (4): 354–359.

Commission on the Social Determinants of Health. 2008. Closing the Gap in a Generation. Geneva: World Health Organization.

Cormier, Loretta. 2010. "The Historical Ecology of Human and Wild Primate Malarias in the New World." *Diversity* 2: 256–280.

Crosby, Alfred. 2004. *Ecological Imperialism: The Biological Expansion of Europe, 900–1900.* Cambridge: Cambridge University Press.

Crosby, Molly. 2006. *The American Plague: The Untold Story of Yellow Fever, the Epidemic That Shaped Our History.* New York: Berkeley Books.

Crowl, Todd, Thomas Crist, Robert Parmenter, Gary Belovsky, and Ariel Lugo. 2008. "The Spread of Invasive Species and Infectious Disease as Drivers of Ecosystem Change." *Frontiers in Ecology and the Environment* 6 (5): 238–246.

Crutzen, Paul. and Eugene Stoermer. 2000. "The Anthropocene." *Global Change Newsletter* 41: 17–18.

Cunningham, Andrew, Peter Daszak, and P. Rodriguez. 2003. "Pathogen Pollution: Defining a Parasitological Threat to Biodiversity Conservation." *Journal of Parasitology* 88 (Supplement 1): S78–S83.

Curriero, Frank, Jonathan Patz, Joan Rose, and Jsubhash Lele. 2001. The Association Between Extreme Precipitation and Waterborne Disease Outbreaks in the United States, 1948–1994." *American Journal of Public Health* 91 (8): 1194–1199.

Curtis, Thomas, William Sloan, and Jack Scannell. 2002. "Estimating Prokaryotic Diversity and Its Limits." *Proceedings of the National Academy of Science* (USA) 99 (16): 10494–10499.

Dabbs, Gretchin. 2009. "Resuscitating the Epidemiological Model of Differential Diagnosis: Tuberculosis at Prehistoric Point Hope, Alaska." *Paleopathology Association Newsletter* 148: 11–24.

Daszak, Peter, Andrew Cunningham, and Alex Hyatt. 2001. "Anthropogenic Environmental Change and the Emergence of Infectious Diseases in Wildlife." *Acta Tropica* 78: 103–116.

Daszak, Peter, Andrew Cunningham, and Alex Hyatt. 2003. "Infectious Disease and Amphibian Population Declines." *Diversity and Distributions* 9: 141–150.

Davies, Dame Sally. 2013. Chief Medical Officer's Summary. Annual Report of the Chief Medical Officer, vol. 2, Infections and the Rise of Antimicrobial Resistance, 11–25. London: Department of Health.

Davies, Julie-Anne. 2013. "Superbug Showdown: The Time Is Nigh to Get Serious About Antibiotics." *Sydney Morning Herald*. December 28. www.smh.com.au/national/health /superbug-showdown-the-time-is-nigh-to-get-serious-about-antibiotics-20131227 -2zzjc.html.

Davis, Mike. 2005. *The Monster at Our Door: The Global Threat of Avian Flu*. New York: New Press.

de Aguilar, Francisco. 1993. *The Conquistadors: First Person Account of the Conquest of Mexico*. Edited and translated by Patricia de Fuentes. Oklahoma City: University of Oklahoma Press.

de Barra, Mícheál, and Val Curtis. 2012. "Are Pathogens of Put-Groups More Dangerous?" *Behavioral and Brain Sciences* 35 (2): 25–26.

De Chiara, Giovanna, Maria Marcocci, Rossella Sgarbanti et al. 2012. "Infectious Agents and Neurodegeneration." *Molecular Neurobiology* 46 (3): 614–638.

Delaporte, François. 2012. *Chagas Disease: History of a Continent's Scourge*. New York: Fordham University Press.

Dell'Arciprete, Ana, José Braunstein, Cecilia Touris, Graciela Dinardi, Ignacio Llovet, and Sergio Sosa-Esani. 2014. "Cultural Barriers to Effective Communication Between Indigenous Communities and Health Care Providers in Northern Argentina: An Anthropological Contribution to Chagas Disease Prevention and Control." *International Journal for Equity in Health* 13: 6. doi:10.1186/1475-9276-13-6.

De Martel, Catherine, Jacques Ferlay, Silvia Franceschi et al. 2012. "Global Burden of Cancers Attributable to Infections in 2008: A Review and Synthetic Analysis." *Lancet Oncology* 13 (6): 605–615.

Department of Aerobiological Engineering. 1998. *The Spread of Respiratory Disease in Office Buildings*. Pennsylvania State University.

Department of Health and Human Services. n.d. The Great Pandemic: The United States in 1918–1999. www.flu.gov/pandemic/history/1918/your_state/northwest/utah /index.html.

de Souza Gomes, Elainne, Onicio Leal-Neto, Jones Albuquerque, Hernande da Silva, and Constança Barbosa. 2012. "Schistosomiasis Transmission and Environmental Change: A Spatio-Temporal Analysis in Porto de Galinhas, Pernambuco, Brazil." *International Journal of Health Geographics* 11: 51 doi:10.1186/1476-072X-11-51.

Diderichsen, Finn, Timothy Evans and Margaret Whitehead. 2001. The Social Basis of Disparities in Health. In *Challenging Inequities in Health: From Ethics to Action* edited by Timothy Evans, Margaret Whitehead, Finn Diderichsen, Abbas Bhuiya and Meg Wirth, p. 13-23. New York: Oxford University Press.

Didierlaurent, Arnaud, John Goulding, and Tracy Hussell. 2007. "The Impact of Successive Infections on the Lung Microenvironment." *Immunology* 122 (4): 457–485.

Dixon-Woods, Mary, Myles Leslie, Julian Bion, and Carolyn Tarrant. 2012. "What Counts? An Ethnographic Study of Infection Data Reported to a Patient Safety Program." *Milbank Quarterly* 90 (3): 548–591.

Dobyns, Henry. 1963. "An Outline of Andean Epidemic History to 1720." *Bulletin of the History of Medicine* 33.

Dove, Alan. 2013. "The Microbiome in Health, Disease, and Therapeutics: Bugs, Guts, and Drugs, Overview." New York Academy of Sciences. www.nyas.org/Publications /EBriefings/Detail.aspx?cid=71e5d453-304b-42d5-9adb-0d6f3f16943c.

Doyal, Lesley, and Len Doyal. 2013. *Living with HIV and Dying with AIDS: Diversity, Inequality and Human Rights in the Global Pandemic*. Surrey, UK: Ashgate Publishing.

Dressler, William, and James Bindon. 2000. "The Health Consequences of Cultural Consonance: Cultural Dimensions of Lifestyle, Social Support, and Arterial Blood Pressure in an African American Community." *American Anthropologist* 102: 244–260.

Dubos, René. 1959. *Mirage of Health*. London: Allen and Unwin.

Dunitz, Jack, and Gerald Joyce. 2013. *Leslie E. Orgel, 1927–2007: A Biological Memoir*. Washington, DC: National Academy of Sciences.

Dunn, Elizabeth. 2008. "Postsocialist Spores: Disease, Bodies, and the State in the Republic of Georgia." *American Ethnologist* 35 (2): 243–258.

Dunn, Rob. 2011. *The Wild Life of Our Bodies: Predators, Parasites and Partners That Shape Who We Are Today*. New York: HarperCollins.

Dunn, Rob. 2012. "After 2 Years Scientists Still Can't Solve Belly Button Mystery, Continue Navel-Gazing." Guest Blog, *Scientific American*, November 7. http://blogs.scientific american.com/guest-blog/2012/11/07/after-two-years-scientists-still-cant-solve-belly -button-mystery-continue-navel-gazing.

Dunn, Rob, Noah Fierer, Jessica Henley, Jonathan Leff, and H. Menninger. 2013. "Home Life: Factors Structuring the Bacterial Diversity Found Within and Between Homes." *PLoS ONE* 8 (5): e64133. doi:10.1371/journal.pone.0064133.

Dunne, Eileen, Carrie Nielson, Katherine Stone, Lauri Markowitz, and Anna Giuliano. 2006. "Prevalence of HPV Infection Among Men: A Systematic Review of the Literature." *Journal of Infectious Diseases* 194 (8): 1044–1057.

Dutt, Asim and William Stead. 1999. "Epidemiology and host factors." In D. Schlossberg (Ed.), *Tuberculosis and nontuberculosis Mycobacterial infections* (4th ed). Philadelphia: W.B. Saunders.

Eardley, W., K. Brown, A. Bonner, D. Green, and J. Clasper. 2010. "Infection in Conflict Wounded." *Philosophical Transactions of the Royal Society B, Biological Sciences* 366 (1562): 204–218.

Ebi, Kristie, K. Alex Exuzides, Edumnd Lau, Michael Kelsh, and Anthony Barnston. 2001. "Association of Normal Weather Periods and El Nino Events with Hospitalization for Viral Pneumonia in Females: California, 1983–1998." *American Journal of Public Health* 91: 1200–1208.

Eckburg, Paul, Paul Lepp, and David Relman. 2003. "Archaea and Their Potential Role in Human Disease." *Infection and Immunity* 7 (2): 591–596.

Editor (no name listed). 2011. "Microbiology by Numbers." *Nature Reviews Microbiology* 9: 628.

Ege, Markus, Melanie Mayer, Ann-Cécile Normand et al. 2011. "Exposure to Environmental Microorganisms and Childhood Asthma." *New England Journal of Medicine* 364: 701–709.

Eisenberg, Joseph, Manish Desai, Karen Levy, Sarah Bates, Song Liang, Kyra Naumoff, and James Scott. 2007. "Environmental Determinants of Infectious Disease: A Framework for Tracking Causal Links and Guiding Public Health Research." *Environmental Health Perspectives* 115 (8): 1216–1223.

Emmer, Chris. 2006. *The Dutch Slave Trade, 1500–1850*. New York: Berghahn Books.

Environmental Protection Agency. 2013. *Literature Review of Contaminants in Livestock and Poultry Manure and Implications for Water Quality*. Washington, DC: EPA, Office of Water.

Epstein, Paul. 2005. "Climate Change and Public Health." *New England Journal of Medicine* 353 (14): 1433–1436.

Estes, Adam. 2013. "The Fascinating Story of Why U.S. Parks Are Full of Squirrels." Gizmodo. http://gizmodo.com/the-fascinating-story-of-why-u-s-parks-are-full-of -squ-1478182563.

Ewald, Paul. 1994. *Evolution of Infectious Disease.* Oxford: Oxford University Press.

Farmer, Paul. 1992. *AIDS and Accusation: Haiti and the Geography of Blame.* Berkeley: University of California Press.

Farmer, Paul. 1996. "Social Inequalities and Emerging Infectious Diseases." *Emerging Infectious Disease* 2 (4): 259–269.

Farmer, Paul. 1999. *Infections and Inequalities.* Berkeley: University of California Press.

Farmer, Paul. 2004. *Pathologies of Power: Health, Human Rights, and the New War on the Poor.* Berkeley: University of California Press.

Fassin, Didier. 2004. "Public Health as Culture: The Social Construction of the Childhood Lead Poisoning Epidemic in France." *British Medical Bulletin* 69 (1): 167–177.

Fassin, Didier. 2007. *When Bodies Remember: Experiences and Politics of AIDS in South Africa.* Berkeley: University of California Press.

Fassin, Didier. 2012. "That Obscure Object of Global Health." In *Medical Anthropology at the Intersections,* edited by Marcia Inhorn and Emily Wentzell, 95–115. Durham, NC: Duke University Press.

Faulkner, Jason, Mark Schaller, Justin Park, and Lesley Duncan. 2004. "Evolved Disease Avoidance Mechanisms and Contemporary Xenophobic Attitudes." *Group Processes and Intergroup Relations* 7: 333–353.

Feazel, Leah, Laura Baumgartner, Kristen Peterson, Daniel Frank, and Kirk Harris, and Norman Pace. 2009. "Opportunistic Pathogens Enriched in Showerhead Biofilms." *Proceedings of the National Academy of Sciences* (USA) 106 (38): 16393–16399.

Fidler, David. 2005. "From International Sanitary Conventions to Global Health Security: The New International Health Regulations." *Chinese Journal of International Law* 4 (2): 325–392.

Fidler, David. 2010. "The H5N1 Virus Sharing Controversy and Its Implications for Global Health Governance." In *Infectious Disease Movement in a Borderless World,* edited by David Relman, Eileen Choffnes and Alison Mack, 210–228. Washington, DC: National Academies Press.

Figueroa-Bossi, Nara, Sergio Uzzau, Daniéla Maloriol, and Lionello Bossi. 2001. "Variable Assortment of Prophages Provides A transferable Repertoire of Pathogenic Determinants in Salmonella." *Molecular Microbiology* 39 (2): 260–270.

Fincher, Corey, and Randy Thornhill. 2008. "A Parasite-Driven Wedge: Infectious Diseases May Explain Language and Other Biodiversity." *Oikos* 117 (9): 1289–1297.

Fincher, Corey, and Richard Thornhill. 2012. "Parasite-Stress Promotes In-Group Assortative Sociality: The Cases of Strong Family Ties and Heightened Religiosity." *Behavioral and Brain Sciences* 35 (2): 61–79.

Fitzgerald, Daniel, Moïse Desvarieux, Patrice Severe, Patrice Joseph, Warren Johnson, and Jean Pape. 2000. "Effect of Post-Treatment Isoniazid on Prevention of Recurrent Tuberculosis in HIV-1-Infected Individuals: A Randomised Trial." *Lancet* 356 (9240): 1470–1474.

Fontes, Gilberto, Anderson Leite, Ana Vasconcelos de Lima, Helen Freitas, John Ehrenberg, and Eliana Mauricio da Rocha. 2012. "Lymphatic Filariasis in Brazil: Epidemiological Situation and Outlook for Elimination." *Parasites and Vectors* 5: 272. doi:10.1186/1756-3305-5-272.

Food and Drug Administration. 2013. Phasing Out Certain Antibiotic Use in Farm Animals. www.fda.gov/forconsumers/consumerupdates/ucm378100.htm.

Foran, Shiela. 2012. "Controlling Japanese Barberry Helps Stop Spread of Tick-Borne Diseases." *UCONN Today.* http://today.uconn.edu/blog/2012/02/controlling-japanese-barberry -helps-stop-spread-of-tick-borne-diseases.

Foster, John Bellamy. 2002. *Ecology Against Capitalism.* New York: Monthly Review Press.

Foucault, Michel. 1976. *The History of Sexuality,* vol. 1. *The Will to Know.* London: Penguin.

Foucault, Michel. 2003. *Society Must Be Defended: Lectures at the Collége de France, 1975–1976.* Edited by Maruo Bertani and Alessandro Fontana. New York: Picador.

France, Anatole. 1894. *The Red Lily.* Paris: Maison Mazarin.

Franco, Crystal, and Tara Sell. 2011. "Federal Agency Biodefense Funding, FY2011–FY2012." *Biosecurity and Bioterrorism* 9 (2): doi:10.1089/bsp.2011.0018.

Frankenberg, Ronald. 1980. "Medical Anthropology and Development: A Theoretical Perspective." *Social Science and Medicine* 14B: 197–202.

Fredricks, David, Tina Fiedler, and Jeanne Marrazzo. 2005. "Molecular Identification of Bacteria Associated with Bacterial Vaginosis." *New England Journal of Medicine* 353: 1899–1911.

Freeman, M., and M. Motsei. 1992. "Planning Health Care in South Africa—Is There a Role for Traditional Healers?" *Social Science and Medicine* 34 (11): 1183–1190.

Fuchs, Martina. 2008. "Egypt: Water Pipe Smoking a Significant TB Risk." IRIN: Humanitarian News and Analysis, UN Office for the Coordination of Humanitarian Affairs. www .irinnews.org/report/77426/egypt-water-pipe-smoking-a-significant-tb-risk.

Fuentes, Austin. 2013. "Blurring the Biology and Social in Human Becomings." In *Biosocial Becomings: Integrating Social and Biological Anthropology,* edited by Tim Ingold and Gisli Palsson, 42–58. Cambridge: Cambridge University Press.

Fuller, George, and Diane Fuller. 1981. "Hydatid Disease in Ethiopia: Epidemiological Findings and Ethnographic Observations of Disease Transmission in Southwestern Ethiopia." *Medical Anthropology* 5: 293–312.

Funkhouser, Lisa, and Seth Bordenstein. 2013. "Mom Knows Best: The Universality of Maternal Microbial Transmission." *PLoS Biology* 11 (8): e1001631. doi:10.1371/journal .pbio.1001631.

Gado, Mark. 2010. "Typoid Mary." Crime Library. www.trutv.com/library/crime/criminal_mind/forensics/typhoid_mary/2.html.

Gage, Kenneth, Thomas Burkot, Rebecca Eisen, Edward Hayes. 2008. "Climate and Vector-borne Diseases." *American Journal of Preventive Medicine* 35(5): 436–450.

Gairdner, William. 1992. *The War Against the Family: A Parent Speaks Out.* Toronto: General Publishing.

Gajdusek, D. Carleton. 1976. "Unconventional Viruses and the Origin and Disappearance of Kuru." Nobel Prize Lecture, December 3. Bethesda, MD: National Institutes of Health.

Gallagher, James. 2014. Ebola response lethally inadequate, says MSF. BBC News, Health. http://www.bbc.com/news/health-29031987.

Gallagher, Kathleen, Michele Jara, Alfred Demaria, George Seage, and Timothy Heeren. 2003. "The Reliability of Passively Collected AIDS Surveillance Data in Massachusetts." *Annals of Epidemiology* 13 (2): 100–104.

Gallagher, Maggie. 1998. Day Careless. National Review, Jan. 26: 37-39.

Gao, Feng, Elizabeth Bailes, David Robertson et al. 1998. "Origin of HIV-1 in the Chimpanzee Pan Troglodytes Troglodytes." *Nature* 397: 436–441.

Garely, Elinor. 2012. "When Bugs Swim." *Global Travel Industry News.* www.eturbonews .com/27225/when-bugs-swim.

Geissler, P. Wenzel. 1998. "Worms Are Our Life, Part I. Understandings of Worms and the Body Among the Luo of Western Kenya." *Anthropology and Medicine* 5 (1): 63–79.

Geneva Declaration Secretariat. 2008. Global Burden of Armed Violence. Geneva, Switzerland: Geneva Declaration Secretariat.

Gérard, Hervé, Ute Dreses-Werringloer, Kristin Wildt et al. 2006. "*Chlamydophila* (Chlamydia) *Penumoniae* in the Alzheimer's Brain." *FEMS Immunolology and Medical Microbiology* 48 (3): 355–366.

Gershwin, Eric, Penelope Nestel, and Carl Keen, eds. 2004. *Handbook of Nutrition and Immunity*. New York: Humana Press.

GIDEON (Global Infectious Diseases and Epidemiology Online Network). 2008. Emergence of Infectious Diseases in the 21st Century. www.gideononline.com/blog/2008/03/05/emergence-of-infectious-diseases-in-the-21st-century.

Gilbert, Hannah. 2013. "Re-visioning Local Biologies: HIV-2 and the Pattern of Differential Valuation in Biomedical Research." *Medical Anthropology* 32: 343–358.

Giuliano, Marina, and Stefano Vella. 2007. "Inequalities in Health: Access to Treatment for HIV/AIDS." *Annali dell'Istituto Superiore di Sanità* 43 (4): 313–316.

Glass, Thomas, and Monica Schoch-Spana. 2002. "Bioterrorism and the People: How to Vaccinate a City Against Panic." *Clinical Infectious Diseases* 34 (2): 217–223.

Godlee, Fiona. 2010. "Conflicts of Interest and Pandemic Flu." *British Medical Journal* 340 doi:http://dx.doi.org/10.1136/bmj.c2947.

Goffman. Erving. 1961. *Asylums: Essays on the Social Situation of Mental Patients and Other Inmates*. Garden City, NY: Anchor Books.

Good, Alan and Thomas Leatherman. 1998. *Building a New Biocultural Synthesis: Political-Economic Perspectives on Human Biology*. Ann Arbor, MI: University of Michigan Press.

Goodale, Mark. 2006. "Toward a Critical Anthropology of Human Rights." *Current Anthropology* 47 (3): 485–511.

Goodman, Alan, and Thomas Leatherman, eds. 1998. *Building a New Biocultural Synthesis*. Lansing: University of Michigan Press.

Gorak, Edward, Stephen Yamada, and Joel Brown. 1999. "Community-Acquired Methicillin-Resistant Staphylococcus Aureus in Hospitalized Adults and Children Without Known Risk Factors." *Clinical Infectious Diseases* 29: 797–800.

Government Accounting Office. 2008. *Indoor Mold: Better Coordination of Research on Health Effects and More Consistent Guidance Would Improve Federal Efforts*. Washington, DC: GAO.

Gracey, Michael, and Malcolm King. 2009. "Indigenous Health Part 1: Determinants and Disease Patterns." *Lancet* 374: 65–75.

Graden, Dale. 2014. *Disease, Resistance, and Lies: The Demise of the Transatlantic Slave Trade to Brazil and Cuba*. Baton Rouge: Louisiana State University Press.

Gramsci, Antonio. 1970. *Prison Notebooks*. London: Lawrence and Wishart.

Grann, David. 2001. "Stalking Dr. Steere Over Lyme Disease." *New York Times*. June 17. www.nytimes.com/2001/06/17/magazine/17LYMEDISEASE.html.

Grant, James. 1982. *The State of the World's Children 1982–83*. Oxford: Oxford University Press.

Grau, Lauretta, Traci Green, Merrill Singer, Ricky Bluthenthal, Patricia Marshall, and Robert Heimer. 2009. "Getting the Message Straight: Effects of a Brief Hepatitis Prevention Intervention among Injection Drug Users." *Harm Reduction Journal* (online journal) 6: 36.

Gray, Michael, Gertraud Burger, and B. Franz Lang. 1999. "Mitochondrial Evolution." *Science* 283: 1476–1481.

Green, Edward. 1999. *Indigenous Theories of Contagious Disease*. Lanham, MD: AltaMira Press.

Greer, Amy, Victoria Ng, and David Fisman. 2008. "Climate Change and Infectious Diseases in North America: The Road Ahead." *Canadian Medical Association Journal* 178 (6): 715–722.

Griffiths, Sian, and Xiao-Nong Zhou. 2012. "Why Research Infectious Diseases of Poverty?" In *Global Report for Research on Infectious Diseases of Poverty*, 11–43. Special Programme for Research and Training in Tropical Diseases. Geneva: World Health Organization.

Grove, David. 1994. *A History of Human Helminthology*. Oxon, UK: C.A.B. International.

Guerrant, Richard, Mark DeBoer, Sean Moore, Rebecca Scharf, and Aldo Lima. 2013. "The

Impoverished Gut: A Triple Burden of Diarrhea, Stunting and Chronic Disease." *Nature Reviews Gastroenterology and Hepatology* 10: 220–229.

Guerrant, Richard, Reinaldo Oría, Sean Moore, Mônica Oría, and Aldo Lima. 2008. "Malnutrition as an Enteric Infectious Disease with Long-Term Effects on Child Development." *Nutrition Reviews* 66 (9): 487–505.

Gürtler, Ricardo, Maria Cécere, D. Rubel et al. 1991. "Chagas Disease in North-West Argentina: Infected Dogs as a Risk Factor for the Domestic Transmission of Trypanosoma cruzi." *Transactions of the Royal Society of Tropical Medicine and Hygiene* 85 (6): 741–745.

Gustavsen, Ken, Adrian Hopkins, and Mauricio Sauerbrey. 2011. "Onchocerciasis in the Americas: From Arrival to (Near) Elimination." *Parasites and Vectors* 4: 205 doi:10.1186/1756-3305-4-205.

Hales, Simon, Phil Weinstein, Yvan Souares, and Alistair Woodward. 1999. "El Nino and the Dynamics of Vectorborne Disease Transmission." *Environmental Health Perspectives* 107: 99–102.

Halkitis, Perry. 2012. "Obama, Marriage Equity, and the Health of Gay Men." *American Journal of Public Health* 102 (9): 1628–1629.

Halkitis, Perry, Robert Moeller, Daniel Siconolfi, Erik Storholm, Todd Solomon, and Kristen Bub. 2013. "Measurement Model Exploring a Syndemic in Emerging Adult Gay and Bisexual Men." *AIDS and Behavior* 17 (2): 662–673.

Hall-Stoodley, Luanne, J. William Costerton, and Paul Stoodley. 2004. "Bacterial Biofilms: From the Natural Environment to Infectious Disease." *Nature Reviews Microbiology* 2: 95–108.

Hamon, Mélanie, Hélène Bierne, and Pascale Cossart. 2006. "Listeria Monocytogenes: A Multifaceted Model." *Nature Reviews Microbiology* 4: 423–434.

Hardy, Anne. 1993. *The Epidemic Streets: Infectious Diseases and the Rise of Preventive Medicine, 1856–1900.* Oxford: Clarendon Press.

Hardy, Chloe, and Marlise Richter. 2006. "Disability Grants or Antiretrovirals?: A Quandary for People with HIV/AIDS in South Africa." *African Journal of AIDS Research* 5 (1): 85–96.

Hargreaves, James, Christopher Bonell, Tania Boler et al. 2008. "Systematic Review Exploring Time Trends in the Association Between Educational Attainment and Risk of HIV Infection in Sub-Saharan Africa." *AIDS* 22: 403–414.

Harper, Ian. 2006. "Anthropology, DOTS and Understanding Tuberculosis Control in Nepal." *Journal of Bioscience* 38: 57–67.

Hayes, R, K. Shulz, and F. Plummer. 1995. "The Cofactor Effect of Genital Ulcers on the Per-Exposure Risk of HIV Transmission in Sub-Saharan Africa." *Journal of Tropical Medicine and Hygiene* 96 (1): 1–8l.

Hays, J. N. 2009. *The Burdens of Disease: Epidemics and Human Response in Western History.* New Brunswick, NJ: Rutgers University Press.

Heggenhougen, Kris. 2009. "Planting 'Seeds of Health' in the Fields of Structural Violence: The Life and Death of Francisco Curruchici." In *Global Health in Times of Violence,* edited by Barbara Rylko-Bauer, Linda Whiteford, and Paul Farmer, 181–199. Santa Fe, NM: School of Advanced Research Press.

Hehemann, Jan-Hendrink, Gaëlle Correc, Tristan Barbeyron, William Helbert, Mirjam Czjzek, and Gurvan Michel. 2010. "Transfer of Carbohydrate-Active Enzymes from Marine Bacteria to Japanese Gut Microbiota." *Nature* 464: 908–U123.

Heinitz, Maxine, Ramona Ruble, Dean Wagner, and Sita Tatini. 2000. "Incidence of Salmonella in Fish and Seafood." *Journal of Food Protection* 63 (5): 579–592.

Helmreich, Stefan. 2009. *Alien Ocean: Anthropological Voyages in Microbial Seas.* Berkeley: University of California Press.

Hemida, M., R. Perera, P. Wang et al. 2013. "Middle Eastern Respiratory Syndrome (MERS)

Coronavirus Seroprevalence in Domestic Livestock in Saudi Arabia, 2010–2013." *Eurosurveillance* 18 (50): 20659.

Hemmaid, Kamel, Amira Awadalla, Essam Elsawy et al. 2013. "Impact of Hepatitis C Virus (HCV) Infection on Biomolecular Markers Influencing the Pathogenesis of Bladder Cancer." *Infectious Agents and Cancer* 8 (1): 24. doi:10.1186/1750-9378-8-24.

Herring, Ann, and Stacy Lockerbie. 2009. "The Coming Plague of Avian Influenza." In *Plagues and Epidemics: Infected Spaces Past and Present*, edited by Ann Herring and Alan Swedlund, 179–191. Oxford: Berg.

Herring, Ann, and Alan Swedlund. 2010. "Plagues and Epidemics in Anthropological Perspective." In *Plagues and Epidemics: Infected Spaces Past and Present*, edited by Ann Herring and Alan Swedlund, 1–19. Oxford: Berg.

Hesser, Jana, ed. 1982. "Part I: Studies of Infectious Disease in an Anthropological Context." *Medical Anthropology* 6 (1): 1–10.

Heuer, Ole, Hilde Kruse, Kari Grave, P. Collignon, Iddya Karunasagar, and Frederick Angulo. 2009. "Human Health Consequences of Use of Antimicrobial Agents in Aquaculture." *Clinical Infectious Diseases* 49 (8): 1248–1253.

Hewitt Krissi, Gerba Charles, Maxwell Sheri, and Kelley, Scott. 2012. "Office Space Bacterial Abundance and Diversity in Three Metropolitan Areas." *PLoS ONE* 7 (5): e37849.

Hewlett, Barry, and Bonnie Hewlett. 2008. *Ebola, Culture, and Politics: The Anthropology of An Emerging Disease*. Belmont, CA: Thompson Wadsworth.

Heymann, David, and Guénaël Rodier. 1997. "Reemerging Pathogens and Diseases Out of Control." *Lancet* 349 (Supplement 3): 8–10.

Hippisley-Cox, Julia, and Mike Pringle. 1998. "Are Spouses of Patients with Hypertension at Increased Risk of Hypertension? A Population Based Case-Control Study." *British Journal of General Practice* 46: 580–1584.

Ho, Ming-Jung. 2004. "Sociocultural Aspects of Tuberculosis: A Literature Review and a Case Study of Immigrant Tuberculosis." *Social Science and Medicine* 59: 753–762.

Hoff, Rani, Joseph Beam-Goulet, and Robert Rosenheck. 1997. "Mental Disorder as a Risk Factor for Human Immunodeficiency Virus Infection in a Sample of Veterans." *Journal of Nervous and Mental Disorders* 185 (9): 556–560.

Hong, Yan, Shannon Mitchell, James Peterson, Carl Latkin, Karin Tobin, and Donald Gann. 2005. "Ethnographic Process Evaluation: Piloting an HIV Prevention Intervention Program Among Injection Drug Users." *International Journal of Qualitative Methods* 4 (1): 1–10.

Hopkins, Donald. 2013. "Disease Eradication." *New England Journal of Medicine* 368: 54–63.

Hotez, Peter. 2008. "Neglected Infections of Poverty in the United States of America." *PLoS Neglected Tropical Diseases* 2 (6): e256. doi:10.1371/journal.pntd.0000256.

Hotez, Peter. 2014. "Aboriginal Populations and Their Neglected Tropical Diseases." *PLoS Neglected Tropical Diseases* 8 (1): e2286. doi:10.1371/journal.pntd.0002286.

Hotez, Peter, Maria E. Bottazzi, Carlos Franco-Paredes, Steven K. Ault, and Mirta R. Periago 2008. "The Neglected Tropical Diseases of Latin America and the Caribbean: A Review of Disease Burden and Distribution and a Roadmap for Control and Elimination." *PLoS Neglected Tropical Diseases* 2 (9): e300. doi:10.1371/journal.pntd.0000300.

Hotez, Peter, Donald A. P. Bundy, Kathleen Beegle et al. 2006. "Helminth Infections: Soil-transmitted Helminth Infections and Schistosomiasis." In *Disease Control Priorities in Developing Countries*. 2nd ed., edited by Dean T. Jamison, Joel G. Breman, Anthony R. Measham et al., 467–482. Oxford: Oxford University Press.

Huttunen, Reetta, and Jaana Syrjanen. 2010. "Obesity and the Outcome of Infection." *Lancet Infectious Diseases* 10: 442—443.

Infectious Disease Society of America. 2004. *Bad Bugs, No Drugs as Antibiotic Discovery Stagnates.* Alexandria, VA: IDSA.

Ingold, Tim. 2013. "Prospect." In *Biosocial Becomings: Integrating Social and Biological Anthropology*, edited by Tim Ingold and Gisli Plasson, 1–21. Cambridge: Cambridge University Press.

Ingold, Tim and Palsson, Gisli (eds.). 2013. *Biosocial Becomings: Integrating Social and Biological Anthropology.* Cambridge: Cambridge University Press.

Inhorn, Marcia, and Peter Brown. 1990. "The Anthropology of Infectious Disease." *Annual Review of Anthropology* 19: 89–117.

Inhorn, Marcia, and Kimberly Buss. 2010. "Infertility, Infection, and Iatrogenesis in Egypt: The Anthropological Epidemiology of Blocked Tubes." *Medical Anthropology* 15 (3): 217–244.

Institute of Science and Society. 2005. Why Genomics Won't Deliver. www.i-sis.org.uk /WGWD.php.

Irfan, Umair. 2012. "Valley Fever on the Rise in U.S. Southwest, with Links to Climate Change." *Scientific American.* September 14. www.scientificamerican.com/article.cfm?id=valley-fever-on-the-rise-in-us-southwest.

Jablonka, Eva, and Marion Lamb. 2005. *Evolution in Four Dimensions: Genetic, Epigenetic, Behavioral, and Symbolic Variation in the History of Life.* Cambridge, MA: MIT Press.

Jakab, George. 1988. "Modulation of Pulmonary Defense Mechanisms Against Viral and Bacterial Infections by Acute Exposures to Nitrogen Dioxide." *Research Report of the Health Effects Institute* 20: 1–38.

Jegede, Ayodele. 2007. "What Led to the Nigerian Boycott of the Polio Vaccination Campaign?" *PLoS Med* 4 (3): e73. doi:10.1371/journal.pmed.0040073.

Johnson, Alex. 2008. "Floodwaters Breed Hidden Health Dangers: West Nile, E. coli Among Deadly Concerns in Swamped Midwest." *MSNBC, Health.* June 20. www.msnbc.msn .com/id/25287816.

Jones, Chaunettta. 2011. "'If I Take My Pills I'll go Hungry': The Choice Between Economic Security and HIV/AIDS Treatment in Grahamstown, South Africa." *Annals of Anthropological Practice* 35: 67–80.

Jones, Kate, Nikita Patel, Mark Levy et al. 2008. "Global Trends in Emerging Infectious Diseases." *Nature* 451 (7181): 990–993.

Kalichman, Seth, Jennifer Pellowski, and Christina Turner. 2011. "Prevalence of Sexually Transmitted Co-infections in People Living with HIV/AIDS." *Sexually Transmitted Infections* 87 (3): 183–190.

Kalm, Pehr. 1773. "Travels into North America," vol. 1. American Journeys: Eye Witnessed Accounts of Early American Explorations and Settlement. www.americanjourneys.org /aj-117a/summary/index.asp.

Kamat, Vinay. 2009. "The Anthropology of Childhood Malaria in Tanzania." In *Anthropology and Public Health: Bridging Differences in Culture and Society,* edited by Robert Hahn and Marcia Inhorn, 35–63. Oxford: Oxford University Press.

Kamat, Vinay. 2013. *Silent Violence: Global Health, Malaria, and Child Survival in Tanzania.* Tucson: University of Arizona Press.

Kaneda, Atsushi, Keisuke Matsusaka, Hiroyuki Aburatani, and Masashi Fukayama. 2012. "Epstein–Barr Virus Infection as an Epigenetic Driver of Tumorigenesis." *Cancer Research* 72 (14): 3445–3450.

Karesh, William, and Eric Noble. 2009. "The Bushmeat Trade: Increased Opportunities for Transmission of Zoonotic Disease." *Mount Sinai Journal of Medicine* 76 (5): 429–434.

Karlsson, Erik, and Melinda Beck. 2010. "The Burden of Obesity on Infectious Disease." *Experimental Biology and Medicine* 235 (12): 1412–1424.

Kaushik, Rajni, Rajasekhar Balasubramanian, and Armah de la Cruz. 2012. "Influence of Air Quality on the Composition of Microbial Pathogens in Fresh Rainwater." *Applied Environmental Microbiology* 78 (8): 2813–2818. doi:10.1128/AEM.07695-11.

Katz, Michael. 1990. *The Undeserving Poor: From the War on Poverty to the War on Welfare.* New York: Pantheon Books.

Keesing, Felicia, Lisa Belden, Peter Daszak et al. 2010. "Impacts of Biodiversity on the Emergence and Transmission of Infectious Diseases." *Nature* 468: 647–652.

Kelleher, S. 1994. "Tuberculosis: A Legacy of Fear." *Buffalo News*, 3.

Kendall, Carl, Hudelson Patricia, Elli Leontsini, Peter Winch, Linda Lloyd, and Fernando Cruz. 1991. "Urbanization, Dengue, and the Health Transition: Anthropological Contributions to International Health." *Medical Anthropology Quarterly* 5 (3): 257–268.

Khalifa, Mohammed, Radwa Sharaf, and Ramy Zaiz. 2010. "Helicobacter pylori: A Poor Man's Gut Pathogen?" *Gut Pathogens* 2: 2.

Khun, Sokrin, and Lenore Manderson. 2007. "Health Seeking and Access to Care for Children with Suspected Dengue in Cambodia: An Ethnographic Study." *BMC Public Health* 7: 262. doi:10.1186/1471-2458-7-262.

Kinney, Patrick. 2008. "Climate Change, Air Quality, and Human Health." *American Journal of Preventive Medicine* 35 (5): 459–467.

Kippax, Susan, Niamh Stephenson, Richard Parker, and Peter Aggleton. 2013. "Between Individual Agency and Structure in HIV Prevention: Understanding the Middle Ground of Social Practice." *American Journal of Public Health* 103 (8): 1367–1375.

Kirton, Adam, Elaine Wirrell, James Zhang and Lorie Hamiwka. 2004. "Seizure-alerting and -response behaviors in dogs living with epileptic children." *Neurology* 62(12): 2303-2305.

Knishkowy, Barry. 2005. "Water-Pipe (Narghile) Smoking: An Emerging Health Risk Behavior." *Pediatrics* 116 (1): e113–e119.

Koch, Erin. 2006. "Beyond Suspicion: Evidence, (Un)Certainty, and Tuberculosis in Georgian Prisons." *American Ethnologist* 33 (1): 50–62.

Koch, Erin. 2013a. *Free Market Tuberculosis: Managing Epidemics in Post-Soviet Georgia.* Nashville, TN: Vanderbilt University Press.

Koch, Erin. 2013b. "Tuberculosis Is a Threshold: The Making of a Social Disease in Post-Soviet Georgia." *Medical Anthropology* 32 (4): 309–324.

Koester, Stephen, and Lee Hoffer. 1994. "Indirect Sharing: Additional HIV Risks Associated with Drug Injection." *AIDS and Public Policy Journal* 9 (2): 100–105.

Köndgen, Sophie, Hjalmar Kuhl, Paul N'Goran et al. 2008. "Pandemic Human Viruses Cause Decline of Endangered Great Apes." *Current Biology* 18 (4): 260–264.

Krieger, Nancy. 2005. *Health Disparities and the Body.* Boston: Harvard School of Public Health.

Krieger, Nancy. 2007. "Ecosocial Theory." In *Encyclopedia of Health and Behavior,* edited by Norman Anderson, p. 293-294. Thousand Oaks, CA: Sage.

Krimsky, Sheldon, and Jeremony Gruber, eds. 2013. *Genetic Explanations: Sense and Nonsense.* Cambridge, MA: Harvard University Press.

Kroeger, Karen. 2008. "AIDS Rumors, Imaginary Enemies, and the Body Politic in Indonesia." *American Ethnologist* 30 (2): 243–257.

Kwa, B. H. 2008. "Environmental Change, Development and Vector Borne Disease: Malaysia Experience with Filariasis, Scrub Typhus and Dengue." *Environment, Development and Sustainability* 10 (2): 209–217.

Kwan, Candice, and Joel Ernst. 2011. "HIV and Tuberculosis: A Deadly Human Syndemic." *Clinical Microbiology Reviews* 24 (2): 351–376.

Lakoff, Andrew. 2008. "The Generic Biothreat, or, How We Became Unprepared." *Cultural Anthropology* 23 (3): 399–428.

Lam, Clarence, Crystal Franco, and Ari Schuler. 2006. "Billions for Biodefense: Federal Agency Biodefense Funding, FY2006–FY2007." *Biosecurity and Bioterrorism: Biodefense Strategy, Practice, and Science* 4 (2): 113–127.

Lammie, Patrick, John Lindo, W. Even Secor, Javier Vasquez, Steven Ault, and Mark Eberhard. 2007. "Eliminating Lymphatic Filariasis, Onchocerciasis, and Schistosomiasis from the Americas: Breaking a Historical Legacy of Slavery." *PLoS Neglected Tropical Diseases* 1 (2): e71. doi:10.1371/journal.pntd.0000071.

Larsen, Clark, and George Milner, eds. 1994. *In the Wake of Contact: Biological Responses to Conquest*. New York: WileyLiss.

Latour, Bruno. 1993. *The Pasteurization of France*. Cambridge, MA: Harvard University Press.

Lazzarini, Zita, Carol Galletly, Eric Mykhalovskiy et al. 2013. "Criminalization of HIV Transmission and Exposure: Research and Policy Agenda." *American Journal of Public Health* 103 (8): 1350–1353.

Leake, Jonathan, David Johnson, Damian Donnelly, Gemma Muckle, Lynne Boddy, and David Read. 2004. "Networks of Power and Influence: The Role of Mycorrhizal Mycelium in Controlling Plant Communities and Agroecosystem Functioning." *Canadian Journal of Botany* 82 (8): 1016–1045.

Leavitt, Judith. 1996. *Typhoid Mary: Captive to the Public's Health*. Boston: Beacon Press.

Leclerc-Madlala, Suzanne. 2006. "'We Will Eat When I Get the Grant': Negotiating AIDS, Poverty and Antiretroviral Treatment in South Africa." *African Journal of AIDS Research* 5 (3): 249–256.

Lederberg, Joshua, Robert Shope, and Stanley Oaks, eds. 1992. *Emerging Infections: Microbial Threats to Health in the United States*. Washington, DC: National Academies Press.

Leicester, John. 2013. "Earth's Atmosphere to Take Beating at World Cup." Associated Press. December 9. http://bigstory.ap.org/article/earths-atmosphere-take-beating-world-cup.

Lello, Joanne, Stephanie Knopp, Khalfan Mohammed, I. Simba Khamis, Jürg Utzinger, and Mark Viney. 2013. "The Relative Contribution of Co-infection to Focal Infection Risk in Children." *Proceedings of the Royal Society* B 280: 20122813.

Leon, Kyla, Marian McDonald, Barbara Moore, and George Rust. 2009. "Disparities in Influenza Treatment Among Disabled Medicaid Patients in Georgia." *American Journal of Public Health* 99 (S2): S378–S382.

Lepani, Katherine. 2013. *Islands of Love, Islands of Risk: Culture and HIV in the Trobriands*. Nashville, TN: Vanderbelt University Press.

Levins, Richard, and Richard Lewontin. 1985. *The Dialectical Biologist*. Cambridge, MA: Harvard University Press.

Levy, Barry, and Victor Sidel, eds. 2008. *War and Public Health*. New York: Oxford University Press.

Lewis, Kim. 2007. "Persister Cells, Dormancy and Infectious Disease." *Nature Reviews Microbiology* 5: 48–56.

Lewis, Kim. 2013. "Platforms for Antibiotic Discovery." *Nature Reviews Microbiology* 12: 371–387.

Ley, Ruth, Daniel Peterson, and Jeffrey Gordon. 2006. "Ecological and Evolutionary Forces Shaping Microbial Diversity in the Human Intestine." *Cell* 124 (4): 837–848.

Lindenbaum, Shirley. 1978. *Kuru Sorcery: Disease and Danger in the New Guinea Highlands*. New York: Mayfield.

Lindenbaum, Shirley. 2001. "Kuru, Prions, and Human Affairs: Thinking About Epidemics." *Annual Review of Anthropology* 30: 363–385.

Lindenbaum, Shirley. 2013. *Kuru Sorcery: Disease and Danger in the New Guinea Highlands*, 2nd ed. London: Paradigm.

Little, C. Scott, Christine Hammond, Angela MacIntyre, Brian Balin, and Denah Appelt. 2004. "Chlamydia Pneumoniae Induces Alzheimer-like Amyloid Plaques in Brains of BALB/c Mice." *Neurobiology of Aging* 25 (4): 419–429.

Liu, Jenny, Sepideh Modrek, Roly Gosling, and Richard Feachem. 2013. "Malaria Eradication: Is It Possible? Is It Worth It? Should We Do It?" *Lancet Global Health* 1 (1): e3.

Livingstone, Frank. 1958. "Anthropological Implications of Sickle Cell Gene Distribution in West Africa." *American Anthropologist* 60: 533–562.

Lock, Margaret. 2001. "The Tempering of Medical Anthropology: Troubling Natural Categories." *Medical Anthropology Quarterly* 15 (4): 478–492.

Lockman, S., N. Hone, T. Kenyon et al. 2003. "Etiology of Pulmonary Infections in Predominantly HIV-Infected Adults with Suspected Tuberculosis, Botswana." *International Journal of Tuberculosis and Lung Disease* 7: 714–723.

Lopez, Liza, Kerry Sexton, and Phil Carter. 2012. *The Epidemiology of Meningococcal Disease in New Zealand in 2011*. Wellington, NZ: Institute of Environmental Science and Research.

Louis, Elan. 1989. "Review of the *Pasteurization of France*." *Yale Journal of Biology and Medicine* 62 (1): 47–48.

Lowe, Celia. 2010. "Viral Clouds: Becoming H5N1 in Indonesia." *Cultural Anthropology* 25 (4): 625–649.

Luby, S., M. Rahman, M. Hossain et al. 2006. "Foodborne Transmission of Nipah Virus, Bangladesh." *Emerging Infectious Diseases* 12 (12): 1888–1894. http://dx.doi.org/10.3201/eid1212.060732.

Lye, Dennis. 2002. "Health Risks Associated with Consumption of Untreated Water from Household Roof Catchment Systems." *Journal of the American Water Resources Association* 38: 1301–1306.

Macauda, Mark, Pamela Erickson, Janice Miller, Paul Mann, Linda Closter, and Peter Krause. 2011. "Long-Term Lyme Disease Antibiotic Therapy Beliefs Among New England Residents." *Vector-Borne and Zoonotic Diseases* 11 (7): 857–862.

MacCormack, Carol. 1985. "Anthropology and the Control of Tropical Disease." *Anthropology Today* 1 (3): 14–16.

Macqueen, S. 1995. "Anthropology and Germ Theory." *Journal of Hospital Infection* 30 (Supplement): 116–126.

Magambo, Japhet, Ernest Njoroge, and Eberhard Zeyhle. 2006. "Epidemiology and Control of Echinococcosis in Sub-Saharan Africa." *Parasitology International* 55 (Supplement): S193–S195.

Malaty, Hoda M. , Jong G. Kim, Soon D. Kim, and David Y. Graham. 1996. "Prevalence of Helicobacter pylori Infection in Korean Children: Inverse Relation to Socioeconomic Status Despite a Uniformly High Prevalence in Adults." *American Journal of Epidemiology* 143 (3): 257–262.

Maloney, Neal, Rebecca Britt, Gregory Rushing et al. 2008. "Insulin Requirements in the Intensive Care Unit in Response to Infection." *American Surgeon* 74 (9): 845–848.

Manchester, Keith. 1991. "Tuberculosis and Leprosy: Evidence for Interaction of Disease." In *Human Paleopathology: Current Synthesis and Future Options*, edited by Donald Ortner and Arthur Aufderheide, 23–35. Washington, DC: Smithsonian Institution Press.

Manderson, Lenore. 1998. "Applying Medical Anthropology in the Control of Infectious Disease." *Tropical Medicine and International Health* 3 (12): 1020–1027.

Manderson, Lenore. 2012. "Neglected Diseases of Poverty." *Medical Anthropology* 31 (4): 283–286.

Manderson, Lenore, Jens Aagaard-Hansen, Pascale Allotey, Marget Gyapong, and Johannes Sommersfeld. 2009. "Social Research on Neglected Diseases of Poverty: Continuing and Emerging Themes." *PLoS Neglected Tropical Disease* 3 (2): e332.

Mann, Jonathan. 1987. Statement at an Informal Briefing on AIDS to the 42nd Session of the United Nations General Assembly. October 20. http://apps.who.int/iris/bitstream/10665/61546/1/WHO_SPA_INF_87.12.pdf.

Margos, Garbriele, Anne Gatewood, David Aanensen et al. 2008. "MLST of Housekeeping Genes Captures Geographic Population Structure and Suggests a European Origin of Borrelia burgdorferi." *PNAS* 105 (25): 8730–8735.

Marshall, Barry. 2006. "Barry, J.Marshall—Biographical." In *Nobel Prizes 2005,* edited by Karl Grandin. Nobelprize.org http://www.nobelprize.org/nobel_prizes/medicine/laureates/2005/marshall-bio.html.

Martin, Emily. 1990. "Toward an Anthropology of Immunology: The Body as Nation State." *Medical Anthropology Quarterly* 4 (4): 410–426.

Martin, R. Shayn, Judy Smith, Jason Hoth, Preston Miller, J. Wayne Meredith, and Michael Chang. 2007. "Increased Insulin Requirements Are Associated with Pneumonia After Severe Injury." *Journal of Trauma* 63 (2): 358–364.

Mascie-Taylor, C. G. N., ed. 1993. *The Anthropology of Disease.* Oxford: Oxford University Press.

Mason, Andrew, Johnson Lau, Nicole Hoang et al. 1999. "Association of Diabetes Mellitus and Chronic Hepatitis C Virus Infection." *Hepatology* 29 (2): 328–333.

Masood, Salman. 2013. "Vaccine Aide Gunned Down in Pakistan." *New York Times.* December 29. www.nytimes.com/2013/12/29/world/asia/vaccine-worker-killed-in-pakistan-amid-taliban-hostility.html?_r=0.

Mathews, John, Robert Glasse, and Shirley Lindenbaum. 1968. "Kuru and Cannibalism." *Lancet* 292: 449–452.

Mayer, Jonathan. 2000. "Geography, Ecology and Emerging Infectious Diseases." *Social Science and Medicine* 50: 937–952.

Mayr, Ernst. 1982. *The Growth of Biological Thought: Diversity, Evolution, and Inheritance.* Cambridge, MA: Belknap Press.

McCaa, Robert. 1995. "Spanish and Nahuatl Views on Smallpox and Demographic Catastrophe in the Conquest of Mexico." *Journal of Interdisciplinary History* 25 (3): 397–431.

McCullers, Jonathan. 2006. "Insights into the Interaction Between Influenza Virus and Pneumococcus." *Clinical Microbiology Reviews* 19 (3): 571–582.

McDade, Thomas. 2002. "Status Incongruity in Samoan Youth: A Biocultural Analysis of Culture Change, Stress, and Immune Function." *Medical Anthropology Quarterly* 16 (2): 123–150.

McFall-Ngai, Margaret, Michael Hadfield, Thomas Bosch et al. 2013. "Animals in a Bacterial World: A New Imperative for the Life Sciences. *PNAS* 110 (9): 3229–3236.

McGowan, John. 2000. "The Impact of Changing Pathogens of Serious Infections in Hospitalized Patients." *Clincial Infectious Diseases* 31 (S4): S124–S130.

McKibben, Bill. 2006. *The End of Nature.* New York: Random House.

McMichael, Anthony. 2013. "Globalization, Climate Change, and Human Health." *New England Journal of Medicine* 368: 1335–1343.

McMichael, Anthony, and Pim Martens. 2002. *Environmental Change, Climate and Health: Issues and Research Methods.* Cambridge: Cambridge University Press.

McMichael, Anthony, Martin McKee, Vladimir Shkolnikov, and Tapani Volonen. 2004. "Mortality Trends and Setbacks: Global Convergence or Divergence?" *Lancet* 363: 1155–1159.

McNeil, William. 1976. *Plagues and Peoples*. Garden City, NY: Anchor Books.

Medecins Sans Frontieres. 2010. *Fighting a Dual Epidemic: Treating TB in a High HIV Prevalence Setting in Rural Swaziland, January 2008–June 2010*. Mbabane, Swaziland: Medecins San Frontieres.

Mehta, Shruti, Fredrick Brancati, Mark Sulkowski, Steffanie Strathdee, Moyses Szklo, and David Thomas. 2001. "Prevalence of Type 2 Diabetes Mellitus Among Persons with Hepatitis C Virus Infection in the United States." *Hepatology* 3 (6): 1554.

Menon, Meena. 2013. "Another Polio Worker Gunned Down in Pakistan." *The Hindu*. December 29. www.thehindu.com/news/international/south-asia/another-polio-worker-gunned-down-in-pakistan/article5511849.ece.

Merkler, D., E. Horvath, W. Bruck, R. Zinkernagel, J. Del la Torre, and D. Pinschewer. 2006. "'Viral Déjà vu' Elicits Organ-Specific Immune Disease Independent of Reactivity to Self." *Journal of Clinical Investigation* 116 (5): 1254–1263.

Meyers, Wayne. 1995. "Mycobacterial Infections of the Skin." In *Tropical Pathology*, edited by S. Doerr and G. Seifert, 292–377. Berlin Springer-Verlag.

Millen, Joyce, Alec Irwin, and Jim Yong Kim. 2000. "Introduction: What Is Growing? Who Is Dying?" In *Dying for Growth: Global Inequality and the Health of the Poor*, edited by Jim Yong Kim, Joyce Millen, Alec Irwin, and John Gershman, 3–10. Monroe, ME: Common Courage Press.

Mills, David. 2000. *Science Shams and Bible Bloopers*. Huntington, WV: Xlibris.

Molina, Natalie. 2006. *Fit to Be Citizens?: Public Health and Race in Los Angeles, 1879–1939*. Berkeley: University of California Press.

Møller-Christiansen, Vilhelm. 1978. *Leprosy Changes of the Skull*. Odense, Denmark: Odense University Press.

Mooney, Chris. 2007. *Storm World: Hurricanes, Politics and the Battle Over Global Warming*. Orlando, FL: Houghton Mifflin Harcourt.

Moore, Maria, M. Goita, and John Finley. 2014. "Impact of the Microbiome on Cocoa Polyphenolic Compounds." 247th National Meeting & Exposition of the American Chemical Society, Dallas, TX.

Moore, P., A. Marfin, L. Quenemoen et al. 1993. "Mortality Rates in Displaced and Resident Populations of Central Somalia During 1992 Famine." *Lancet* 341 (8850): 935–938.

Moorman, Ann, Kiprotich Chelimo, Odada Sumba et al. 2005. "Exposure to Holoendemic Malaria Results in Elevated Epstein-Barr Virus Loads in Children." *Journal of Infectious Diseases* 191 (8): 1233–1238.

Moorman, Ann, Kiprotich Chelimo, Peter Sumba, Daniel Tisch, Rosemary Rochford, and James Kazura. 2007. "Exposure to Holoendemic Malaria Results in Suppression of Epstein-Barr Virus-Specific T Cell Immunosurveillance in Kenyan Children." *Journal of Infectious Diseases* 195 (6): 799–808.

Moran-Thomas, Amy. 2013. "A Salvage Ethnography of the Guinea worm: Witchcraft, Oracles and Magic in a Disease Eradication Program." In *When People Come First: Critical Studies in Global Health*, edited by Joāb Biehl and Adriana Petranya, 207–239. Princeton, NJ: Princeton University Press.

Morens, David, Jeffery Taubenberger, and Anthony Fauci. 2009. "The Persistent Legacy of the 1918 Influenza Virus." *New England Journal of Medicine*, 361 (3): 225–229.

Morin, Stephan, Jeffery Kelly, Edwin Charlebois et al. 2011. "Responding to the National HIV/ AIDS Strategy—Setting the Research Agenda." *Journal of Acquired Deficiency Syndrome* 57 (3): 175–180.

Morrison, Rosemary, Natalie Hall, Mina Said et al. 2011. "Risk Factors Associated with Complications and Mortality in Patients with Clostridium Difficile Infection." *Clinical Infectious Diseases* 52 (12): 1173–1178.

Morse, Stephen. 1992. "Global Microbial Traffic and the Interchange of Disease." *American Journal of Public Health* 82 (10): 1326–1327.

Mosack, Katie, Maryann Abbott, Merrill Singer, Margaret Weeks, and Lucy Rohena. 2005. "If I Didn't Have HIV, I'd Be Dead Now: Illness Narratives of Drug Users Living with HIV/AIDS." *Qualitative Health Research* 15 (5): 586–605.

Moxon, E. Richard, Paul Rainey, Martin Nowak, and Richard Lenski. 1994. "Adaptive Evolution of Highly Mutable Loci in Pathogenic Bacteria." *Current Biology* 4 (1): 24–33.

Muirhead, M., and Thomas Alexander. 1997. *Managing Pig Health and the Treatment of Disease: A Reference for the Farm.* Sheffield, UK: 5M Publishing.

Murphy, Ellen, Y. Chistov, R. Hopkins, P. Rutland, and G. Taylor. 2009. "Tuberculosis Among Iron Age Individuals from Tyva, South Siberia: Palaeopathological and Biomolecular Findings." *Journal of Archaeological Science* 36: 2029–2038.

Murray, Christopher, and Alan Lopez. 1996. *The Global Burden of Disease: A Comprehensive Assessment of Mortality and Disability from Diseases, Injuries and Risk Factors in 1990 and Projected to 2020.* Cambridge, MA: Harvard School of Public Health.

Murray, C., G. Poletti, T. Kebadze et al. 2006. "Study of Modifiable Risk Factors for Asthma Exacerbations: Virus Infection and Allergen Exposure Increase the Risk of Asthma Hospital Admissions in Children." *Thorax* 61: 376–382

Murray, Polly. 1996. *The Widening Circle: A Lyme Disease Pioneer Tells Her Story.* New York: St. Martin's Press.

Mwangi, Tabitha, Jeffrey Bethony, and Simon Brooker. 2007. "Malaria and Helminth Interactions in Humans: An Epidemiological Viewpoint." *Annals of Tropical Medicine and Parasitology* 100 (7): 551–570.

Myers, Norman. 1980. Conversion of Tropical Moist Forests: A Report for the Committee Research Priorities in Tropical Biology of the National Research Council. Washington, DC: National Academy of Sciences.

Nakashima, Ellen. 2004. "Mandela Tells of TB's Peril." *Washington Post.* July 15. www.washingtonpost.com/wp-dyn/articles/A53142-2004Jul15.html.

Nash, Linda. 2006. *Inescapable Ecologies: A History of Environmental Disease, and Knowledge.* Berkeley: University of California Press.

National Institute of Mental Health Collaborative HIV/STD Prevention Trial Group. 2007. "Design and Integration of Ethnography Within an International Behavior Change HIV/Sexually Transmitted Disease Prevention Trial." *AIDS* 21 (S2): S37–S48.

National Wildlife Federation. 2008. Telspan Conference. www.nwf.org/nwfwebadmin/binaryVault/Transcript_Global_Warming_Flooding1.pdf.

Navarrete, Carlos, and Daniel Fessler. 2006. "Disease Avoidance and Ethnocentrism: The Effects of Disease Vulnerability and Disgust Sensitivity on Intergroup Attitudes." *Evolution and Human Behavior* 27: 270–282.

Navarro, Vicente. 2009. "What We Mean by Social Determinants of Health." *International Journal of Health Services* 39 (3): 423–441.

Needle, Richard, Susan Coyle, Helen Cesari et al. 1998. "HIV Risk Behaviors Associated with the Injection Process: Multiperson Use of Drug Injection Equipment and Paraphernalia in Injection Drug User Networks." *Substance Use and Misuse* 33 (12): 2403–2423.

Needle, Richard, Robert Trotter, Merrill Singer et al. 2003. "Rapid Assessment of the HIV/AIDS Crisis in Racial and Ethnic Minority Communities: An Approach for Timely Community Interventions." *American Journal of Public Health* 93 (6): 970–979.

Neuman, Eric, James Kiebenstein, Colin Johnson et al. 2005. "Assessment of the Economic Impact of Porcine Reproductive and Respiratory Syndrome on Swine Production in the United States." *Journal of the American Veterinary Medical Association* 227 (3): 385–392.

Nichter, Mark. 2008. *Global Health: Why Cultural Perceptions, Social Representations, and Biopolitics Matter.* Tucson: University of Arizona Press.

Nguyen, Vinh-Kim, and Karine Peschard. 2003. "Anthropology, Inequality, and Disease: A Review." *Annual Review of Anthropology* 32: 447–474.

Niewöhner, Jörg. 2011. "Epigenetics: Embedded Bodies and the Molecularisation of Biography and Milieu." *BioSocieties* 6: 279–298.

Oertli, Mathias, and Anne Müller. 2012. "Helicobacter pylori Targets Dendritic Cells to Induce Immune Tolerance, Promote Persistence and Confer Protection Against Allergic Asthma." *Gut Microbers* 3 (6): 566–571.

Ostfeld, Richard. 2011. *Lyme Disease: The Ecology of a Complex System.* Oxford: Oxford University Press.

Ostrach, Bayla, and Merrill Singer. 2012. "At Special Risk: Biopolitical Vulnerability and HIV Syndemics Among Women." *Health Sociology Review* 21 (3): 258–271.

Ostrach, Bayla, and Merrill Singer. 2013. "Syndemics of War: Malnutrition-Infectious Disease Interactions and the Unintended Health Consequences of Intentional War Policies." *Annals of Applied Anthropology* 36 (2): 256–272.

Ostry, Jonathan, Andrew Berg and Charlalambos Tsangarides. 2014. Redistribution, Inequality, and Growth. International Monetary Fund. http://www.imf.org/external/pubs/ft/sdn/2014/sdn1402.pdf.

Packard, Randall. 1989. *White Plague, Black Labor: Tuberculosis and the Political Economy of Health and Disease in South Africa.* Berkeley: University of California Press.

Padmawati, Siwi and Mark Nichter. 2008. "Community Response to Avian Flu in Central Java, Indonesia." *Anthropology and Medicine* 15 (1): 31–51.

Page, J. Bryan, Dale Chitwood, Prince Smith, Normie Kane, and Duane McBride. 1990. "Intravenous Drug Abuse and HIV Infection in Miami." *Medical Anthropology Quarterly* 4 (1): 56–71.

Page, J. Bryan, S. Lai, Dale Chitwood, N. Klimas, Prince Smith, and M. Fletcher. 1990. "HTLV-I/II Seropositivity and Death from AIDS Among HIV-1 Seropositive Intravenous Drug Users." *Lancet* 335: 1439–1441.

Palefsky, Joel, Elizabeth Holly, Mary Ralston, and Naomi Jay. 1998. "Prevalence and Risk Factors for Human Papillomavirus Infection of the Anal Canal in Human Immunodeficiency Virus (HIV)-Positive and HIV-Negative Homosexual Men." *Journal of Infectious Diseases* 177 (2): 361–367.

Palefsky, Joel, and Mary Rubin. 2009. "The Epidemiology of Anal Human Papillomavirus and Related Neoplasia." *Obstetrics and Gynecology Clinics of North America* 36 (1): 187–200.

Pandey, M., R. Neupane, A. Gautam, and I. Shrestha. 1989. "Domestic Smoke Pollution and Acute Respiratory Infections in a Rural Community of the Hill Region of Nepal." *Environment International* 15: 337–340.

Parashar, Umesh, Erik Hummelman, Joseph Bresee, Mark Miller, and Roger Glass. 2003. "Global Illness and Deaths Caused by Rotavirus Disease in Children." *Emerging Infectious Diseases* 9 (5): 565–572.

Parenti, Michael. 2007. "Mystery: How Wealth Creates Poverty in the World." Common Dreams. www.commondreams.org/views07/0216-30.htm.

Parker, Richard. 2009. *Bodies, Pleasures, and Passions: Sexual Culture in Contemporary Brazil.* Nashville, TN: Vanderbilt University Press.

Parker, Richard, and Aggleton, Peter. 2003. "HIV and AIDS-Related Stigma and Discrimination: A Conceptual Framework and Implications for Action." *Social Science and Medicine* 57: 13–24.

Parks, L. 2009. "Blacks and Latinos Suffering the Brunt of H1N1 in Boston." *Iconoculture.*

http://blog.iconoculture.com/2009/09/21/blacks-and-latinos-suffering-the-brunt -of-h1n1-in-boston.

Parmenter, Robert, Ekta Yadav, Ceryl Parmenter, Paul Ettestad and Kenneth Gage. 1999. "Incidence of Plague Associated with Increased Winter-Spring Precipitation in New Mexico." *American Journal of Tropical Medicine and Hygiene* 61: 814–821.

Parry, Charles, Tara Carney, Petal Petersen, Sarah Dewing, and Richard Needle. 2009. HIV-Risk Behavior Among Injecting or Non-Injecting Drug Users in Cape Town, Pretoria, and Durban, South Africa." *Substance Use and Misuse* 44 (6): 886–904.

Parry, Charles, Andreas Plüddemann, Hilton Donson, Anesh Sukhai, Sandra Marais, and Carl Lombard. 2005. "Cannabis and Other Drug Use Among Trauma Patients in Three South African Cities, 1999–2001." *South African Medical Journal* 95: 428–431.

Pascual, Mercedes, Xavier Rodo, Stephen Ellner, Rita Colwell, and Menno Bouma. 2000. "Cholera Dynamics and El Nino-Southern Oscillation." *Science 2000* 289: 1766–1769.

Paul, Benjamin. 1955. "Introduction." In *Health, Culture and Community: Case Studies of Public Reactions to Health Programs,* edited by Benjamin Paul, 1–11. New York: Russell Sage Foundation.

Paxson, Heather. 2008. "Post-Pasteurian Cultures: The Microbiopolitics of Raw-Milk Cheese in the United States." *Cultural Anthropology* 23 (1): 15–47.

Perlman, Robert. 2013. *Evolution and Medicine.* Oxford: Oxford University Press.

Perrone, Matthew. 2013. "FDA: Anti-Bacterial Soaps May Not Curb Bacteria." *The Big Story.* AP News. http://bigstory.ap.org/article/fda-says-germ-killing-soap-could-pose-health-risks.

Perry, Robert and Neal Halsey. 2004. "The Clinical Significance of Measles: A Review." *Journal of Infectious Disease* 189 (S1): S4–S16.

Petryna, Adriana, and Arthur Kleinman. 2006. "The Pharmaceutical Nexus." In *Global Pharmaceuticals: Ethics, Markets, Practices,* edited by Adriana Petryna, Andrew Lakoff, and Arthur Kleinman, 1–32. Durham: Duke University Press.

Piot, Peter. 2012/ *No Time to Lose: A Life in Pursuit of Deadly Viruses.* New York: W. W. Norton.

Pisani, Paola, D. Maxwell Parkin, Nubia Muñoz, and Jacques Ferlay. 1997. "Cancer and Infection: Estimates of the Attributable Fraction in 1990." *Cancer Epidemiology, Biomarkers and Prevention* 6 (6): 387–400.

Platt, Orah, Donald Brambilia, Wendell Rosse et al. 1994. "Mortality in Sickle Cell Disease: Life Expectancy and Risk Factors for Early Death." *New England of Journal of Medicine* 330: 1639–1644.

Playfair, John. 2004. *Living with Germs in Health and Disease.* Oxford: Oxford University Press.

Ploetz, Randy. 2005. "Panama Disease: An Old Nemesis Rears its Ugly Head Part 2: The Cavendish Era and Beyond." APSnet Features doi: 10.1094/APSnetFeature-2005-1005. http://www.apsnet.org/publications/apsnetfeatures/Pages/PanamaDiseasePart2.aspx.

Pongsiri, Montira, Joe Roman, Vanessa Ezenwa et al. 2009. "Biodiversity Loss Affects the New Global Disease Ecology." *Bioscience* 59: 945–954.

Pounds, J. Alan, Michael Fogden, and John Campbell. 1999. "Biological Response to Climate Change on a Tropical Mountain." *Nature* 398: 611–615.

Prasad, Simon, and Phillippa Smith. 2013. Meeting the Threat of Antibiotic Resistance: Building a New Frontline Defence. Canberra City, Australia: Office of the Chief Scientist, Occasion Paper Series.

Proto: Dispatches from the Frontiers of Medicine. 2010. "Paul Ehrlich and the Salvarsan Wars." Massachusetts General Hospital. http://protomag.com/assets/paul-ehrlich-and -the-salvarsan-wars.

Pylpa, Jen. 2004. *Healing Herbs and Dangerous Doctors: Local Models and Response to Fevers in Northeast Thailand.* Doctoral Dissertation, Department of Anthropology, University of Arizona.

Qiu, Chengxuan, Milia Kivipelto, and Eva von Strauss. 2009. "Epidemiology of Alzheimer's Disease: Occurrence, Determinants, and Strategies Toward Intervention." *Diagnoses in Clinical Neuroscience* 11 (2): 111–128.

Randolph, Sarah, and Andrew Dobson. 2012. "Pangloss Revisited: A Critique of the Dilution Effect and the Biodiversity-Buffers-Disease Paradigm." *Parasitology* 139 (7): 847–863.

Rantala, Markus. 1999. "Human Nakedness: Adaptation Against Ectoparasites?" *International Journal for Parasitology* 29: 1987–1989.

Ratard, R., C. Brown, J. Ferdinands et al. 2006. "Health Concerns Associated with Mold in Water-Damaged Homes After Hurricanes Katrina and Rita—New Orleans Area, Louisiana, October 2005." *Morbidity and Mortality Weekly Report* 55 (2): 41–44.

Redfield, Peter. 2013. *Life in Crisis: The Ethical Journey of Doctors Without Borders.* Berkeley: University of California Press.

Reidpath, Daniel, Pascale Allotey, and Subhash Pokhre. 2011. "Social Sciences Research in Neglected Tropical Diseases: A Bibliographic Analysis." *Health Research Policy and Systems* 9: 1, doi:10.1186/1478-4505-9-1.

Renne, Elisha. 2009. "Anthropological and Public Health Perspectives on the Global Polio Eradication Initiative in Northern Nigeria." In *Anthropology and Public Health: Bridging Differences in Culture and Society,* edited by Robert A Hahn and Marcia Inborn, 512–538. Oxford: Oxford University Press.

Ribera, Joan, Koen Grietens, Elizabeth Toomer, and Susanna Hausmann-Muela. 2009. "A Word of Caution Against the Stigma Trend in Neglected Tropical Disease Research and Control." *PLoS Neglected Tropical Diseases* 3 (10): e445.

Richards, Frank. 2000. "Using a GIS to Target River Blindness Control Activities in Guatemala." In *Geographical Targeting for Poverty Alleviation: Methodology and Applications,* edited by Fofack Hippolyte and David Bigman, 235–257. New York: World Bank Publications.

Riley, Lee, Eva Raphael, and Eduardo Faerstein. 2012. "Obesity in the United States: Dysbiosis from Exposure to Low-Dose Antibiotics?" *Frontiers in Public Health* 1: 69, doi:10.3389/fpubh.2013.00069.

Roberts, J. Timmons, and Bradley Parks. 2006. *A Climate of Injustice: Global Inequality, North-South Politics, and Climate Policy.* Cambridge, MA: MIT Press.

Roberts, Leslie, and Martin Enserink. 2007. "Did They Really Say . . . Eradication?" *Science* 318 (5856): 1544–1545.

Robertson, Brian. 2003. *Day Care Deception: What the Child Care Establishment Isn't Telling Us.* San Francisco: Encounter Books.

Rock, Melanie. 2013. "Connecting Lives: Reflections on a Syndemic Approach to Prevention Involving Research on How People Relate to Pets." *Annals of Applied Anthropology* 36 (2): 310–325.

Rock, Melanie, Bonnie Buntain, Jennifer Hatfield, and Benedikt Hallgrimsson. 2009. "Animal–Human Connections, 'one health,' and the Syndemic Approach to Prevention." *Social Science and Medicine* 68: 991–995.

Romney, Kimball, William Batchelder, and Susan Weller. 1987. "Recent Applications of Cultural Consensus Theory." *American Behavioral Scientist* 31 (2): 163–177.

Roossinck, Marilyn. 2011. "The Good Viruses: Viral Mutualistic Symbioses." *Nature Reviews Microbiology* 9: 99–108.

Rose, Geoffrey. 1992. *The Strategy of Preventive Medicine.* Oxford: Oxford University Press.

Rose, Nikolas. 2007. *The Politics of Life Itself: Biomedicine, Power, and Subjectivity in the Twenty-First Century.* Princeton, NJ: Princeton University Press.

Rothman, Daniel, Gregory Fournier, Katherine French et al. 2014. "Methanogenic Burst in the End-Permian Carbon Cycle." *Proceedings of the National Academy of Sciences of the United States of America* 111 (13): 5462–5467. www.pnas.org/cgi/doi/10.1073/pnas.1318106111.

Røttingen, John-Arne, William Cameron, and Geoffrey Garnett. 2001. "A Systematic Review of the Epidemiologic Interactions Between Classic Sexually Transmitted Diseases and HIV: How Much Really Is Known?" *Sexually Transmitted Disease* 28 (10): 579–597.

Royster, Deirdre. 2003. *Race and the Invisible Hand: How White Networks Exclude Black Men from Blue-Collar Jobs.* Berkeley: University of California Press.

Ruiez-Tiben, Ernesto, and Donald Hopkins. 2006. "Dracunculiasis (Guinea worm disease) Eradication." *Advances in Parasitology* 61: 275–309.

Rylko-Bauer, Barbara, Merrill Singer, and John van Willigin. 2006. "Reclaiming Applied Anthropology: Its Past, Present, and Future." *American Anthropologist* 108 (1): 178–190.

Sabbatani, S., R. Manfredi, and S. Fiorino. 2010. "Malaria Infection and Human Evolution." *Le Infezioni in Medicina* 18 (1): 56–74.

Salkeld, Daniel, Kerry Padgett, and James Jones. 2013. "A Meta-Analysis Suggesting That the Relationship Between Biodiversity and Risk of Zoonotic Pathogen Transmission Is Idiosyncratic." *Ecology Letters* 16 (5): 679–686.

Samet, Jeffrey, Nicholas Horton, Elizabeth Traphagen, Sarah Lyon, and Kenneth Freedberg. 2003. "Alcohol Consumption and HIV Disease Progression: Are They Related?" *Alcoholism: Clinical and Experimental Research* 27 (5): 862–867.

Santiago, Mario, Magdalena Lukasik, Shadrack Kamenya et al. 2003. "Foci of Endemic Simian Immunodeficiency Virus Infection in Wild-Living Eastern Chimpanzees (*Pan troglodytes schweinfurthii*)." *Journal of Virology* 77 (13): 7545–7562.

Sawchuk, Lawrence. 2010. "Deconstructing an Epidemic: Cholera in Gibraltar." In *Plagues and Epidemics: Infected Spaces Past and Present,* edited by Ann Herring and Alan Swedlund, 95–117. Oxford: Berg.

Schacker, Timothy. 2001. "The Role of HSV in the Transmission and Progression of HIV." *Herpes* 8 (2): 46–49.

Schoch-Spana, Monica, Crystal Franco, Jennifer Nuzzo, and Christiana Usenza. 2007. "Community Engagement: Leadership Tool for Catastrophic Health Events." *Biosecurity and Bioterrorism: Biodefense Strategy, Practice, and Science* 5 (1): 8–25.

Scott, Susan and Christopher Duncan. 2004. *Return of the Black Death: The World's Greatest Serial Killer.* Malden, MA: Wiley.

Sedivy, John, Jill Kreilling, Nicola Neretti et al. 2013. "Death by Transposition: The Enemy Within?" *BioEssays* 35 (12): 1035–1043.

Shapiro, Howard. 2000. "Microbial Analysis at the Single-Cell Level: Tasks and Techniques." *Journal of Microbiological Methods* 42: 3–16.

Sharp, Paul, and Beatrice Hahn. 2010. "The Evolution of HIV-1 and the Origin of AIDS." *Philosophical Transactions of the Royal Society* B 365 (1552): 2487–2494.

Sheppard, Samuel, Noel McCarthy, Daniel Falush, and Martin Maiden. 2008. "Convergence of Campylobacter Species: Implications for Bacterial Evolution." *Science* 320 (5873): 237–239.

Sherman, Irwin. 2007. *Twelve Diseases That Changed Our World.* Herndon, VA: ASM Press.

Shoreman-Ouimet, Eleanor, and Helen Kopnina. 2011. "Introduction: Environmental Anthropology of Yesterday and Today." In *Environmental Anthropology Today,* edited by Helen Kopnina and Eleanor Shoreman-Ouimet, 1–33. London: Routledge.

Silbergeld, Ellen, Jay Graham, and Lance Price. 2008. "Industrial Food Animal Production, Antimicrobial Resistance, and Human Health." *Annual Review of Public Health* 29: 151–169.

Simmons, G., V. Hope, G. Lewis, J. Whitmore, and W. Gao. 2001. "Contamination of Potable Roof-collected Rainwater in Auckland, New Zealand." *Water Resources* 35 (6): 1518–1524.

Singer, Merrill. 1996. "A Dose of Drugs, a Touch of Violence, a Case of AIDS: Conceptualizing the SAVA Syndemic." *Free Inquiry in Creative Sociology* 24: 99–110.

Singer, Merrill. 2004. The Social Origins and Expressions of Illness. In Cultures of Health, Cultures of Illness, George Davey Smith and Mary Shaw, Eds., pp. 9-20. Oxford: Oxford University Press.

Singer, Merrill. 2008. "The Perfect Epidemiological Storm: Food Insecurity, HIV/AIDS and Poverty in Southern Africa." *Anthropology News* (October): 12, 15.

Singer, Merrill. 2009a. "Beyond Global Warming: Interacting Ecocrises and the Critical Anthropology of Health." *Anthropology Quarterly* 82 (3): 795–820.

Singer, Merrill. 2009b. "Pathogens Gone Wild?: Medical Anthropology and the 'Swine Flu' Pandemic." *Medical Anthropology* 28 (3): 199–206.

Singer, Merrill. 2009c. *Introduction to Syndemics: A Systems Approach to Public and Community Health*. San Francisco: Jossey-Bass.

Singer, Merrill. 2010a. "Atmospheric and Marine Pluralea Interactions and Species Extinction Risks." *Journal of Cosmology* 8: 1832–1837.

Singer, Merrill. 2010b. "Ecosyndemics: Global Warming and the Coming Plagues of the 21st Century." In *Plagues and Epidemics: Infected Spaces Past and Present,* edited by Alan Swedlund and Ann Herring, 21–37. London: Berg.

Singer, Merrill. 2011. "Toward a Critical Biosocial Model of Ecohealth in Southern Africa: The HIV/AIDS and Nutrition Insecurity Syndemic." *Annals of Anthropology Practice* 35 (1): 8–27.

Singer, Merrill. 2013a. "Development, Coinfection, and the Syndemics of Pregnancy in Sub-Saharan Africa." *Infectious Diseases of Poverty* 2: 26.

Singer, Merrill. 2013b. "Respiratory Health and Ecosyndemics in a Time of Global Warming." *Health Sociology Review* 22 (1): 98–11.

Singer, Merrill. 2014. "Zoonotic Ecosyndemics and Multispecies Ethnography." *Anthropological Quarterly* 87(4): 1273–1303.

Singer, Merrill, Scott Clair, Monica Malta, Francisco Bastos, Neilane Bertoni, and Claudia Santelices. 2011. "Doubts Remain, Risks Persist: HIV Prevention Knowledge and HIV Testing Among Drug Users in Rio de Janeiro, Brazil." *Substance Use and Misuse* 46: 511–522.

Singer, Merrill, and Julie Eiserman. 2007. "Twilight's Last Gleaning: Rapid Assessment of Late Night HIV Risk in Hartford, CT." In *Communities Assessing Their AIDS Epidemics: Results of the Rapid Assessment of HIV/AIDS in Eleven U.S. Cities,* edited by Ben Bowser, Ernest Quimby and Merrill Singer, 193–208. Lanham, MD: Lexington Books.

Singer, Merrill, and Pamela Erickson. 2013. *Global Health: Anthropological Perspectives.* Walnut Creek, CA: Left Coast Press.

Siraj, Amir, Mauricio Santos-Vega, Menno Bouma, M. Yadeta, Daniel Ruiz Carrascal, and Mercedes Pascual. 2014. "Altitudinal Changes in Malaria Incidence in Highlands of Ethiopia and Colombia." *Science* 343 (6175): 1154–1158.

Skaar, Eric. 2010. "The Battle for Iron Between Bacterial Pathogens and Their Vertebrate Hosts." *PLoS Pathogens* 6 (8): e1000949.

Smallegange, Renate, Geert-Jan van Gemert, Marga van de Vegte-Bolmer, Willem Gezan, Robert Sauerwein, and James Logan. 2013. "Malaria Infected Mosquitoes Express Enhanced Attraction to Human Odor." *PLos One* 8 (5): e63602. doi:10.1371/journal.pone.0063602.

Smallman-Raynor, Matthew, and Andrew Cliff. 2004. "Impact of Infectious Diseases on War." *Infectious Disease Clinics of North America* 18: 341–368.

Smart, Rose. 2005. "HIV/AIDS-related Stigma and Discrimination, Module 1.4." In *Setting the Scene,* vol. 1, *Educational Planning and Management in a World with AIDS,* 117–148. Paris: UNESCO.

Smolinski, Mark, Margaret Hamburg, and Joshua Lederberg. 2003. *Microbial Threats to Health: Emergence, Detection, and Response.* Washington, DC: National Academies Press.

Solar, O., and A. Irwin. 2007. "A Conceptual Framework for Action on the Social Determinants of Health: Discussion Paper for the Commission on Social Determinants of Health, Draft, April 2007. Geneva: WHO Secretariat Commission on Social Determinants of Health, 2007, 7–9. www.who.int/social_determinants/resources/csdh_framework_action_05_07.pdf.

Soto, Basilio, Armandó Sanchez-Quijano, Luis Rodrigo et al. 1997. "Human Immunodeficiency Virus Infection Modifies the Natural History of Chronic Parenterally-Acquired Hepatitis C with an Unusually Rapid Progression to Cirrhosis." *Journal of Hepatology* 26 (1): 1–5.

South African Department of Health. 2006. HIV and STI Strategic Plan for South Africa, 2007–2011. Un AIDS. http://data.unaids.org/pub/ExternalDocument/2007/20070604_sa_nsp_final_en.pdf.

Spellberg, Brad, and Bonnie Taylor-Blake. 2013. "On the Exoneration of Dr. William H. Stewart: Debunking an Urban Legend." *Infectious Diseases of Poverty* 2: 3. doi:10.1186/2049-9957-2-3.

Spratt, David, and Philip Sutton. 2008. *Climate Code Red: The Case for Emergency Action.* Carlton North, Australia: Scribe Publications.

Stall, Ron, M. S. Friedman, and J. Catania. 2007. "Interacting Epidemics and Gay Men's Health: A Theory of Syndemic Production Among Urban Gay Men." In *Unequal Opportunity: Health Disparities Affecting Gay and Bisexual Men in the United States,* edited by Richard J. Wolitski, Ron Stall, and Ronald O. Valdiserri p. 251-274. Oxford: Oxford University Press.

Stapleton, Jack, Carolyn Williams, and Jinhua Xiang. 2004. "GB Type C: A Beneficial Infection?" *Journal of Clinical Microbiology* 42 (9): 3915–3919.

Steele, Russell, Rajasekharan Warrier, Patrick Unkel et al. 1996. "Colonization with Antibiotic-Resistant Streptococcus Pneumoniae in Children with Sickle Cell Disease." *Journal of Pediatrics* 128 (4): 531–535.

Steere, Alan, Stephen Malawista, John Hardin, Shaun Ruddy, Philip Askenase, and Warren Andiman. 1977. "Erythema Chronicum Migrans and Lyme Arthritis: The Enlarging Clinical Spectrum." *Annals of Internal Medicine* 86 (6): 685–698.

Stern, Rachel. 2003. "Hong Kong Haze: Air Pollution as a Social Class Issue." *Asian Survey* 43 (5): 780–800.

Steward, Julian. 1955. *Theory of Culture Change: The Methodology of Multilinear Evolution.* Urbana: University of Illinois Press.

Stillwagon, Eileen. 2002. "HIV/AIDS in Africa: Fertile Terrain." *Journal of Development Studies* 38 (6): 1–22.

Stine, Kathleen. 1999. "Human Papillomavirus Infection: The Most Common Sexually Transmitted Infection." *Journal of the Gay and Lesbian Medical Association* 3 (1): 21–22.

Stokes, J., and J. Peterson. 1998. "Homophobia, Self-Esteem, and Risk for HIV Among African American Men Who Have Sex with Men." *AIDS Education and Prevention* 10 (3): 278–292.

Strachan, David. 1989. "Hay Fever, Hygiene, and Household Size." *BMJ* 299 (6710): 1259–1260.

Stratton, Leanne, Marie O'Neill, Margaret Kruk, and Michelle Bell. 2008. "The Persistent Problem of Malaria: Addressing the Fundamental Causes of a Global Killer." *Social Science and Medicine* 67: 854–862.

Suarez, Mariana, Marcela Raffaelli, and Ann O'Leary. 1996. "Use of Folk Healing Practices by HIV-Infected Hispanics Living in the United States." *AIDS Care* 8 (6): 683–690.

Sumartojo. Esther. 1993. "When Tuberculosis Treatment Fails: A Social Behavioral Account of Patient Adherence." *American Review of respiratory Diseases* 147 (5): 1311–1320.

Swaddle, John, and Stavros Calos. 2008. "Increased Avian Diversity Is Associated with Lower Incidence of Human West Nile Infection: Observation of the Dilution Effect." *PLoS ONE* 396: e2488 doi:10.1371/journal.pone.0002488.

Swerdlow, Joel, and Ari Johnson. 2002. "Living with Microbes." *Wilson Quarterly* 26 (2): 42–60.

Tapp, E. 1979. "Disease in the Manchester Mummies." In *Science in Egyptology,* edited by Rosalie David, 95–102. Manchester, UK: Manchester University Press.

Tatem, A., D. Rogers, and S. Hay. 2006. "Global Transport Networks and Infectious Disease Spread." *Advances in Parasitology* 62: 293–343.

Telfer, Sandra, Xavier Lambin, Richard Birtles et al. 2010. "Species Interactions in a Parasite Community Drive Infection Risk in a Wildlife Population." *Science* 330: 243–246.

Terris, Milton. 1979. "The Epidemiologic Tradition." *Public Health Reports* 94 (3): 203–209.

Thio, C., E. Seaberg , R. Skolasky et al. 2002. "HIV-1, Hepatitis B Virus, and Risk of Liver-Related Mortality in the Multicenter Cohort Study (MACS)." *Lancet* 14: 1921–1926.

Thompson, Mark, Robert Breiman, Mary Hamel et al. 2012. "Influenza and Malaria Coinfection Among Young Children in Western Kenya, 2009–2011." *Journal of Infectious Diseases* 206 (11): 1674–1684.

Thompson, William, David K. Shay, Eric Weintraub, Lynnette Brammer, Nancy Cox, Larry Anderson, and Keiji Fukuda. 2003. "Mortality Associated With Influenza and Respiratory Syncytial Virus in the United States." *Journal of the American Medical Association* 289(2): 179-186.

Tice, D. 1997. "Flu Deaths Rivaled, Ran Alongside World War I." *Pioneer Planet.* March 10.

Timberg, Craig, and Daniel Halperin. 2012. *Tinderbox: How the West Sparked the AIDS Epidemic and How the World Can Finally Overcome It.* New York: Penguin Press.

Ting, Chao-Nan, Michael Rosenberg, Claudette Snow, Linda Samuelson, and Miriam Meisler. 1992. "Endogenous Retroviral Sequences Are Required for Tissue-Specific Expression of a Human Salivary Amylase Gene." *Genes Development* 6: 1457–1465.

Tishkoff, Sarah, and Brian Verrelli. 2003. "Patterns of Human Genetic Diversity: Implications for Human Evolutionary History and Disease." *Annual Review of Genomics and Human Genetics* 4: 293–340.

Tomley, Fiona, and Martin Shirley. 2009. "Livestock Infectious Diseases and Zoonoses." *Philosopical Transactions of the Royal Society* B 364 (1530): 2637–2642.

Tomori, Oyewale. 2010. "Implementing the Revised International Health Regulations in Resource-Poor Countries: Intentional and Unintentional Realities." In *Infectious Disease Movement in a Borderless World,* edited by David Relman, Eileen Choffnes and Alison Mack, 204–210. Washington, DC: National Academies Press.

Torgbor, Charles, Peter Awuah, Kirk Deitsch, Parisa Kalantari, Karen Duca, and David Thorley-Lawson. 2014. "A Multifactorial Role for P. falciparum Malaria in Endemic Burkitt's Lymphoma Pathogenesis." *PLOS Pathogens* 10: e1004170.

Towghi, Fouzieyha. 2013. "The Biopolitics of Reproductive Technologies Beyond the Clinic: Localizing HPV Vaccines in India." *Medical Anthropology* 32 (4): 325–342.

Trafzer, Clifford. 1990. *The Kit Carson Campaign: The Last Great Navajo War.* Oklahoma City: University of Oklahoma Press.

Trotter, Robert, and Merrill Singer. 2005. "Rapid Assessment Strategies for Public Health: Promise and Problems." In *Community Interventions and AIDS,* edited by Edison Trickett and Willo Pequegnat, 130–152. Oxford: Oxford University Press.

Tully, Damien, and Mario Fares. 2008. "The Tale of a Modern Animal Plague: Tracing the Evolutionary History and Determining the Time-Scale for Foot and Mouth Disease Virus." *Virology* 382 (2): 250–256.

Turnbaugh, Peter, Ruth Ley, Micah Hamady, Claire Fraser-Liggett, Rob Knight, and Jeffrey Gordon. 2007. "The Human Microbiome Project." *Nature* 449 (7164): 804–810.

Turnbaugh, Peter, Ruth Ley, Michael Mahowald, Vincent Magrini, Elaine Mardis, and Jeffrey Gordon. 2006. "An Obesity-Associated Gut Microbiome with Increased Capacity for Energy Harvest." *Nature* 444 (7122): 1027–1031.

Udwadia, Zarirk, Rohit Amale, Kanchan Ajbani, and Camilia Rodriquests. 2011. "Totally Drug-Resistant Tuberculosis in India." *Clinical Infectious Diseases* 54 (4); 579–581. doi:10.1093/cid/cir889.

UNICEF. 2013. "Japan Steps Up to Help Stop Polio Outbreak in Somalia." Press Release. www.unicef.org/media/media_70084.html.

United Nations. 1948. *The Universal Declaration of Human Rights.* Geneva: United Nations.

United Nations Secretariat. 2012. The Millennium Development Goals Report. New York: United Nations. www.undp.org/content/dam/undp/library/MDG/english/The_MDG_Report_2012.pdf.

Vajdic, Claire, Marina van Leeuwen, F. Jin et al. 2009. "Anal Human Papillomavirus Genotype Diversity and Co-infection in a Community-Based Sample of Homosexual Men." *Sexually Transmitted Infections* 85 (5): 330–335.

Van Hollen, Cecilia. 2013. *Birth in the Age of AIDS: Women, Reproduction, and HIV/AIDS in India.* Stanford, CA: Stanford University Press.

Vecchiato, Norbert. 1997. "Sociocultural Aspects of Tuberculosis Control in Ethiopia." *Medical Anthropology Quarterly* 11 (2): 183–201.

Ventura-Garcia, Laia, Maria Roura, Christopher Pell et al. 2013. "Socio-Cultural Aspects of Chagas Disease: A Systematic Review of Qualitative Research." *PLoS Neglected Tropical Diseases* 7 (9): e2410.

Viboud, Cécile, Khashayar Pakdaman, Pierre-Yves Boëlle et al. 2004. "Association of Influenza Epidemics with Global Climate Variability." *European Journal of Epidemiology* 19: 1055–1059.

Vieira, Antonio, Peter Collignon, Frank Aarestrup et al. 2011. "Association Between Antimicrobial Resistance in Escherichia coli Isolates from Food Animals and Blood Stream Isolates from Humans in Europe: An Ecological Study." *Pathogens and Disease* 8 (12): 1295–1301.

Virchow, Rudolf. 2006 (original 1849). "Report on the Typhus Epidemic in Upper Silesia." *American Journal of Public Health* 96 (2): 2012–2105.

Vlassoff, Carol, Mitchell Weiss, E. Ovuga, E. et al. 2000. "Gender and the Stigma of Onchocercal Skin Disease in Africa." *Social Science and Medicine* 50 (10): 1353–1368.

Waitzkin, Howard. 2000. *The Second Sickness: Contradictions of Capitalist Health Care.* Lanham, MA: Rowman and Littlefield.

Waldman, Carl. 1985. *Atlas of the North American Indian.* New York: Infobase Publishing.

Waldman, Ronald, Eric Mintz, and Heather Papowitz. 2013. "The Cure for Cholera: Improving Access to Safe Water and Sanitation." *New England Journal of Medicine* 368: 592–594.

Walker, Alan, Jennifer Ince, Sylvia Duncan et al. 2011. "Dominant and Diet-Responsive Groups of Bacteria Within the Human Colonic Microbiota." *Isme Journal* 5 (2): 220–230.

Walker, Christa, Igor Rudan, Li Liu et al. 2013. "Global Burden of Childhood Pneumonia and Diarrhea." *Lancet* 381: 1405–1415.

Walsh, Matthew, Nangsung Kim, Yuho Kadono et al. 2004. "Osteoimmunology: Interplay Between the Immune System and Bone Metabolism." *Annual Review of Immunology* 24: 33–63.

Walsh, Douglas, Francoise Portaels, and Wayne Meyers. 2008. "Buruli ulcer (Mycobacterium ulcerans infection)." *Transactions of the Royal Society of Tropical Medicine and Hygiene* 102 (10): 969–978.

Walsh, J., David Molyneux, and Martin Birley. 1993. "Deforestation: Rffects on Vector-Borne Disease." *Parasitology* 106 (S1): S55–S75.

Ward, Helen, and Minttu Rönn. 2010. "Contribution of Sexually Transmitted Infections to the Sexual Transmission of HIV." *Current Opinion in HIV and AIDS* 5: 305–310.

Washer, Peter. 2010. *Emerging Infectious Diseases.* New York: Palgrave Macmillan.

Wassenaar, Trudy. 2012. *Bacteria: The Benign, the Bad, and the Beautiful.* Hoboken, NJ: Wiley-Blackwell.

Watanapa, P., and W. Watanapa. 2002. "Liver Fluke-Associated Cholangiocarcinoma." *British Journal of Surgery* 89 (2): 962–970.

Watson, Emma, Allan Templeton, Ian Russell et al. 2002. "The Accuracy and Efficacy of Screening Tests for Chlamydia trachomatis: A Systematic Review." *Journal of Medical Microbiology* 51 (12): 1021–1031.

Watts, Luisa, Naima Joseph, Maria Wallace et al. 2009. "HPV Vaccine: A Comparison of Attitudes and Behavioral Perspectives Between Latino and Non-Latino Women." *Gynecological Oncology* 112 (3): 577–582.

Webb, Steven, Ville Pettila, Ian Seppelt et al. 2009. "Critical Care Services and 2009 H1N1 Influenza in Australia and New Zealand." *New England Journal of Medicine* 361, 1925–1934.

Wellin, Edward. 1955. "Water Boiling in a Peruvian Town." In *Health, Culture and Community,* edited by Benjamin. Paul, 71–103. New York: Russell Sage Foundation.

Welshman, John. 2010. Importation, deprivation, and susceptibility: tuberculosis narratives in postwar Britain. In *Tuberculosis Then and Now: Perspectives on the History of an Infectious Disease,* edited by F. Condrau, F. and M. Worboys, p. 123-147. Montreal: McGill-Queens University Press.

Wessner, David. 2010. "The Origin of Viruses." *Nature Education* 3 (9): 37.

West, Stuart, Stephen Diggle, Angus Buckling, Andy Gardner, and Ashleigh Griffin. 2007. "The Social Lives of Microbes." *Annual Review of Ecology, Evolution and Systematics* 38: 53–77.

Whiteford, Linda. 1997. "The Ethnoecology of Dengue Fever." *Medical Anthropology Quarterly* 11 (2): 202–223.

Wierenga, Klaas, Ian Hambleton, and Norma Lewis. 2001. "Survival Estimates for Patients with Homozygous Sickle-Cell Disease in Jamaica: A Clinic-Based Population Study." *Lancet* 357 (9257): 680–683.

Wilbur, A, A. Farnbach, K. Knudson, and Jane Buikstra. 2008. "Diet, Tuberculosis, and the Paleopathological Record." *Current Anthropology* 49 (6): 963–991.

Williams, Carolyn, Donna Kinzman, Traci Yashita et al. 2004. "Persistent GB Virus C Infection and Survival in HIV-Infected Men." *New England Journal of Medicine* 350: 981–990.

Williams, Paul, Klaus Winzer, Weng Chan, and Miquel Cámara. 2007. "Look Who's Talking: Communication and Quorum Sensing in the Bacterial World." *Philosophical Transactions of the Royal Society B: Biological Sciences* 362 (1483): 1119–1134.

Williamson, Heather, Mark Benbow, Lindsay Campbell, Christian Johnson, Ghislain Sopoh, Yves Barogui, Richard Merritt and Pamela Small. 2012. "Detection of Mycobacterium ulcerans in the Environment Predicts Prevalence of Buruli Ulcer in Benin." *PLOS Neglected Tropical Disease* 6(1): e1506. doi:10.1371/journal.pntd.0001506.

Wilson, M., R. Cheke, S. Flasse et al. 2002. "Deforestation and the Spatio-Temporal Distribution of Savannah and Forest Members of the Simulium damnosum Complex in Southern Ghana and Southwestern Togo." *Transactions of the Royal Society of Tropical Medicine and Hygiene* 96 (6): 632–639.

Winskell, Kate, Peter Brown, Amy Patterson, Camilla Burkot, and Benjamin Mbakwem. 2013.

"Making Sense of HIV in Southeastern Nigeria: Fictional Narratives, Cultural Meanings, and Methodologies in Medical Anthropology." *Medical Anthropology Quarterly* 27 (2): 193–214.

Wolfe, Nathan. 2013. "Small, Small World." *National Geographic*. http://ngm.national geographic.com/2013/01/microbes/wolfe-text.

Wolfe, Nathan, Claire Dunavan and Jared Diamond. 2007. "Origins of major human infectious diseases." *Nature* 447: 279–s283.

Wolfe, Nathan, Eitel Mpoudi-Ngole, Jim Gockowski et al. 2000. "Deforestation, Hunting and the Ecology of Microbial Emergence." *Global Changer and Human Health* 1 (1): 10–25.

Wolfe, Nathan, Tassy Prosser, Jean Carr et al. 2004a. "Exposure to Nonhuman Primates in Rural Cameroon." *Emerging Infectious Diseases* 10 (12): 2094–2099.

Wolfe, Nathan, W. Switzer, Bhullar Carr Jean et al. 2004b. "Naturally Acquired Simian Retrovirus Infections in Central African Hunters." *Lancet* 363: 932–937.

Won, K., D. Kruszon-Moran, P. Schantz, and J. Jones. 2008. "National Seroprevalence and Risk Factors for Zoonotic Toxocara spp. Infection." *American Journal of Tropical Medicine and Hygiene* 79: 552–557.

Work, John. 1945. *Fur Brigade to the Bonaventura: John Work's California Expedition, 1832–1833, for the Hudson's Bay Company*. Edited by Alice Bay Maloney. San Francisco: California Historical Society.

World Health Organization. 1946. Preamble to the Constitution of the World Health Organization as adopted by the International Health Conference, New York, 19–22 (Official Records of the World Health Organization, no. 2, 100) and entered into force on April 7, 1948.

World Health Organization. 1995. The World Health Report 1995: Bridging the Gaps. Geneva: World Health Organization.

World Health Organization. 2011. Global Tuberculosis Control: WHO Report. Geneva: World Health Organization.

World Health Organization. 2012a. Global Tuberculosis Report 2012. Geneva: World Health Organiation.

World Health Organization. 2012b. Polio Global Eradication Initiative, Annual Report. Geneva: World Health Organization.

World Health Organization. 2013a. "HIV/AIDS." WHO. www.who.int/gho/hiv/en.

World Health Organization. 2013b. "WHO Report on Global Surveillance of Epidemic Prone Infectious Diseases." WHO. www.who.int/csr/resources/publications/introduction/en/index4.htmlduction/en/index4.html.

World Health Organization. 2013c. "Trypanosomiasis, Human African (Sleeping Sickness). Fact Sheet No. 259." WHO. www.who.int/mediacentre/factsheets/fs259/en.

World Health Organization. 2013d. "Pneumonia. Fact Sheet N331." WHO. www.who.int/mediacentre/factsheets/fs331/en.

World Health Organization. 2014a. "Middle East Respiratory Syndrome Coronavirus (MERS-CoV) Summary and Literature Update, as of June 11, 2014." WHO. www.who.int/csr/disease/coronavirus_infections/MERS-CoV_summary_update_20140611.pdf?ua=1.

World Health Organization. 2014b. "WHO Report on Global Surveillance of Epidemic-Prone Infectious Diseases: Introduction." WHO. www.who.int/csr/resources/publications/introduction/en/index5.html.

World Wildlife Fund. 2014. "Deforestation." World Wildlife Fund. https://worldwildlife.org/threats/deforestation.

Worobey, M., M. Gemmel, D. Teuwen et al. 2008. Direct Evidence of Extensive Diversity of HIV-1 in Kinshasa by 1960." *Nature* 455 (7213): 661–664.

Wrangham, Richard, James Jones, Greg Laden, David Pilbeam, and NancyLou Conklin-Brittain.

1999. "The Raw and the Stolen: Cooking and the Ecology of Human Origins." *Current Anthropology* 40 (5): 567–594.

Wright, Barbara. 2000. "A Biochemical Mechanism for Nonrandom Mutations and Evolution." *Journal of Bacteriology* 182911): 2993–3001.

Yamin, Alicia. 2009. "Shades of Dignity: Exploring the Demands of Equality in Applying Human Rights Frameworks to Health." *Health and Human Rights* 11 (2): 1–18.

Yanni, Emid, Scott Grosse, Quan Yang, and Richard Olney. 2009. "Trends in Pediatric Sickle Cell disease-Related Mortality in the United States, 1983–2002." *Journal of Pediatrics* 154 (4): 541–455.

Yazdanbakhsh, Maria, Anita van der Biggelaar, and Rick Maizels. 2001. "Th2 Responses Without Atopy: Immunoregulation in Chronic Helminth Infections and Reduced Allergic Disease." *Trends in Immunology* 22: 373–377.

Yeganeh, Nava, Donna Curtis, and Alice Kuo. 2010. "Factors Influencing HPV Vaccination Status in a Latino Population; and Parental Attitudes Towards Vaccine Mandates." *Vaccine* 28 (25): 4186–4191.

Zabarenko, Deborah. 2008. "U.S. Midwest Floods Show Impact of Global Warming, Say Conservationists." *Insurance Journal* (July). www.insurancejournal.com/news/national/2008/07/03/91589.htm.

Zalar, P., M. Novak, and N. de Hoog. 2011. "Dishwashers: A Man-Made Ecological Niche Accommodating Human Opportunistic Fungal Pathogens." *Fungal Biology* 115 (10): 997–1007.

Zangwill, Kenneth, Douglas Hamilton, Bradley Perkins et al. 1993. "Cat Scratch Disease in Connecticut: Epidemiology, Risk Factors, and Evaluation of a New Diagnostic Test." *New England Journal of Medicine* 329 (1): 8–13.

Zarychanski, Ryan, Tammy Stuart, Anand Kumar et al. 2010. "Correlates of Severe Disease in Patients with 2009 Pandemic Influenza (H1N1) Virus Infection." *Canadian Medical Association Journal* 182 (3): 257–264.

Zeba, Augustin, Hermann Sorgho, Noel Rouamba et al. 2008. "Major Reduction of Malaria Morbidity with Combined Vitamin A and Zinc Supplementation in Young Children in Burkina Faso: A Randomized Double Blind Trial." *Nutrition Journal* 7: 7. doi:10.1186/1475-2891-7-7.

Zettler, Erik, Tracy Mincer, and Linda Amal-Zettler. 2013. "Life in the 'Plastisphere': Microbial Communities on Plastic Marine Debris." *Environmental Science and Technology* 47: 7137–7146.

Zhang, Mingming, Yaoquo Yang, Xinchun Yang, and Jun Cai. 2011. "Human Cytomegalovirus Infection Is a Novel Etiology for Essential Hypertension." *Medical Hypotheses* 76 (5): 682–684.

Zhang, Qianyi, Jianzhong Shi, Guohua Deng et al. 2013. "H7N9 Influenza Viruses Are Transmissible in Ferrets by Respiratory Droplet." *Science* 341 (6144): 410–414.

Zinnser, Hans. 1935. *Rats, Lice and History.* Boston: Little, Brown.

Zyga, Lisa. 2013. "We Are Living in a Bacterial World, And It's Impacting Us More Than Previously Thought." *Science X Network.* http://phys.org/news/2013-02-bacterial-world-impacting-previously-thought.html.

INDEX

ABOUT THE AUTHOR

Merrill Singer, PhD, a medical and cultural anthropologist, is a Professor in the Departments of Anthropology and Community Medicine at the University of Connecticut. He is affiliated with both the Center for Health, Intervention and Prevention and the Center for Interdisciplinary Research on AIDS. Over his career, his research and writing have focused on HIV/AIDS and other infectious diseases in highly vulnerable and disadvantaged populations, illicit drug use and drinking behavior, community and structural violence, health disparities, and the political ecology of health. His current research focuses on the nature and impact of both syndemics (interacting epidemics) and pluralea (intersecting ecocrises) on health. Dr. Singer has published over 265 scholarly articles and book chapters and has authored or edited 29 books. He is a recipient of the Rudolph Virchow Prize, the George Foster Memorial Award for Practicing Anthropology, the AIDS and Anthropology Paper Prize, the Prize for Distinguished Achievement in the Critical Study of North America, the Solon T. Kimball Award for Public and Applied Anthropology, and the AIDS and Anthropology Research Group's Distinguished Service Award.